Nutrition in
pregnancy and lactation

Nutrition in pregnancy and lactation

Bonnie S. Worthington, Ph.D.

Chief Nutritionist, Child Development and Mental
Retardation Center; Associate Professor,
Nutrition, University of Washington,
Seattle, Washington

Joyce Vermeersch, Dr.P.H.

Assistant Professor, Department of Nutrition,
University of California at Davis,
Davis, California

Sue Rodwell Williams, M.P.H., M.R.Ed., Ph.D.

Chief, Nutrition Program, Kaiser-Permanente Medical Center,
Oakland, California; Instructor, Human Nutrition, Chabot College,
Hayward, California; Field Faculty, M.P.H.—Dietetic Internship
Program and Coordinated Undergraduate Program
in Dietetics, University of California,
Berkeley, California

with 34 illustrations

The C. V. Mosby Company

Saint Louis   1977

Copyright © 1977 by The C. V. Mosby Company

All rights reserved. No part of this book may be reproduced
in any manner without written permission of the publisher.

Printed in the United States of America

Distributed in Great Britain by Henry Kimpton, London

The C. V. Mosby Company
11830 Westline Industrial Drive, St. Louis, Missouri 63141

Library of Congress Cataloging in Publication Data

Worthington, Bonnie S   1943-
    Nutrition in pregnancy and lactation.

    Includes bibliographical references and index.
    1. Pregnancy—Nutritional aspects.   2.   Mothers—
Nutrition. 3. Lactation. I. Vermeersch, Joyce,
1945-   joint author. II. Williams, Sue Rodwell,
1922-   joint author. III. Title.
RG559.W67   618.2′4   76-57760
ISBN 0-8016-5237-5

GW/CB/CB   9 8 7 6 5 4 3·2 1

Contributing authors

Roscius N. Doan, M.D.

Clinical Instructor, Pediatrics,
Child Development and Mental Retardation Center,
University of Washington,
Seattle, Washington

Jane M. Rees, M.S.

Clinical Nutritionist,
Child Development and Mental Retardation Center,
University of Washington,
Seattle, Washington

Lynda E. Taylor, M.S.

Clinical Nutritionist,
Seattle, Washington

Preface

The purpose of this book is to provide in concise format basic information on nutritional considerations as they relate to pregnancy, lactation, and the periods before and between development of these special physiological conditions. It is our intention to direct this presentation to health professionals in a variety of disciplines who relate in their clinical activities to expectant families and to children of all ages who eventually will enter reproductive life. Because it is our wish to provide information that is practical for application in a variety of clinical settings, an effort has been made to approach all topics with the major goal of providing useful information accompanied by *essential* supportive research data. Consequently, detailed literature reviews have been replaced by concise summaries of major research findings in significant areas.

The topics selected for discussion in this book are presented in what we believe is the most logical sequence. After preliminary review of the status of maternal health in the United States, the subject of nutrition and pregnancy is discussed in a series of chapters. The role of nutrition in determining pregnancy outcome is first reviewed, and this is followed by a careful consideration of the physiology of pregnancy as it relates specifically to nutritional requirements and diet. The subsequent chapter attempts to provide practical recommendations about how our knowledge of the relationship between nutrition and pregnancy can be applied skillfully and sensibly in the clinical setting. Considerable detail is included in this area, since the focus of this text is to provide *applicable* information for exemplary clinical work. The remaining two chapters related to pregnancy include explanations of the special conditions of pregnancy that elicit concern and may require special nutritional counseling. Included in these discussions are the problems of anemia, toxemia, diabetes mellitus, heart disease, pulmonary disease, and adolescent pregnancy.

The remaining topics considered in this book include lactation, family planning, and a generalized discussion of nutrition education as it relates to the preparation of today's youth for the experience of reproductive life. Lactation is considered in two parts, with the first summarizing the physiological basis of the process and the nutritional support required to maintain milk production and maternal health. The second part considers in depth the practical issues of concern during lactation and specifies for the health professional how greatest assistance and support can be provided to lactating mothers. The chapter on family planning attempts to define the interrelationships between nutrition and family planning in underdeveloped as well as in developed societies; the known effects of oral contraceptives on nutritional status are also discussed at this time. The final chapter presents a strong case for preparing today's youth for the reproductive experience long before pregnancy is ever considered. Recommendations are provided as to how, when, and where this should be done and what the ultimate benefits to maternal and child health in the United States might be.

In summary, then, a sincere effort has been made to construct for the health professional a useful textbook related to nutritional support of women during pregnancy and lactation. Consideration of the interconceptional period is also provided, and emphasis is placed on the importance of "quality" nutrition education in preparing for the reproductive period. Hopefully this book provides under one cover all significant nutrition information pertinent to health professionals involved in clinical management of "mamas" and "babies."

Bonnie S. Worthington
Joyce Vermeersch
Sue Rodwell Williams

Contents

1

Health problems of mothers and infants

Joyce Vermeersch

GOAL OF PRENATAL CARE

Of all periods in the life cycle, pregnancy is one of the most critical and unique. When a woman becomes pregnant, all the experiences of her past join with those of the present to lay the foundations of a new life, whose potential, in turn, will influence the welfare of generations to come. The critical place that pregnancy occupies in the chain of life has health and social importance for individuals, families, and society as a whole.

The unique nature of pregnancy lies in the fact that at no other time is the well-being of one individual so directly dependent on the well-being of another. During the gestational period, the mother and child have an intimate and inseparable relationship. The physical and mental health of the mother before and during her pregnancy have profound effects on the status of her infant in utero and at birth. It is only through efforts directed at the mother herself that advantages can be provided to assure that her infant will be well born.

The vulnerability and dependence of the infant and the intergenerational significance of pregnancy in the life cycle have led all societies throughout history to recognize the special needs of pregnant women and to make provisions for their care. In a modern world the goal is no longer simply to produce a living infant from a living mother. As society struggles with problems of overpopulation amid limited resources, it is increasingly faced with the moral and social responsibility to make sure that every woman who chooses to conceive has the opportunity for a safe and successful pregnancy and the ability to deliver and care for an infant whose maximum physical and mental potential is not impaired.

INDEXES OF MATERNAL AND INFANT HEALTH

The goal of prenatal care is so important that the extent to which it is achieved is often used as a measure of social and economic development among nations throughout the world. International comparisons of maternal and infant health statistics reveal that promoting the health of mothers and infants requires solutions to problems which still affect a sizeable proportion of the population. Much of this book will focus on the contribution that nutrition can make toward solving these problems. The importance of nutrition to the course and outcome of pregnancy can be better appreciated when the incidence of reproductive casualties and factors associated with them are understood.

Maternal mortality and morbidity

At the turn of the century, childbearing was one of the leading causes of mortality among women in all countries of the world. It is still a major cause of death in developing countries, and the statistics show that, even in places like the United States, an unacceptable number of women continue to have problems.

The maternal mortality rate expresses the number of all women who die of conditions related to pregnancy during the gestational period, labor and birth, and the puerperium (i.e., 90 days following birth) in a given year over the number of infants born alive in that same year. In spite of a dramatic drop in maternal mortality since 1900, the rate in the United States was still 15.2 per 100,000 live births in 1973.

Maternal deaths are most frequently due to the toxemias of pregnancy, abortion, hemorrhage, and infection. Most health authorities believe that these are preventable conditions whose incidence can be reduced through early and continued high-quality prenatal care.

Fetal and infant death and disability

For purposes of presenting vital statistics, prenatal and infant life are usually divided into developmental stages. These help to identify the periods when the developing child is particularly at risk. The stages are diagrammed in Fig. 1-1.

The forty weeks of gestation from conception to birth are separated into two twenty-week parts. These are termed the early fetal period and the late fetal period, respectively.

Infancy includes the time from birth to 1 year of age. The first 28 days of infant life are called the neonatal period. The postneonatal period extends from 28 days of age to the infant's first birthday.

Recently another period has been adopted to recognize that fetal and infant life are parts of an inseparable continuum. This is the perinatal period, which includes the two periods—late fetal and neonatal— that immediately surround birth.

Deaths in the early fetal period are difficult to estimate because loss may occur before the mother realizes that she is pregnant. Consequently, the statistic most often reported is for deaths in the late fetal period. This is called the fetal death ratio or sometimes the stillbirth ratio. In 1973 fetal deaths in the United States were 12.2 per 1000 live births.

Compared with other developed coun-

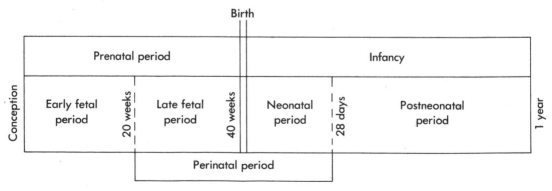

Fig. 1-1. Periods of prenatal and infant life. (Modified from Wilner, D. M., Walkley, R. P., and Goerke, L. S.: Introduction to public health, ed. 6, New York, 1973, The Macmillan Co.)

tries, the United States occupies an inferior position with respect to the number of babies who die in their first year of life. Although the infant mortality rate has been steadily declining and is presently at an all-time low, 16.5 deaths per 1000 live births occurred in 1974. This is approximately the rate that Sweden had fifteen years ago. Furthermore, over the past twenty-five years, several countries have experienced more rapid declines in infant mortality than the United States and have overtaken it in international rankings. In 1950 the United States had the sixth lowest infant mortality rate in the world; by 1972 it ranked at the bottom of a list of sixteen countries with vital records of sufficient quality to allow international comparisons to be made. Thus, in spite of its wealth and sophisticated systems of health care, the United States has yet to discover the means of assuring the survival of its youngest citizens. It has been suggested that if the United States had an infant mortality rate similar to that of Sweden in 1967, nearly 40,000 infant deaths could have been prevented in that year alone.[5]

Some clues to the problem are gained by looking more closely at when and how these infants die. By far, the largest number die within the first 28 days of life. Neonatal deaths in the United States were 12.2 per 1000 live births in 1974 compared with 4.5 in the postneonatal period.

Postneonatal deaths are related to conditions in the infant's *immediate environment*. Rates are particularly high in poor countries without safe and hygienic conditions in the hospital and in the home. Neonatal deaths are more often associated with *prenatal* factors. The relatively high infant mortality rate in the United States can therefore be traced to conditions that influence or are concurrent with the mother's state during pregnancy. To emphasize this point, it has been noted that of all infant deaths in the United States in a given year, about 65% occur in the first 5 days of life, before most infants even leave the hospital

and in spite of the intensive care which modern hospitals are able to provide.[6] The conditions most often responsible are congenital anomalies, birth injuries, erythroblastosis fetalis, infection, and immaturity unqualified as to cause.

High rate of early infant death is the worst possible outcome of pregnancy, but the casualties of reproduction also include the thousands of children who are impaired but do not die. These suffer from the same conditions that cause death in their most severe forms, as well as disorders such as cerebral palsy, epilepsy, and mental retardation. Still more have physical handicaps and developmental disabilities that may be prenatal in origin but may not be detected until later in life.

RISKS OF LOW BIRTH WEIGHT

Infants who weigh less than 2500 grams (5½ pounds) represent about 8% of all live births in the United States each year. Although the word *premature* is sometimes used to describe these infants, the term is confusing because low birth weight infants are really of two different types. There are those who are born too small because they are born too soon, and there are those who are born on time but are too small for their gestational age. To avoid confusion, the word *preterm* is used for infants born under thirty-seven weeks' gestation; full-term but underweight infants are called *growth retarded* or *small-for-date*.

The risks for preterm and growth-retarded infants are so well documented that low birth weight itself is considered an unfavorable outcome of pregnancy. For example, deaths of low birth weight infants in the neonatal period are thirty times more frequent than deaths of newborns of normal weight.

Bergner and Susser[2] examined the records of infants born in New York City between 1958 and 1961 and found that perinatal mortality varied to a much greater extent with birth weight than with the length of gestation. It is now widely held that if the birth weight distribution could be improved, this alone would produce a substantial reduction in mortality.

A number of studies have also shown an increased incidence of handicapping conditions among infants who have the misfortune of being born too small. Low birth weight is a known etiological factor in cerebral palsy,[10,13] and it has been implicated in epilepsy and various forms of mental retardation as well.[7,16,22] There is also evidence that, as a group, children who were extremely undersized at birth have more frequent hospitalizations for illness,[12] more visual and hearing disabilities,[12,17] more behavioral disorders,[19,25] and more learning problems when they enter school.[8,9]

EPIDEMIOLOGICAL FACTORS

If progress is to be made in the prevention of death and disability associated with reproduction, specific factors that place women and their infants at risk must be determined. Much has been learned about predisposing conditions by studying the distribution of reproductive casualties among population groups. Epidemiological investigations of this type have revealed the influences of age, parity, past obstetrical performance, race, and social class on the course and outcome of pregnancy.

Age

It has become axiomatic that the age of the mother is a determinant of her reproductive efficiency. Very young mothers do not have the physiological maturity to withstand the additional stresses of pregnancy. At the other end of the spectrum, older women are beginning to show the effects of the aging process. Consequently, the pattern of reproductive loss by age is a U-shaped curve, with mortality elevated in those below 17 and over 35 years of age. Mothers who are between 20 and 29 years of age have the best performance and outcome of pregnancy.

Age of the mother is also related to age-specific death rates and causes of death in the offspring. Young mothers have the highest number of infants who die in the neonatal period, and more deaths are caused by infection, parasitic disease, and unqualified immaturity or low birth weight. Older mothers experience a greater incidence of fetal loss. Their babies more frequently die of congenital malformations, birth injuries, and hemolytic disease.

Parity

The number of previous pregnancies a woman has had is, in some ways, a function of her age, but there is sufficient evidence that birth order itself exerts an influence on reproductive performance.

First pregnancies are often difficult, regardless of maternal age. They are more frequently complicated by toxemia and problems of labor and delivery. First-born infants also show higher rates of mortality and morbidity, but in the opinion of some investigators, this may be due to sociological rather than physiological factors. A national study of infant mortality conducted by the United States Center for Health Statistics found the *lowest* mortality among first-born infants. Infants who ranked sixth or more in birth order had the highest mortality, and no consistent trend was observed for birth orders two through five. The investigators speculate that their data may differ from previous studies because their sample contained only infants of married mothers. Infants born to unwed mothers are known to have high mortality, and they are usually disproportionately represented among the first-born infants.[14]

There is no doubt, however, about the risks imposed by high parity, especially when the pregnancies are closely spaced. Perinatal mortality and morbidity are both greater among high birth order infants of mothers whose pregnancies have come in rapid succession.

Past obstetrical performance

Poor performance in a prior pregnancy increases the chance of problems in subsequent ones. As long ago as 1939, Gardiner and Yerushalmy[11] noted a tendency for women who experienced specific reproductive losses to repeat them.

More recently, data from the National Infant Mortality Survey (1964-1966) and the National Natality Survey (1965) showed that 5.4% of mothers of single, live-born infants reported previous infant deaths. Infant mortality is two and one-half times greater among the infants of mothers who had a previous infant death than among mothers whose earlier pregnancies all had favorable outcomes. The same tendencies were noted for mothers who had experienced previous fetal loss.[14]

The chance of having a low birth weight infant is also greater when past pregnancy performance is poor. The surveys revealed that the proportion of mothers who had a previous infant death was approximately twice as high when surveyed infants weighed 2500 grams or less at birth.

These and other studies imply that reproductive casualties are not merely chance occurrences. History *does* repeat itself, suggesting that there are underlying circumstances which place some women at the continual risk of developing problems each time they are pregnant.

Race

Maternal and perinatal mortality and morbidity rates are two to three times higher among nonwhites compared with whites in the United States. Fig. 1-2 shows the difference in infant mortality between whites and nonwhites that has persisted over the last fifty years.

It is difficult to determine how much of the difference in mortality and morbidity is truly racial in origin or the result of socioeconomic circumstances. As a group, racial minorities in the United States have always had the least favored position with respect to income, education, and occupation, which have traditionally been the gates of access to general medical and prenatal care. In addition, nonwhite women are overrepresented in some of the categories that impose pregnancy risk. More nonwhite women have babies at an early age,

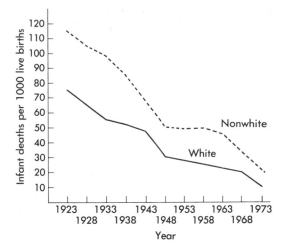

Fig. 1-2. Infant mortality, white and nonwhite, United States, 1923-1973. (From National Center for Health Statistics: Vital statistics of the United States, 1970, and Monthly Vital Statistics Report, Feb. 10, 1975.)

and more continue to have their sixth, seventh, or eighth child after they are 35 years old.

There is also a distinct birth weight variation according to race. Compared with the 8% incidence for the United States as a whole, the rate for nonwhites is 13% to 14%. Although some researchers have failed to find significant socioeconomic explanations, there is evidence that lower birth weights among nonwhite infants may not be a totally genetic phenomenon.

Williams has recently studied intrauterine growth curves among four major ethnic groups in California. Intrauterine growth curves express the relationship between median birth weights and the stage of gestation. Their construction is based on the assumption that the weights of babies born at each stage of gestation are representative of all babies both in and out of the uterus. Williams' analysis of over 1.5 million births in California from 1966 to 1970 showed that at twenty-six weeks' gestation black and white-Spanish infants are actually heavier than non-Spanish whites and Orientals. Beginning at about thirty-five or thirty-six weeks' gestation, however, their growth slows so that by term they have lost their initial advantage and weigh considerably less than non-Spanish whites.[23]

Bergner and Susser[1] found essentially the same pattern for black infants in New York City—that is, they are born heavier than whites up to twenty-eight to thirty weeks' gestation and are born lighter thereafter.

These studies lead to the speculation that genetic potential is not responsible for the higher incidence of low birth weight among certain ethnic groups. Instead, it is possible that the variations which are observed are due to fetal growth retardation in the last trimester of pregnancy. If this retardation could be modified, perinatal loss among nonwhite infants might be substantially reduced.

Social class

Social class in Western countries is usually determined by income, occupation, and education. According to government estimates, 750,000 infants in the United States are born each year to families whose incomes fall below the poverty line. As shown in Fig. 1-3, nonwhite infants have a much greater chance of being born poor. The National Natality and Infant Mortality Surveys found that whereas only one sixth of the white births in their sample were in the lowest income category, nearly one half of the black babies were born to families with incomes of $3000 or less. The same difference, although less marked, was found for parental education.[15]

Since social class is so confounded by race, attempts to isolate the effects of socioeconomic variables on reproductive performance must look at variations within racial groups. A number of studies from around the world have confirmed a distinct socioeconomic gradient in the course and outcome of pregnancy.

Some of the most striking data come from Great Britain—a country that is relatively homogeneous as far as race and ethnic background are concerned. The British Perinatal Mortality Survey (1958)[4] and the British Births Survey (1970)[3] found that death rates for babies from the fifth month of gestation through the first week of life increased consistently as families moved

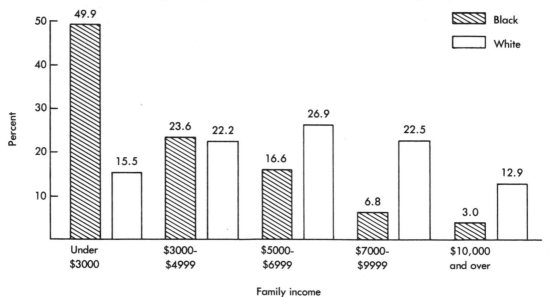

Fig. 1-3. Percent of legitimate live births by family income and race, United States National Natality and Infant Mortality Surveys, 1964-1966. (From MacMahon, B., Kovar, M. G., and Feldman, J. J.: Infant mortality rates: socio-economic factors, DHEW Pub. No. [HSM] 72-1045, March, 1972, Rockville, Md., National Center for Health Statistics.)

down the social ladder. The lowest mortality rates were observed among the professional classes, whereas the highest rates were found among the unskilled labor class. Furthermore, mortality rates were associated with the social mobility of the mother. Those women who had married men from a higher social class than their own had better obstetrical outcomes than women who married men from a lower social class.

Birth weight has also been shown to vary with social class. This was found in the British study and has been confirmed in other countries. For example, Table 1-1 is adapted from data compiled by the World Health Organization from studies by different investigators in several locations in India. Although Indian infants are usually born lighter than their European and American counterparts, their weights are consistently higher among the well-to-do classes and, in some cases, approach the mean weights of newborns in the West.[24]

Table 1-1. Mean birth weights by social class from selected studies in India*

Place	Social class	Mean birth weight (g)	Source of data
Madras	Well-to-do	2985	Achar and Yankauer (1962)
	Mostly poor	2736	
South India	Wealthy	3182	Venkatachalam (1962)
	Poor	2810	
Bombay	Upper class	3247	Udani (1963)
	Upper middle class	2945	
	Lower middle class	2796	
	Lower class	2578	
Calcutta	Paying patients	2857	Mukerjee and Biswas (1959)
	Poor class	2656	

*Modified from World Health Organization: Nutrition in pregnancy and lactation, WHO Technical Report Series No. 302, Geneva, 1965.

Table 1-2. Estimated number of infant deaths per 1000 live births by race, education of father, and family income, United States, 1964-1966*

Family income	Education of father				
	8 years or less	9-11 years	12 years	13-15 years	16 or more years
White					
Under $3000	34.0	25.6	25.1	23.3	†
$3000-4999	30.0	24.2	18.4	18.1	15.3
$5000-6999	25.9	23.3	15.6	14.6	13.0
$7000-9999	24.8	22.1	16.8	22.9	17.4
$10,000 and over	†	23.1	15.3	19.2	19.8
Black					
Under $3000	40.5	52.1	35.0	†	†
$3000-4999	†	51.6	40.3	†	†
$5000-6999	†	†	15.0	†	†
$7000-9999	†	†	†	†	†
$10,000 and over	†	†	†	†	†

*From MacMahon, B., Kovar, M. G., and Feldman, J. J.: Infant mortality rates: socio-economic factors, U.S. Department of Health, Education and Welfare Pub. No. (HSM) 72-1045, Rockville, Md., March, 1972, National Center for Health Statistics.
†Too few in sample to calculate rates.

In the United States the relationships between infant mortality, birth weight, and social class exhibit the same general trends. Even among white infants, the incidence of mortality and low birth weight is higher in the lower socioeconomic groups no matter what indicator—income, occupation, or education—is used to define social class. An important finding, however, is that one does not always see a continuous decline from the highest to the lowest social classes in the United States which is observed in Great Britain and other countries. Whether family income and parental education are considered separately or in combination, there is substantially more infant mortality in the two lowest groups but there are no significant differences among the three upper strata. Table 1-2 presents evidence from the National Natality and Infant Mortality Surveys with respect to family income and parental education for both blacks and whites.[15] The data suggest that, by living standards in the 1960s, a high school diploma and a family income of at least $6000 per year were critical dividing lines between high and low rates of infant mortality in the United States.

Why the rates do not continue to decline in the highest socioeconomic groups is open to speculation. Again the possibility arises that there are underlying factors, independent of social class, exerting influences on reproductive performance.

TARGETS FOR HEALTH INTERVENTION: THE CHALLENGE AHEAD

The epidemiological data provide a profile of women who have the greatest risk of developing problems in pregnancy:

    Race: nonwhite
    Poverty
    Lack of education
    Age: under 17 or over 35 years
    First pregnancy or high parity
    Pregnancies less than one year apart
    Prior obstetrical complications
    Previous fetal-infant death or disability
    Unwed mother

Women with one or more of these characteristics are also more likely to produce a low birth weight infant who has physical or mental impairments or who will die in the first year of life. These women must be the targets of special intervention if recurrent tragedies of reproductive loss are to be prevented.

A closer look at Fig. 1-2 shows that much progress has been made in recent years. After a period of virtual stagnation at midcentury, the reduction in infant mortality has begun to accelerate and the gap between whites and nonwhites in 1973 is the narrowest it has ever been.

What this chapter has attempted to demonstrate is that these morbidity and mortality rates are the end results of a number of complex and interrelated factors. Any attempt to explain them in terms of a single cause or a simple solution will only confound efforts to find answers to the problems that still remain. Nonetheless, it is not unreasonable to assert that the extension of better prenatal care to disadvantaged women and the wider availability and acceptance of family planning have greatly contributed to the overall decline in reproductive casualties over the last ten years.

These measures should continue to improve pregnancy outcomes. It is doubtful, however, that they alone can equalize the risks for white and nonwhite women and their infants. For example, in 1973 only 3.4% of nonwhite births occurred without the benefits of prenatal care—a figure which is still about twice that of whites but not great enough to account totally for the differences in mortality and morbidity. It is also unlikely that bringing the nonwhite infant mortality rate into line with that of whites will automatically move the United States from its present basement position to the top of the list of international rankings. We have already stated that infant mortality in the United States cannot be completely explained by either race or socioeconomic status. Chase[6] has demonstrated that when infant mortality in Sweden and Norway is compared with just three states—Minnesota, North Dakota, and South Dakota, whose populations are largely derived from Swedish and Norwegian stock—the United States remains in an inferior position. This implies that there is still room for improvement even among those who currently have a better-than-average chance for a favorable outcome of pregnancy.

Williams[23] came to the same conclusion for birth weight. His intrauterine growth curves for the relatively prosperous non-Spanish whites in California were, on the average, 150 grams lower than Norwegian infants whose growth was assessed by similar methods.

The implications are that if further progress is to be made in promoting maternal and infant health, health professionals must now go beyond the obvious solutions and seek ways to identify and modify the underlying risk factors in reproduction. This is the challenge that has begun to focus increased attention on the role of nutrition in the course and outcome of pregnancy. With this perspective in mind, we can proceed to an understanding of the importance of nutrition in prenatal care.

REFERENCES

1. Achar, S. T., and Yankauer, A.: Studies on the birth weight South Indian infants, Indian J. Child Health **11:**157-167, 1962.
2. Bergner, L., and Susser, M. W.: Low birth weight and prenatal nutrition: an interpretive review, Pediatrics **46:**946, 1970.
3. Born in Britain 1970, Lancet **1:** April 3, 1976.
4. Butler, N. R., and Bonham, D. G.: Perinatal mortality: the first report of the 1958 British Perinatal Mortality Survey, Edinburgh, 1963, E. & S. Livingstone, Ltd.
5. Chase, H.: Perinatal and infant mortality in the United States and six West European countries, Am. J. Public Health **57:**1735, 1967.
6. Chase, H.: The position of the United States in international comparisons of health status, Am. J. Public Health **62:**581, 1972.
7. Drillien, C. M.: Prematures in school, Pediatr. Dig., p. 75, Sept., 1965.
8. Douglas, J. W. B.: Mental ability and school achievement of premature children at 8 years of age, Br. Med. J. **1:**1210, 1956.
9. Douglas, J. W. B.: Premature children at primary schools, Br. Med. J. **1**(2):1008, 1960.
10. Eastman, N. J., and DeLeon, M.: Etiology of cerebral palsy, Am. J. Obstet. Gynecol. **69:**950, 1955.
11. Gardiner, E. M., and Yerushalmy, I.: Familial susceptibility to stillbirths and neonatal deaths, Am. J. Hyg. **30:**11, 1939.
12. Harper, P. A., and Wiener, G.: Sequelae of low birth weight, Annu. Rev. Med. **16:**405, 1965.
13. Lilienfeld, A. M., and Pasamanick, B.: The association of prenatal factors with the development of cerebral palsy and epilepsy, Am. J. Obstet. Gynecol. **70:**93, 1955.
14. MacMahon, B., Kovar, M. G., and Feldman, J. J.: Infant mortality rates: relationships with mother's reproductive history. DHEW Pub. No. (HSM) 73-1976, Rockville, Md., April, 1973, National Center for Health Statistics.
15. MacMahon, B., Kovar, M. G., and Feldman, J. J.: Infant mortality rates: socio-economic factors, DHEW Pub. No. (HSM) 72-1045, Rockville, Md., March, 1972, National Center for Health Statistics.
16. McDonald, A. D.: Intelligence in children of very low birth weight, Br. J. Prev. Soc. Med. **18:**59, 1964.
17. McDonald, A. D.: Neurological and ophthalmic disorders in children of very low birth weight, Br. Med. J. **1:**895, 1962.
18. Mukherjee, S., and Biswas, S.: Duration of labour and its relationship to maternal age and parity—a statistical approach, J. Indian Med. Assoc. **33:** 173, 1959.
19. Pasamanick, B., Rogers, M. E., and Lilienfeld, A. M.: Pregnancy experience and the development of behavior disorder in children, Am. J. Psychiatry **112:**613, 1956.
20. Udani, P. M.: Physical growth of children in different socio-economic groups in Bombay, Indian J. Child Health **12:**594, 1963.
21. Venkatachalam, P. S.: Maternal nutritional status and its effect on the newborn, WHO Bull. **26:**193, 1962.
22. Wiener, G., Rider, R. V., Oppel, W. C., and Harper, P. A.: Correlates of low birth weight. Psychological status at eight to ten years of age, Pediatr. Res. **2:**110, 1968.
23. Williams, R. L.: Intrauterine growth curves: intra- and international comparisons with different ethnic groups in California, Prev. Med. **4:**163, 1975.
24. World Health Organization: Nutrition in pregnancy and lactation, WHO Techn. Rep. Series No. 302, Geneva, 1965.
25. Wortis, H., Braine, M., Cutler, R., and Freedman, A.: Deviant behavior in 2½-year-old premature children, Child. Dev. **35:**871, 1964.

2
Maternal nutrition and the outcome of pregnancy

Joyce Vermeersch

NUTRITION IN PERSPECTIVE

Food is essential to life and growth. Without an adequate supply of food and the nutrients it contains, an organism cannot grow and develop normally. Eventually, it dies.

In spite of these simple and well-established facts, the role that nutrition plays in the course and outcome of pregnancy has not always been appreciated. In the controlled conditions of the laboratory, researchers have been able to demonstrate harmful effects of deficient diets on pregnant animals and their offspring in a number of species. But when studies are made on free-living human populations, direct relationships between what a mother eats during the nine months of gestation and the course and outcome of her pregnancy have not always been shown. Consequently, the emphasis that nutrition has received in prenatal care has varied over the years. At times when researchers have been able to show positive effects, nutrition has received a great deal of attention. At other times, when studies produced equivocal results, nutrition has slipped to a position of indifference and neglect.

Part of the problem is that the changes which occur during pregnancy, their influence on nutritional needs, and the effects of long-term nutritional status on reproductive performance are not fully understood. As a science, the application of nutrition principles to pregnancy has had to depend on progress in a knowledge of reproduction itself, and as in any science, one of the most important advances is simply learning to ask the right questions. By reviewing how the emphasis of research has changed as more has become known about nutrition, reproduction, and human growth, health professionals can gain a sense of perspective that helps in understanding why different dietary recommendations for pregnant women have been made.

Early beliefs and practices

During the nineteenth century, much of what was known and recommended about diet during pregnancy was based on empiricism, that is, on casual observation rather than controlled studies. Since little information was available on the nutrient composition of foods or their biological values, dietary advice was influenced by beliefs that obvious physical properties of different foods could produce specific effects on the mother or child. The beliefs were often colored by the emotional and mystical aura surrounding the pregnant state. For example, pregnant women were sometimes forbidden to eat salty, acid, or sour foods for fear the infant would be born with a "sour" disposition. Eggs were sometimes restricted because of their association with the reproductive function. On the other hand, certain foods were encouraged for their presumed beneficial effects. Pregnant women were often advised to eat broths, warm milk, and ripe fruits to soothe the fetus and ease the birth process.

At this time dietary recommendations for pregnancy were also influenced by problems current in obstetrical practice. In the days of the Industrial Revolution, children in Europe had poor diets and worked long hours in dark factories. Rickets was a common nutritional disorder that impaired normal bone formation during the growing years. When women became pregnant, contracted pelvis presented a major obstetrical risk. Physicians did not have the modern means of delivering infants from these mothers that are available today. Mortality of both mother and child during childbirth was very high.

Experience with his own patients in the 1880s led a German physician, Prochownick, to advocate a fluid-restricted, low-carbohydrate, high-protein diet for women with contracted pelvis to be followed for six weeks prior to the birth. Women using such a diet produced smaller infants who were easier to deliver. The diet may have had some justification in the 1880s, but it later gained in popularity and became a standard recommendation for women throughout pregnancy even when the original rationale for it no longer applied. Remnants of the Prochownick diet, restricting fluid or carbohydrate, persist today.

Clinical studies

Empiricism gave way to a more scientific approach at the turn of the century. In the first four decades of the 1900s, great dis-

coveries were made about the functions of vitamins in health and disease. It was only natural that attention should turn to the role of these "protective" nutrients in the diets of pregnant women. Three studies, all published in the 1940s, have become classical examples of methods used to demonstrate a relationship between diet in pregnancy and the incidence of reproductive problems whose etiologies were poorly understood.

Burke's[4] study at the Boston Lying-In Hospital addressed the simple question of whether women who ate diets of different nutritional quality had different experiences and outcomes of pregnancy. After obtaining dietary histories from 216 pregnant women, Burke and her associates rated the intakes as good, fair, or poor according to the Recommended Dietary Allowances. When the infants were born, obstetricians and pediatricians who did not know the mothers' diet ratings were asked to judge the performance of the mothers during pregnancy and the conditions of their infants at birth. When the ratings were compared, there was a significant tendency for the diet ratings and the ratings of the infants to correspond. Those with good diets tended to have superior infants, whereas those with poor diets had infants who were more often rated inferior. A similar but less striking correspondence was found between diet ratings and the mother's own course of pregnancy.

Ebbs and his co-workers[10] in Toronto were interested in a different question. They wanted to know whether supplementing the diets of pregnant women could improve pregnancy performance. Ebbs had three groups to study: 170 women who had good diets and therefore were given only dietary advice during pregnancy; 90 women with poor diets who were given vitamin and mineral supplements as well as dietary advice; and 120 women with poor diets who were given no supplements and no advice. To rule out the possibility that the supplements might have a beneficial psychological effect, the control groups were given placebos. Results indicated that the incidence of miscarriage, stillbirth, prematurity, and neonatal death were all significantly lower in the group who received the supplements and dietary advice.

In England and Wales food supplements had been distributed to pregnant women in economically depressed areas since 1935. In the 1940s Balfour[3] published a study that assessed the effects of these supplements on stillbirth rates, maternal mortality, and the incidence of toxemia. Over 11,000 women participated in the supplementation program, with another 8000 serving as controls. The supplements were yeast extracts with high amounts of the B vitamins and supplements of vitamins A and D, calcium, phosphorus, and iron.

Although maternal deaths in the study were too few to show statistically significant differences, there was a significant reduction of stillbirths and neonatal deaths in the supplemented group compared with the controls. The incidence of maternal and neonatal deaths in which toxemia was a primary or contributing cause was also lower among those receiving supplements.

These results, along with similar findings by other investigators, did much to encourage dietary counseling and the routine prescription of vitamin and mineral supplements for pregnancy in the 1940s and early 1950s. However, the studies on which these practices were based have been faulted on several counts. One criticism was that dietary intake alone is not a measure of nutritional status, and few of the studies made systematic attempts to determine the actual nutritional status of the women before or during their pregnancies.

In the 1950s a carefully controlled study was undertaken at Vanderbilt University to evaluate the nutriture of pregnant women according to diet, physical findings, and laboratory tests to determine whether a significant relationship could be found between nutritional status and the development of maternal or fetal complications.[15]

Approximately 2300 women and their infants were studied by the Vanderbilt group. All of the women were white; 95% were married; 67% had enrolled for prenatal care during the first trimester of pregnancy. Dietary intakes were recorded, and the women received a clinical examination for signs of nutritional deficiencies. Tests were also made to determine nutrient levels in blood and urine.

The dietary records showed that the average intakes did not always meet the Recommended Dietary Allowances, but in the opinion of the investigators, the levels were "not disturbingly low." Food patterns showed frequent consumption of milk, eggs, green vegetables, and citrus fruits. Some women had low hemoglobin levels, but biochemical values for other nutrients were consistent with health. Except for obesity, there were no signs of even the mildest forms of malnutrition in any of the women.

As in Burke's study, physicians at the hospital were blind to the nutritional evaluations of their patients. The investigators made no attempts to alter the normal care provided to the patients so some physicians prescribed supplemental vitamins and minerals whereas others did not.

The evaluations indicate that the women in the Vanderbilt study were generally in good health and nutritional status. Their socioeconomic backgrounds and the quality of prenatal care should have minimized their risk of reproductive problems, yet maternal and fetal complications did occur. There were no maternal deaths, but 72 infants died in the perinatal period. Prematurity was 5.6%, and 103 women developed acute toxemia during pregnancy. None of these conditions could be attributed to variations in diet or nutritional status. A widely held theory that protein deficiency was a cause of toxemia was discounted when the investigators demonstrated that women consuming less than 50 grams of protein during pregnancy were no more likely to develop toxemia than those with higher intakes. Neither could it be shown that women who had taken vitamin and mineral supplements had a better course or outcome than women who had not received supplements.

Not long after the findings of the Vanderbilt study were released, another carefully controlled investigation involving 489 women in Aberdeen, Scotland, was published by Thomson.[19] Some of Thomson's objections to the earlier studies were that they failed to control for the effects of parity on reproductive performance and that dietary evaluations by the recall method were likely to be unreliable. Using only primigravidas in his study, Thomson had the women keep home-weighed food records for one week during the seventh month of pregnancy. Although he found that nutrient intakes among the women varied considerably, Thomson could find no associations between diet during pregnancy and the length of gestation, antepartum hemorrhage, fetal malformations, or perinatal mortality. Birth weights of the infants and caloric intakes of the mothers were positively correlated, but when the data were adjusted for maternal height and social class, it was found that women from the upper social classes were taller, heavier, and consequently consumed more calories than women from the lower classes. Thomson concluded that height of the mother, as a reflection of life-long nutriture, and social class were more important than dietary intake during pregnancy itself and that women in good nutritional status prior to conception could tolerate relatively wide variations in both the quantity and quality of their diets during pregnancy without clinically apparent effects.

The generally negative results of these two important studies diminished the enthusiasm for diet in pregnancy that was produced in previous years. The general need for good nutrition was not questioned, but the absence of frank nutritional deficiencies encouraged the opinion that women in the Western world were well nourished and could withstand the extra demands of pregnancy without difficulty. Since obesity was more often encountered than undernutrition, weight restriction became a rather routine part of prenatal care. It was common to allow pregnant women to gain only 10 to 15 pounds throughout gestation, and some women were even advised to lose weight. This was not considered dangerous because it seemed as though the fetus was a "perfect parasite" that could easily meet its own nutrient needs by drawing from the reserves of the well-nourished mother. This philosophy regarding the nutritional care of pregnant women became prevalent during the 1960s and is still common today.

Interpreting results

Looking back on the different ideas about the dietary management of pregnant women, one can see the influence of research. When one contrasts the positive findings of the 1940s with the negative results of the 1950s, it is no wonder that some confusion and controversy over the importance of diet during pregnancy has crept into clinical practice. Yet there are a number of methodological difficulties existent in even the more carefully executed studies, which make it hard to draw definite conclusions.

One problem common to all of the studies is that the research questions were oversimplified in view of the complex interrelationships which were assessed. The studies all sought to relate nutrition to the most extreme outcomes of pregnancy without sufficient control of the other factors involved. Reproductive casualties such as stillbirth, fetal malformations, and maternal or neonatal death have been shown to be related to a number of epidemiological factors. A study cannot isolate diet during pregnancy as the only cause and ignore the other factors.

Another problem was rightly identified by the Vanderbilt group—that dietary intake assessed for one day or even one week during pregnancy is not necessarily an indication of nutritional status. Nutritional status reflects not only what people eat but how the nutrients are absorbed, utilized in the body, and stored. It is a continuous process that is influenced by lifetime dietary habits as well as the individual's own physiological and psychological state.

A third problem concerns evaluating the nutritional adequacy of an individual's diet. To say that a person's diet is poor if it does not meet the Recommended Dietary Allowances (RDA) is really a perversion of the purposes for which the allowances were originally devised. According to the National Research Council, the RDA are intended as a planning guide to meet the nutrient needs of almost all healthy persons in the United States. To assure this, the allowances provide margins of safety so that the levels recommended are well above those at which clinical signs of nutrient deficiencies appear. Actual requirements for one individual may differ from those of another according to body size, age, activity, and state of health. The RDA should only be used to evaluate the dietary adequacy of a group of people. If a study shows that a significant percentage of a population fails to meet the RDA, one can say that the group is at nutritional risk but one cannot say that a particular individual within that group necessarily has a poor diet.

These are important technicalities for interpreting studies on diet during pregnancy as well as what nutritionists encounter in daily practice. The variation in individual nutritional requirements means that when a group of pregnant women is generally in good nutritional status, as was the case in the Vanderbilt study, the relatively small differences in dietary intake have marginal significance. Furthermore, it would be impossible to predict an individual woman's pregnancy performance and outcome on the basis of her diet alone. In practice nutritionists frequently encounter a woman whose diet does not meet the RDA but who has a normal pregnancy and a healthy child. Conversely, sometimes

a woman's diet appears adequate but she has a poor performance or outcome. It is only on a population basis that statistically significant relationships can be demonstrated. To have assurance that important epidemiological factors and individual variations in nutritional requirements are randomly distributed, a large number of subjects would have to be studied. Baird[2] has estimated that more than 5000 women and an equal number of controls would have to be used to show that changes in an index like perinatal mortality are attributable to diet in the general population of pregnant women.

In summary, it can be said that the early studies have contributed more to a clarification of the methodological issues in research than to the elaboration of specific influences of diet during pregnancy and nutritional status on reproductive performance or outcome. Whereas it is reasonable to conclude that women in good nutritional status are going to be better off than women in poor nutritional status, it is also reasonable to conclude that not every problem of pregnancy has a nutritional cause. It is likely that there are circumstances in which nutrition does indeed play a direct and critical role. But it is also probable that, for some conditions, nutrition has little or no influence at all. The task of present and future research is to identify what these various conditions are.

Direction of modern research

In 1970 a special Committee on Maternal Nutrition of the National Research Council made recommendations about the kinds of studies that are needed in view of what has been learned from the past.[7] These are (1) studies of maternal-fetal relationships on the molecular level to learn what controls fetal growth and development, the sources of metabolites, and the mechanisms that maintain homeostasis; (2) studies on maternal molecular ecology to learn how nutrient intake at different phases of the life cycle influences the regulation of life processes, including reproduction; and (3) studies of the natural experiments that take place as underdeveloped countries develop economically, as rural people become urban, and as ethnic groups merge and begin to communicate more freely. Concerning the third type of studies, the Committee on Maternal Nutrition emphasized the need to record all of the influences affecting specific groups in a uniform way so that researchers can compare and begin to understand how they interact. These are the directions that research on maternal nutrition and the outcome of pregnancy has taken in recent years.

NUTRITIONAL INFLUENCES ON FETAL GROWTH

It is not possible to examine maternal-fetal relationships directly at the cellular and molecular levels in humans for obvious ethical reasons. Consequently, work toward understanding how maternal nutrition influences growth and development in utero must be done on animals. The technique has usually been to manipulate the diets of pregnant animals and study the effects on cellular morphology and physiology in the offspring at various stages of gestation. Over the past few years much information has accumulated from studies of this type. Nutritional requirements for fetal growth and development will be discussed in Chapter 3, but in this section we will explore some of the recent findings of research that have begun to identify outcomes of pregnancy that are most affected by maternal nutrition. These findings have contributed to a revival of interest in the importance of nutrition in prenatal care.

Experiments with animals

Two types of dietary restrictions have been imposed on laboratory animals to study the effects of maternal nutrition on fetal growth and development. One restriction is simply not giving the animals enough food so that the diet is low in calories. The other restriction holds calories at

an adequate level but reduces or completely eliminates one or more essential nutrients. The effects of deficiencies of almost all of the known nutrients have been studied this way, but restrictions of protein and calories have more relevance to humans than restrictions of vitamins or minerals. All animals need energy and use protein in essentially the same way, but the need for vitamins and minerals and their specific functions differ from species to species.

A number of investigators have demonstrated what can happen to fetuses when pregnant animals are fed calorie- or protein-restricted diets. Maternal malnutrition can interfere with the ability of the mother to conceive, it can produce death and resorption or abortion of the fetuses, and it can produce malformations or retard growth. Of course, the more severe the dietary restrictions are the more serious the effects will be, but Chow and Lee[6] have shown that a reduction of as little as 25% of total calories without an imbalance in the quality of the maternal diet in rats can reduce both the number of pups born and their ability to survive.

Biochemical studies give evidence of why this occurs. One effect of protein-calorie malnutrition is an impairment of energy metabolism in the cells by interfering with the synthesis of deoxyribonucleic acid (DNA) and enzymes involved in glycolysis and the citric acid cycle. Without adequate supplies of amino acids and energy, cell functions break down and normal processes of growth cannot occur. The effects would be most damaging when cells are normally undergoing rapid division. This implies that the timing of the dietary deficiency, as well as its severity, is important.

Stages of cell growth

Basically, all animals grow in one of two ways. They get larger because their cells increase in number or because the number of cells they already have increases in size. Winick and co-workers[25,26] have employed techniques developed by others to determine how these two kinds of growth take place. The method is based on measurements of DNA content of organs and tissues. In a given species all cells of a certain ploidy contain the same amount of DNA. For example, all diploid cells in the human body contain 6.0 pg of DNA. For the rat it is 6.2 pg of DNA per diploid cell. Cells of other ploidy have different amounts of DNA, but it has been shown that the DNA content is proportional to the total amount of cytoplasm. So for practical purposes the amount of DNA in an organ or tissue sample divided by the amount of DNA per cell gives an estimation of the number of cells present. Once this is known, the total weight of the organ or, alternatively, the total protein content, can be divided by the number of cells to give an indication of the average cell size.

By using this technique with rats, Winick has identified a sequence of cell growth common to all organs of the body (Fig. 2-1). In the first stage of this sequence, growth takes place only by an increase in the number of cells; that is, cells are replicating and all are approximately of equal size. This stage of cell proliferation is called hyperplasia. In the second stage new cells continue to be made, but the ones already present now begin to increase in size, which is called hypertrophy; thus the second stage is both hyperplastic and hypertrophic. The third stage is totally hypertrophic. Growth in this stage is taking place only by increases in cell size, and no new cells are being made. The fourth stage is maturity, in which all cell growth stops. In this stage there is further development as enzyme systems are elaborated, and cell functions are integrated.

The stages of cell growth are not really discrete processes but merge into one another. The length of each stage and the periods of maximum cell proliferation differ according to species and in various parts of the body. In most regions there is a continuous increase until equilibrium is reached as old cells die and new ones are made. But in nonregenerating organs like the brain, the number and size of cells

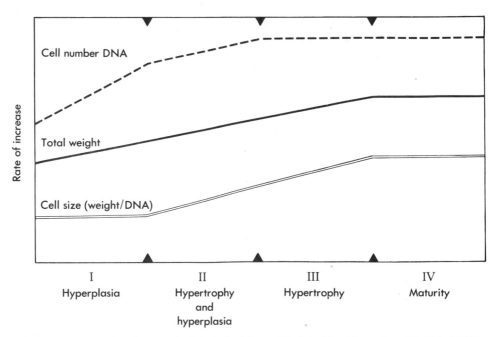

Fig. 2-1. Stages of cell growth. (Modified from Winick, M.: Nutr. Rev. **26:**195, 1968.)

present at maturity must last a lifetime. For this organ in particular, any interference with normal cell growth may have consequences that cannot be repaired.

The rat has a normal gestational period of twenty-one days. Hyperplastic growth of the placenta is complete by seventeen days. Throughout gestation all fetal tissues are increasing in cell number. Most continue to proliferate postnatally until weaning, but certain types of cells, such as neurons of the central nervous system, stop dividing before birth.

The consequences of any interference with normal cell growth would depend on the time at which it occurs. Interference in the hyperplastic phase would result in a decrease in the number of cells produced. If interference occurs when cells are undergoing hypertrophy, cells would be reduced in size. Both types of interference would cause the animal to experience growth failure.

Types of growth failure

It is now clear that a number of things can produce growth failure in utero. The cause can be either "intrinsic" or "extrinsic." The difference may be determined by the condition of the placentas of animals born small for gestational age. In intrinsic intrauterine growth failure, placentas are usually of normal size, which implies that retardation of fetal growth was not due to inadequate maternal-fetal transport but was the result of other factors. Some examples include chromosomal abnormalities, certain drugs that cross the placental barrier, and maternal infections. Extrinsic intrauterine growth failure is usually manifested by placentas that are reduced in size, which indicates that they were incapable of supplying the fetus with adequate nutrition.

Extrinsic intrauterine growth failure can be produced experimentally in a number of ways. One way is to ligate one of the uterine arteries of the mother rat so that blood supplies to one whole side of the uterus are cut off. The procedure is usually applied at seventeen days' gestation in the rat, that is, after hyperplastic growth of the placenta is complete.

Another way of producing extrinsic growth retardation is to impose a severe protein restriction on the mother's diet at different times during pregnancy to reduce the supply of nutrients available for the synthesis of placental and fetal cells.

The techniques for measuring cell number and cell size have made it possible to compare changes that occur in the placenta and fetal organs from these different types of intrauterine growth failure. Re-

Table 2-1. Types of intrauterine growth failure*

| | | Extrinsic | |
	Intrinsic	Asymmetrical	Symmetrical
Placenta			
Cell growth	Normal	Reduced 20%-30%	Reduced 20%-30%
Fetus			
Malformations	Multiple	Absent	Absent
Weight	Reduced	Reduced 20%	Reduced 20%
Head circumference	Variable	Normal	Reduced 20%
Brain			
Cell growth		Normal	Reduced 20%
Liver			
Cell growth		Reduced 50%	Reduced 20%
Glycogen		Reduced 100%	Reduced 20%

*From Winick, M., Brasel, J. A., and Velasco, E. G.: Effects of prenatal nutrition upon pregnancy risk, Clin. Obstet. Gynecol. **16:**184, 1973.

sults from such comparisons are summarized in Table 2-1.

The principal feature of intrinsic growth failure is the presence of multiple malformations in the fetuses. These are absent in growth failure produced by ligation and are variable in maternal malnutrition, depending on the timing of the restriction.

In both vascular and nutritional growth failure, placentas are reduced in proportion to fetal weight. In the ligated animals and in late maternal malnutrition, the reduction is due to a decrease in the average size of the cells. Maternal protein restriction maintained throughout most of gestation, however, decreases both the number and size of placental cells.

The fetuses themselves also show different patterns of growth retardation. Those subjected to vascular insufficiency show an asymmetrical retardation. The fetuses have relatively normal brain sizes and head circumferences, but their livers are greatly reduced, by as much as 50%, and glycogen reserves are completely absent. Proportionally, these animals have bigger brains and heads compared with the rest of their bodies; they are extremely hypoglycemic at birth.

When maternal protein restriction is limited to the last few days of gestation, the fetuses exhibit a pattern of growth retardation which is similar to that produced by vascular insufficiency—proportionally big heads and small bodies. But when the restriction is imposed throughout most of the gestational period, the pattern of fetal growth retardation becomes more symmetrical. There is a decrease in cell number of approximately 15% to 20% in all organs, including the brain; head circumference is also reduced. The reduction in cell number is greatest in those regions of the brain which are undergoing the most rapid rates of cell division.[27]

Consequences of growth failure

These findings make it obvious that fetuses are *not* perfect parasites which can survive intrauterine insults without adverse effects. The data suggest that inadequate maternal nutrition can affect the fetus in ways which are coincident with the stages of cell growth and that the bodily reserves of the mother cannot always insulate the fetus from dietary deficiencies. What happens to animals whose mothers were nutritionally deprived during pregnancy depends to a great extent on how they are fed after birth.

Nutrition of the neonate can be manipulated by altering the number of pups a mother rat must nurse. If the usual litter is reduced from ten to three and the pups are nursed by foster mothers whose diets were not restricted during pregnancy, there is evidence that the deficits in cell numbers can be entirely made up by the time of weaning. Other studies have shown, however, that prenatally malnourished pups nursed in normal litter sizes do not catch up.

Perhaps the finding of most concern is the effect of continued deprivation on the growth of brain cells. If prenatally malnourished pups are restricted after birth by feeding them in litters of eighteen pups per dam, they demonstrate a 60% reduction in brain cell number by the time they are weaned. This is in contrast with the 15% to 20% reduction that is seen in either prenatal or postnatal malnutrition alone. Thus it seems as though malnutrition that is continued throughout the entire time when brain cells are dividing will produce deficits that are much greater than would be expected if the separate effects were simply added together.[24] Experiments by McCance and Widdowson,[14] Chow and Lee,[6] and others have shown that nutritional rehabilitation will not enable these animals to recover their normal size once the period of cell proliferation is passed. They will continue to be small no matter how well fed they are after weaning. Zamenhof and associates[29] have data to suggest that maternal malnutrition may even have intergenerational effects. They found that brain cell numbers were reduced in rats whose mothers were prenatally malnourished, even though these mothers had adequate diets after weaning and during gestation.

These studies would not be so disturbing if size were not related to function. The fact is, however, that alterations in normal biochemical and developmental processes have been shown to accompany fetal and neonatal malnutrition in several species of animals. Changes in the usual constituents of cells are observed as well as the delayed appearance of specific enzyme systems. Depending on the timing of the dietary deficiency, degeneration of the cerebral cortex, the medulla, and the spinal cord can be produced. Muscular development is also impaired because of a reduced number of muscle cells and fibers.

Some investigators have associated these changes with abnormal neuromotor and mental development. For example, Zamenhof and associates[28] have shown that prenatally malnourished rats do not respond normally to stimuli in the environment and have abnormalities in gait. Caldwell and Churchill[5] found that rat pups whose mothers had protein-restricted diets in pregnancy could not learn to run a rat maze as quickly as adequately nourished controls and were slower in avoidance conditioning.

What has been learned

Much can still be learned from experiments with animals about the processes of fetal growth and development and the consequences of maternal malnutrition, but the work to date has produced important results. The general conclusions can be summarized as follows:

1. Although a number of prenatal influences affect fetal growth, maternal malnutrition can be one cause of growth failure that results in small offspring of low birth weight.

2. Animals that are malnourished from restrictions of their mothers' diets throughout most of gestation are characterized by (a) reduced number and size of cells in the placenta, (b) reduced brain cell number and head size, (c) proportional reductions in the size of other organs, and (d) alterations in normal cell constituents and biochemical processes.

3. The consequences of malnutrition for the fetus depend on the timing, severity, and duration of the maternal dietary restriction. These consequences may be reversible if the restriction primarily affects growth in cell size, but a reduction in the number of cells may be permanent if the restriction is maintained throughout the entire period of hyperplastic growth.

Human experience

In view of the risks of early death or permanent disability associated with low birth weight, it is apparent that the research on intrauterine growth failure in laboratory animals may have great implications for human problems. Of the annual incidence of low birth weight infants, it has been estimated that from 10% to 20% are the result of intrauterine growth failure. This means that between 80,000 and 120,000 infants in the United States are born each year who have experienced malnutrition in utero. An important thing to understand when interpreting these statistics is that a number of factors can retard fetal growth. When the term *fetal malnutrition* is applied to human infants, it simply means that there was a reduction in the maternal supply or placental transport of nutrients so that fetal growth is retarded significantly below genetic potential. It does not necessarily mean that the mother's own nutrition was at fault. At present, there is no way to judge how many growth-retarded infants are the result of maternal malnutrition.

Although the animal experiments are highly suggestive, caution must be exercised in making direct applications to humans. A primary reason for doing research on animals is to find out what can *possibly* happen when certain conditions are imposed. The findings do not guarantee that these things *actually* happen in the normal course of human events. There are a number of reasons why the dramatic results of maternal malnutrition demonstrated in animals may not occur as readily in human beings. In effect, the consequences of maternal malnutrition on fetal growth and development are all magnified in the animal studies. This is because (1) relative rates of growth and development are much slower in humans compared with laboratory animals, (2) the timing of maximum growth also differs, (3) the number and size of fetuses a mother must nourish in utero compared with her own body size and nutritional reserves are much smaller in humans than in laboratory animals, and (4) the magnitude of dietary deprivation used for experimentation is rarely encountered in human populations under ordinary circumstances.

Human fetal growth

The techniques for measuring cell number and cell size are now being used to determine the stages of maximum cell growth and development in humans. Although the data are presently limited, a picture that generally parallels the sequence outline for animals is beginning to emerge.

The human placenta grows rapidly throughout gestation. By thirty-four to thirty-six weeks it has completed cell division. From that time until term, growth continues only by an increase in the size of existing cells.

It is known from studies of embryology that growth of the fetus can be divided into three periods. The first is the period of blastogenesis in which the fertilized egg cleaves into cells that fold in on one another. These evolve into an inner cell mass, which gives rise to the embryo and an outer coat, the trophoblast, which becomes the placenta. The process of blastogenesis is complete at about two weeks after fertilization.

The second period is the embryonic stage, the critical time when cells differentiate into three germinal layers. The ecto-

derm gives rise to the brain, nervous system, hair, and skin. The mesoderm produces all of the voluntary muscles, bones, and components of the cardiovascular and excretory systems. The endoderm differentiates to form the digestive system, respiratory system, and glandular organs of the body. By sixty days' gestation all of the major features of the human infant have been achieved.

The fetal stage is the period of most rapid growth. From the third month until term fetal weight increases nearly five-hundred-fold from about 6 grams to 3000 to 3500 grams at birth. Fig. 2-2 shows the average weight curve from ten weeks until term.

Measurements of DNA and protein in embryonic and fetal tissues show that growth in the embryonic stage occurs only by an increase in the number of cells. During the fetal stage, growth in cell number continues, but it is now accompanied by an increase in cell size.

Cells of most organs continue to proliferate after birth. Data derived from cases of therapeutic abortions and accidental

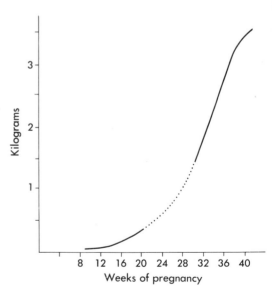

Fig. 2-2. Average curve of fetal growth. (From Hytten, F. E., and Leitch, I.: The physiology of human pregnancy, ed. 2, Oxford, 1971, Blackwell Scientific Publications, Ltd.)

deaths indicate that cell division in the normal human brain is linear throughout gestation, slows after birth, and reaches maximum around 18 months of age. It is believed that growth in cell size begins at about seven months' gestation and may continue into the third year of life. These estimates are for the whole organ and do not identify patterns in specific cells and regions of the central nervous system. There is evidence that growth in cell number stops earlier in the cerebellum. Neuronal cell number is probably complete at birth, whereas growth of glial cells peaks near birth and continues through the first year of life.[8]

Brain and nerve cells are not only composed of protein but also have considerable amounts of lipid materials. These include fatty acids, cholesterol, phospholipids, glycolipids, and other esters. Most lipids in brain and nerve cells are used for the synthesis of myelin, the substance that insulates the cells and aids in the conduction of nerve impulses. Changes in lipid composition are used to measure the rate of myelination occurring at different times.

Lipid deposition is fairly constant in the early part of gestation, but it begins to increase rapidly during the last trimester. In gray matter of the brain, adult composition is reached by about 3 months of age. Myelination is slower in white matter. It attains about 90% of adult composition by 2 years of age and is not completed until the child is approximately 10 years.

The other organs of the body grow prenatally and postnatally at varying rates. DNA measurements show that cell numbers in all organs which have been studied to date increase from thirteen weeks' gestation until term. There are continued increases in cell numbers in heart, liver, kidney, and spleen throughout the first year of life.

No change is observed in the size of cells during the prenatal period in the heart, kidney, spleen, thyroid, thymus, tongue, esophagus, stomach, and intestines. There is a slow increase in cell size beginning at about seven months' gestation in the liver, lungs, adrenal glands, and diaphragm.

Muscle, bone, and adipose cells exhibit patterns similar to the growth of other organs. Cells begin to proliferate rapidly at three to four months' gestation and continue to divide in postnatal life. Growth in the size of cells shows the most rapid increase beginning at about seven months' gestation.

Humans have not been studied well enough to know precisely how long the various stages of growth last. The current hypothesis is that there are only certain times in life when new cells are made. Growth at other times is believed to take place only by an increase in the size of preexisting cells.

Growth-retarded infants

From the sequence of growth that has been described, it is possible to theorize the effects of malnutrition at different stages of gestation. In the very early months of pregnancy, a severe limitation on the supply or transport of nutrients would have to occur because the quantitative requirements of the embryo are extremely small. Nevertheless, a restriction of materials and energy needed for cell synthesis and cell differentiation could produce malformations or cause the embryo to die.

Malnutrition after the third month of gestation would not have teratogenic effects, but it could interfere with fetal growth. Nutrient requirements are greatest in the last trimester of pregnancy, when cells are increasing both in number and in size. Even a relatively mild restriction could be a serious impediment at this time.

The theoretical effects of fetal malnutrition are reflected in the characteristics of small-for-date infants. Their conditions are variable, suggesting the multiple etiologies and importance of timing shown in animals. Among those small-for-date infants who do not have birth anomalies, there are two patterns of growth retardation. One type affects weight more than length; the other affects weight and length equally.

In the first type of retardation, head circumference and skeletal growth are about normal, but the infants have poorly developed muscles and almost no subcutaneous fat. The resemblance of these infants to the large-head, small-body features of animals malnourished during the last weeks of gestation from maternal dietary restrictions or uterine ligation is remarkable.

In the type of growth retardation that affects weight and length equally, the size of all parts of the body, including head circumference and skeleton, is proportionally reduced. The physical characteristics of these infants are similar to those of rat pups whose mothers were maintained on deficient diets throughout most of gestation.

Effects of maternal malnutrition

These observations provide fertile grounds for speculation, but is there any evidence that maternal malnutrition really is a cause of fetal malnutrition in human populations? Of necessity much of the information is circumstantial, but there have been three kinds of studies that have addressed this question with highly significant results. These are (1) natural experiments in which birth statistics before, during, and after periods of acute famine are studied and compared; (2) measurements of organ size and cell numbers in stillbirths and neonatal deaths where all causes not related to maternal malnutrition have been ruled out; and (3) epidemiological studies of the nutritional correlates of birth weight.

Natural experiments. The hardships of war afford researchers an opportunity to study the effects of severe dietary restrictions during pregnancy under conditions that thankfully are seldom duplicated. Throughout most of Europe at various times during World War II, food shortages were commonplace. Reports were made on the effects of these shortages during the 1940s, but they are being considered with

renewed interest today in light of the findings from animal research.

An eighteen-month period of acute starvation was experienced in Russia during the seige of Leningrad in 1942. Antonov[1] compared statistics for infants born before, during, and after the seige. He found that during the famine period there was a twofold increase in fetal mortality and an increase in the number of infants weighing less than 2500 grams at birth.

Similar findings were reported by Smith[21] from Holland. Here the statistics are more insightful because the famine was of sharp onset and limited to approximately six months during the winter of 1944 and 1945. It was not accompanied by other deprivations as severe as those experienced during the seige of Leningrad, and the women of Holland were considered to have eaten fairly good diets prior to the food shortage. During the famine, dietary intake dropped to less than 1000 cal/day and protein was limited to 30 or 40 grams. Since the famine lasted only six months, babies conceived before and during it were exposed for varying lengths of time, but none was exposed for the entire course of gestation. This situation set up natural conditions that are similar to the animal experiments. When evaluating the statistics, Smith was able to consider how the timing of maternal dietary restrictions might affect fetal growth.

On the average, birth weights of infants exposed to the famine were reduced by 200 grams. Weights were lowest for babies exposed to the famine during the entire last half of pregnancy. Added exposure prior to that time did not reduce birth weights further. In fact, babies who were exposed to the famine during the first twenty-seven weeks of gestation but finished their terms after the famine ended had higher average birth weights than those who were only exposed during the last three weeks of gestation.

The data for stillbirths and congenital malformations followed a different pattern.

The rates were lowest for infants conceived before the famine and highest for those conceived during it.

The findings are in line with what is hypothesized from knowledge of the stages of human growth. Poor nutrition in the latter part of pregnancy affects fetal growth, whereas poor nutrition in the early months affects development of the embryo and its capacity to survive.

It is interesting to note that in contrast with the experiences in Russia and Holland, the perinatal mortality rate in Great Britain, which had been fairly constant before the war, actually declined between 1940 and 1945, despite poor environmental conditions and no discernible improvements in prenatal care. One possible explanation is that pregnant and lactating women were given priority status for food rationing in Britain as a matter of national policy.

Organ studies. Studies that attempt to relate the size of organs in human infants to maternal nutrition must control for other conditions known to affect fetal growth. Naeye and associates[17] looked at the organs of 252 United States stillborn infants and infants dying in the first 48 hours of life, excluding all multiple births, maternal complications, and congenital defects. The infants were categorized as coming from poor or nonpoor families according to income. Comparisons of organs between the two groups showed that the mass of adipose tissue as well as the size of individual fat cells were smaller in the poor infants. These infants also had smaller livers, adrenal glands, thymuses, and spleens. Heart, kidney, and skeleton were also reduced but the differences were not as great. The ranking in organ sizes is consistent with reductions noted in animals who have been prenatally malnourished and in humans who have experienced uterine or placental disorders. Since the last two were ruled out, Naeye concluded that undernutrition could be responsible for prenatal growth retardation in infants from low-income families.

The organs of infants who survive intrauterine malnutrition cannot be studied to see if cells are reduced in number or in size, but one organ that is available is the placenta. Winick[24] has reported that the size of placentas and the number of placental cells are 15% to 20% below normal when infants experience intrauterine growth failure. By comparing placentas from different sources, he has shown that those from indigent populations in developing countries have reductions in cell numbers similar to the reductions noted in placentas from United States infants with intrauterine growth failure. In one interesting case in the United States, a mother who was severely undernourished from anorexia nervosa during pregnancy gave birth to an infant weighing less than 2500 grams. When the placenta was examined, it was found to have only 50% of the normal number of cells.[24]

Lechtig and co-workers[13] have also looked at human placentas. The 49 women in their study all came from Guatemala City. Their socioeconomic status was evaluated according to family income, education, and sanitary conditions in the home. Measurements of height, postpartum weight, skin folds, and the ratio of nonessential to essential amino acids in serum all showed significant differences indicative of chronic protein-calorie malnutrition in the low socioeconomic group. The average weight of placentas from women in the low socioeconomic group was 15% below the average weight of placentas from the high socioeconomic group. On microscopic examination it was found that low placental weight was associated with reduced surface area of the placental peripheral villi. The peripheral villi are responsible for the transport of nutrients to the fetus. The reduction in surface area may be what accounts for the observed association between placental weight and the size of the infant at birth.

Nutritional correlates of birth weight. Studies of the relationship between maternal nutrition and the birth weight of the infant have tended to focus directly on the nutrient composition of the diet during pregnancy. Because of variations in the nutritional requirements of individuals, we have seen that these studies have produced conflicting results. However, there are two indicators of long-term and immediate nutritional status that have shown consistent associations with birth weight. These are maternal body size (height and prepregnancy weight) and the amount of weight gained by the mother during pregnancy itself.

It should not be surprising that big mothers have big babies. What is less often appreciated is that the size of the infant at birth is completely dependent on the size of the mother and is not influenced by the size of the father. This was shown years ago in a classical experiment by Walton and Hammond.[23] They bred Shire stallions with Shetland mares and Shetland stallions with Shire mares. The newborn foals were always of a size appropriate to the mothers' breeds, and no intermediate sizes were ever produced. The same effects have since been demonstrated in a number of animals, and there is indirect evidence for the same phenomenon in humans.

It has been further demonstrated that, in humans, height and prepregnancy weight of the mother have independent and additive effects on the birth weight of the child. In an analysis of 4095 mothers in Aberdeen, Thomson and associates[20] found that, on the average, the tallest and heaviest mothers had babies who weighed 500 grams more at birth than babies of the shortest and lightest mothers. It is postulated that maternal size is a conditioning factor on the ultimate size of the placenta and thus controls the blood supply of nutrients which will be available to the fetus.

A relationship is also noted between infant birth weight and the amount of weight the mother gains during pregnancy. Since part of the maternal weight gain is represented by the products of conception, it is logical that such a relationship exists, yet there have been several recent studies which have shown that women who gain more than the combined weight of the fetus, placenta, and amniotic fluid tend to produce heavier infants. One such study by Eastman and Jackson[9] examined the pregnancy weight gains of 25,154 mothers in Baltimore. They excluded all preterm infants and cases of stillbirth, multiple birth, toxemia, and other complicating conditions. The group contained approximately equal numbers of black and white mothers. The investigators found the typical difference in mean birth weight between blacks and whites, but in both racial groups the mean weights of infants consistently increased with maternal weight gain. There was an average difference of 350 to 450 grams between infants of women who gained 10 pounds or less and infants of women who gained 40 pounds or more.

A unique study that demonstrates the combined effects of prepregnancy weight and weight gain during pregnancy on birth weight and size of the infant has been published by Naeye and colleagues.[16] Again, excluding all maternal and fetal incidents that could confound the results, these researchers conducted autopsies on 1044 stillbirths and neonatal deaths at one hospital in New York City. Medical records were also examined to determine the mothers' prepregnancy weights for height and pregnancy weight gains. On the basis of these findings, the mothers were assigned to one of four nutritional categories: (1) overweight prior to pregnancy with a high pregnancy weight gain, (2) overweight prior to pregnancy with a low pregnancy weight gain, (3) underweight prior to pregnancy with a high pregnancy weight gain, and (4) underweight prior to pregnancy with a low pregnancy weight gain. A low pregnancy weight gain was defined as less than the combined weight of the fetus, placenta, and amniotic fluid. A high weight gain was considered to be three and one-half times the weight of these products of conception. Measurements were then made for body weight of the infants, body length, weight of the placentas, and weights of the brain, thymus, heart, lungs, spleen, liver, adrenals, and kidneys. There were no discernible differences for infants less than thirty-three weeks' gestation, but for those carried over thirty-three weeks body and organ weights of the infants decreased progressively from maternal nutritional categories 1 through 4. A statistically significant difference was observed at the extremes; that is, the greatest differences in body size and organ weights of the infants were between the overweight–high gain mothers and the underweight–low gain mothers. Organs that were most reduced in the infants from the underweight–low gain mothers were placentas, livers, and adrenals. Brains and skeletons appeared to be spared, but the brains of infants from the best nourished mothers tended to be larger than the norm.

What is most significant for its practical implications is that the investigators also looked at what kind of dietary management the mothers had received during pregnancy. In all four nutritional categories, infants of mothers who had been placed on 1000- to 1500-calorie diets during pregnancy had smaller body and organ measurements than infants from mothers who had been given general advice with no dietary restrictions. Again, the greatest differences were between overweight–high gain mothers and underweight–low gain mothers.

All of the relationships in this study held, even when factors such as race, marital status, work status, and the interval since the last pregnancy were taken into account. Successive pregnancies in the most poorly nourished mothers led to progressively more undernourished infants, whereas mothers in the highest nutritional category had successively larger offspring. Low-income mothers tended to have small infants, but the authors attributed this to the fact that more of these women were placed on low-calorie diets during pregnancy.

IMPROVING THE OUTCOME OF PREGNANCY

There are sufficient parallels between animal and human research to conclude that maternal nutrition can influence reproductive performance, especially of women who have a high risk of giving birth to low birth weight infants. Birth weight, as a reflection of intrauterine growth, is a determinant of the child's potential for survival and future health. This is true of both physical and mental performance.

Recently there has been much discussion about the possible effects of prenatal nutrition on intelligence and learning ability. Whether an infant whose size and brain cells are reduced at birth from maternal malnutrition is going to have a permanent mental disability is not presently known. Given the understanding of growth and development, however, it is reasonable to suppose that the consequences will depend to some extent on the nutrition of the child in postnatal life as well as the physical and social environment in which he is born. A follow-up study of children born during the World War II famine in Holland could find no evidence of lower than average intelligence or a higher incidence of mental retardation.[22] It is possible that acute dietary deprivation of previously well-nourished women during pregnancy can be compensated by adequate nutrition later on. But the situation in Holland is not what typically occurs. Most women in good nutritional status prior to conception do not suddenly eat poor diets during pregnancy and then try to make up for it by feeding their children well after they are born. The factors that place a pregnant woman at nutritional risk have operated over her lifetime and will continue to affect the nutritional status, growth, and development of her child. These include poverty, poor education, a deprived environment, and poor health. Surveys have shown clear associations between these factors and the nutritional status of infants, children, and women of childbearing age. Although all women need nutritional guidance during pregnancy, those who conceive in poor nutritional status and whose life circumstances impair their ability to secure adequate diets for themselves and their families require special care.

Implications for practice

The studies on weight gain during pregnancy have great importance for clinical practice. There must surely be an upper limit to birth weight that will not be exceeded despite progressively higher maternal weight gains. Furthermore, obesity engenders its own health risks and should not be encouraged. Yet the studies by Eastman and Jackson, Naeye, and others clearly demonstrate that pregnancy is no time for women to try to lose weight. The common practice of restricting weight gain by placing pregnant women on low-calorie diets must be discouraged. There are public health implications that can be shown not only for low-income mothers but for those from the upper socioeconomic strata as well.

A vast body of information on the distribution of birth weights around the world has been summarized by Hytten and Leitch.[11] Data on American infants show that the average birth weights range from 3000 to 3500 grams. However, when perinatal mortality rates are examined, the lowest rates occur when infants weigh between 3501 and 4000 grams. In other words, it would appear that the optimum birth weight for the lowest risk of mortality is somewhat higher than the average birth weight.

We have seen in Chapter 1 that intrauterine growth for nonwhites declines during the last trimester of pregnancy and that curves for even the more affluent white infants are lower in the United States than in Scandinavian countries. When this is compared with the demonstrated effects of

maternal height, prepregnancy weight, and weight gain on the size and weight of infants carried to term, there is reason for believing that improving maternal nutrition before and during pregnancy may be one of the most practical steps that can be taken toward improving the distribution of birth weights and the rate of perinatal death.

Nutritional care for high-risk mothers

Nutritional intervention to improve pregnancy outcomes must be both short and long term. Nutritional status of the mother, as reflected by her height and prepregnancy weight, is a fixed variable not subject to manipulation once pregnancy occurs. Intervention must be directed at future generations of mothers to assure that they receive adequate nutrition to reach their maximum growth potential and maintain optimum weight. Diet and weight gain after conception, however, are factors that can be modified during pregnancy itself. If they are indeed major influences on birth weight and maternal and infant health, special dietary management of women who have a high risk of reproductive problems should produce beneficial results. Two separate groups of researchers in Guatemala and Canada have recently tested this hypothesis.

The study in Guatemala is one of the most comprehensive investigations of the relationship between maternal nutrition and the outcome of pregnancy that has ever been undertaken. It involves all women of childbearing age in four villages in a long-term, prospective study to see what effects nutrition has on physical growth and mental development of their offspring.[12] Before beginning their study, the investigators collected a great deal of information about birth statistics, dietary practices, and nutritional status of the women in the four villages. They found evidence of chronic but moderate malnutrition by measuring heights, weights, and head circumferences. During pregnancy, women averaged a weight gain of only 15 pounds. They typically consumed about 1500 calories and 40 grams of protein per day. This protein-to-calorie ratio is adequate. The moderate degree of malnutrition was primarily the result of insufficient food consumption. Mean birth weights in the population were between 3000 and 3200 grams, but about one third of the infants carried to term were of low birth weight.

The plan of the study included the provision of dietary supplements to all pregnant women who would voluntarily accept them. In two of the villages, the supplement Atole contained both protein and calories. The supplement Fresco was given to women in the other two villages. It contained calories but no protein. Both supplements had approximately equal amounts of vitamins and minerals.

Intakes from the supplements and home diets were recorded in each trimester of pregnancy to make sure that the women were not substituting the supplements for their usual food. The records showed that the supplements did, in fact, increase total intake by an average of 26,820 calories during the entire course of pregnancy. However, since consumption of the supplements was voluntary, there were wide ranges of intakes. The investigators were therefore able to divide the women into a low-supplement group and a high-supplement group according to the total number of additional calories they consumed. The level of 20,000 calories was chosen as the dividing line because this was the median value for all of the women. When the women were divided this way, there was a difference of 34,000 calories between the mean supplemental intakes of the high and low groups.

During the first four years of the study, complete data on maternal supplementation and birth weight were available for 405 infants born in the four villages. The first thing to be noted in the results is that for full-term infants there was a consistent increase in birth weight as the total supplemental calories of the mother increased. The distribution was such that for each 10,000 calories ingested by the mother during pregnancy, birth weight of the infant increased 50 grams. The greatest difference in birth weight was observed between infants whose mothers consumed less than 20,000 supplemental calories and those whose mothers consumed 20,000 supplemental calories or more. The significance of this is shown by the percent of low birth weight babies born to high- and low-supplemented mothers (Fig. 2-3). The rate of low birth weight was roughly two times lower when the mothers consumed 20,000 supplemental calories or more throughout gestation.

The investigators also examined weights of the placentas. They found, on the average, that the group with low maternal supplementation had placentas weighing 11% less than the group with high maternal supplementation. Further analysis showed that most of the association between maternal supplementation and birth weight could be explained statistically by the difference in placental weight. This finding supports the earlier observation that the size of the placenta may be the means by which maternal nutrition affects birth weight.

A most interesting aspect of these findings is that there was no difference in placental weight, mean birth weight, or the percent of low birth weight babies associated with the *type* of supplement used. As long as the calories were equivalent, it did not matter whether the supplement contained protein. This may seem surprising in view of emphasis people tend to place on the importance of protein in the diet and the research that has been done on the effects of protein restriction in animals. The authors of the study concluded that in a population experiencing chronic but moderate malnutrition, the limiting factor in the diet is calories, not protein. The amount of protein may actually be higher

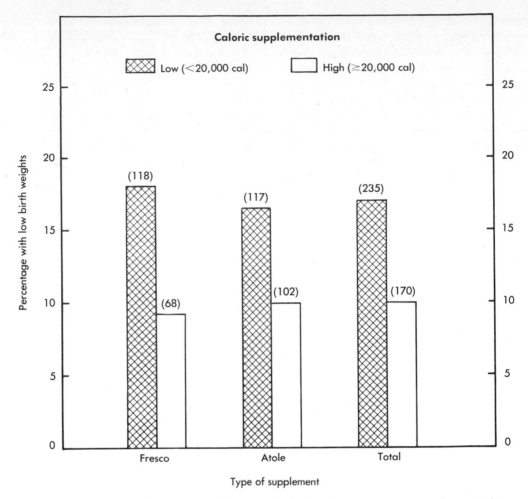

Fig. 2-3. Relationship between supplemented calories during pregnancy and proportion of low birth weight babies (2500 grams). Numbers in parentheses indicate number of cases. (From Lechtig, A., Habict, J. R., Delgado, H., Klein, R. E., Yarbrough, C., and Martorell, R.: Pediatrics **56:**508, 1975.)

than that needed to maintain tissue synthesis, but the women simply do not consume enough calories to spare protein from meeting energy needs. For infants of these women, the increment in birth weight from the consumption of additional calories is mostly due to the accumulation of fetal adipose tissue. The benefits are that the entire birth weight distribution is shifted upward. Low birth weight infants still have greater risks, but the fact that fewer of them are born causes a reduction in the overall rate of neonatal death.

The experiences of Primrose and Higgins[18] at the Montreal Diet Dispensary in Canada show that the benefits of extra calories and special dietary management during pregnancy are not confined to chronically malnourished women in developing countries but can also improve the pregnancy performance of high-risk mothers in the more affluent nations. Knowing the risk of reproductive problems associated with low income, these investigators selected the hospital handling the highest percentage of poor patients in Montreal. All patients from two of the hospital's public maternity clinics were enrolled—a total of 1544 women between 1963 and 1970. A unique feature was that dietary needs for calories and protein were individually calculated for each woman based on her body weight for height with adjustments for protein deficiency, underweight, and other stress conditions. Women whose family incomes fell below specified levels—70% of all women in the study—were given supplies of milk, eggs, and oranges every two weeks. All of the women received counseling on food selection to meet their individual needs every time they visited the clinic, and nutritionists visited all patients at home at least once during their pregnancies.

Such intensive nutritional care enabled the women to average 93% of their total caloric needs and 96% of their total protein requirements throughout gestation. Since the majority started out with large average daily deficits, they all showed significant improvements in the quality of their diets.

Birth statistics indicate how the mothers and their infants benefited from these measures. The incidence of low birth weight in this high-risk study group was brought down to the all-Canada rate and was lower than the rate for Quebec province. Stillbirths, neonatal mortality, and perinatal mortality were also lower than the rates prevailing in Canada and Quebec.

Primrose and Higgins[18] found a direct relationship between maternal weight gains and birth weights, which were, in turn, directly related to the length of time the women had received Diet Dispensary service. No such relationship between birth weights and service was observed for other public patients who were not part of the Montreal Diet Dispensary study but who received prenatal care and gave birth at the same hospital.

It is impossible to know how much of the improvements in pregnancy performance and outcome demonstrated in this study can be attributed to the diets of the women,

the food supplements, or the special attention they received. What is important about the study is that it shows how high-risk mothers, against all odds, can experience successful pregnancies when superior nutritional guidance is a part of their prenatal care.

REFERENCES

1. Antonov, A. N.: Children born during the seige of Leningrad in 1942, J. Pediatr. **30:**250, 1947.
2. Baird, D.: Variations in fertility associated with changes in health statistics, J. Chronic Dis. **18:**1109, 1965.
3. Balfour, M. J.: Supplementary feeding in pregnancy, Lancet **1:**208, 1944.
4. Burke, B. S., Beal, V. A., Kirkwood, S. B., and Stuart, H. C.: The influence of nutrition upon the condition of the infant at birth, J. Nutr. **26:**569, 1943.
5. Caldwell, D. F., and Churchill, J. A.: Learning ability in the progeny of rats administered a protein-deficient diet during the second half of gestation, Neurology **17:**95, 1967.
6. Chow, B. F., and Lee, C. T.: Effect of dietary restriction of pregnant rats on body weight gain of offspring, J. Nutr. **82:**10, 1964.
7. Committee on Maternal Nutrition, Food and Nutrition Board, National Research Council, National Academy of Sciences: Maternal malnutrition and the course of pregnancy, Washington, D.C., 1970, Government Printing Office.
8. Dobbing, J., and Sands, J.: Quantitative growth and development of human brain, Arch. Dis. Child. **48:**757, 1973.
9. Eastman, N. J., and Jackson, E.: Weight relationships in pregnancy. I. The bearing of maternal weight gain and pre-pregnancy weight on birth weight in full term pregnancies, Obstet. Gynecol. Surv. **23:**1003, 1968.
10. Ebbs, J. H., Tisdall, F. F., and Scott, W. A.: The influence of prenatal diet on the mother and child, Milbank Mem. Fund Q. **20:**35, 1942.
11. Hytten, F. E., and Leitch, I.: The physiology of human pregnancy, ed. 2, Oxford, 1971, Blackwell Scientific Publications, Ltd.
12. Lechtig, A., Habict, J. P., Delgado, H., Klein, R. E., Yarbrough, C., and Martorell, R.: Effect of food supplementation during pregnancy on birth weight, Pediatrics **56:**508, 1975.
13. Lechtig, A., Yarbrough, C., Delgado, H., Martorell, R., Klein, R. E., and Behar, M.: Effect of moderate maternal malnutrition on the placenta, Am. J. Obstet. Gynecol. **123:**191, 1975.
14. McCance, R. A., and Widdowson, E. M.: Nutrition and growth, Proc. R. Soc. Biol. **156:**326, 1962.
15. McGanity, W. J., Cannon, R. O., Bridgeforth, E.

B., Martin, M. P., Densen, P. M., Newbill, J. A., McClellan, G. S., Christie, A., Peterson, J. C., and Darby, W. J.: The Vanderbilt Cooperative Study of Maternal and Infant Nutrition. VI. Relationship of obstetric performance to nutrition, Am. J. Obstet. Gynecol. **67:**501, 1954.

16. Naeye, R. L., Blanc, W., and Paul, C.: Effects of maternal nutrition on the human fetus, Pediatrics **52:**494, 1973.
17. Naeye, R. L., Diener, M. M., and Dellinger, W. S.: Urban poverty: effects on prenatal nutrition, Science **166:**1026, 1969.
18. Primrose, T., and Higgins, A.: A study of human antepartum nutrition, J. Reprod. Med. **7:**257, 1971.
19. Thomson, A. M.: Diet in pregnancy, Br. J. Nutr. **13:**509, 1959.
20. Thomson, A. M., Bellewicz, W. Z., and Hytten, F. E.: The assessment of fetal growth, J. Obstet. Gynaecol. Br. Commonw. **75:**903, 1968.
21. Smith, C. A.: Effects of maternal undernutrition upon the newborn infant in Holland, J. Pediatr. **30:**229, 1947.
22. Stein, Z., Susser, M., Saenger, G., and Marolla, F.: Nutrition and mental performance, Science **178:**708, 1972.
23. Walton, A., and Hammond, J.: Maternal effects in growth and conformation in Shire horse–Shetland pony crosses, Proc. R. Soc. Biol. **125:**311, 1938.
24. Winick, M.: Fetal malnutrition, Clin. Obstet. Gynecol. **13:**526, 1970.
25. Winick, M.: Nutrition and cell growth, Nutr. Rev. **26:**195, 1968.
26. Winick, M., Brasel, J. A., and Rosso, P.: Nutrition and cell growth. In Winick, M., editor: Nutrition and development, New York, 1972, John Wiley & Sons, Inc.
27. Winick, M., Brasel, J. A., and Velasco, E. G., Effects of prenatal nutrition upon pregnancy risk, Clin. Obstet. Gynecol. **16:**184, 1973.
28. Zamenhof, S., Van Marthens, E., and Margolis, F. L.: DNA (cell number) and protein in neonatal brain: alterations by maternal dietary protein restriction, Science **160:**322, 1964.
29. Zamenhof, S., Van Marthens, E., and Gravel, L.: DNA (cell number) in neonatal brain: second generation (F2) alteration by maternal (F0) dietary protein restriction, Science **172:**850, 1971.

3
Physiological basis of nutritional needs

Joyce Vermeersch

MATERNAL PHYSIOLOGICAL ADJUSTMENTS

In Chapter 2 most of the discussion was focused on the fetus to show how maternal nutrition can affect its growth. In this chapter more attention will be given to the mother in considering how pregnancy alters her nutritional needs.

Normal pregnancy is accompanied by anatomical and physiological changes that affect almost every function of the body. Many of these changes are apparent in the very early weeks. This indicates that they are not merely a response to the physiological stress imposed by the fetus but are an integral part of the maternal-fetal system which creates the most favorable environment possible for the developing child. The changes are necessary to regulate maternal metabolism, promote fetal growth, and prepare the mother for labor, birth, and lactation.

The changes that occur in pregnancy are too complex to be given full treatment here, but a look at some that have effects on general metabolism will lay the foundation for interpreting nutritional requirements and dietary allowances.

ROLE OF THE PLACENTA

The placenta is not simply a passive barrier between the mother and the fetus but plays an active role in reproduction. It is the principal site of production for several of the hormones that are responsible for the regulation of maternal growth and development. For the fetus it is the only way that nutrients, oxygen, and waste products can be exchanged.

Structure and development

The placenta evolves from a small mass of cells in the first weeks of pregnancy into a complex network of tissue and blood vessels weighing about 650 grams at term. The vital role it plays as a link between mother and child is represented by the two principal parts of the placenta—one uterine and the other fetal.

On the maternal side the placenta is a part of the uterine mucosa. When the tiny blastocyst implants in the uterus six or seven days after fertilization, the uterine tissue and blood vessels break down to form small spaces that fill with blood. These spaces are eventually bounded on the maternal side by the decidua or basal plate.

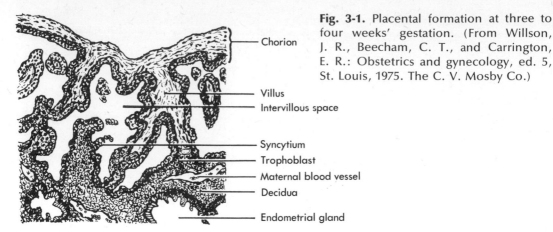

Chorion

Villus
Intervillous space

Syncytium
Trophoblast
Maternal blood vessel
Decidua

Endometrial gland

Fig. 3-1. Placental formation at three to four weeks' gestation. (From Willson, J. R., Beecham, C. T., and Carrington, E. R.: Obstetrics and gynecology, ed. 5, St. Louis, 1975. The C. V. Mosby Co.)

Blood begins to circulate in the spaces at about twelve days' gestation.

Meanwhile, the trophoblast grows and sends out rootlike villi into the pools of maternal blood. The villi contain capillaries, which will exchange nutrients and waste products between the mother and the fetus. In the early weeks of pregnancy, the villi are thick columns of cells, but as they subdivide throughout gestation, the villi become thinner and produce numerous branches. These give the villi a large surface area from which nutrients can be absorbed. On the fetal side the villi merge into the chorion. Inside the chorion are vessels that connect with the vein and two arteries coming from the fetus in the umbilical cord (Fig. 3-1).

Mechanisms of nutrient transfer

The efficiency with which the placenta accomplishes its function of nutrient transfer is a determinant of fetal well-being. Reduced surface area of the villi, insufficient vascularization, or changes in the hydrostatic pressure in the intervillous space can limit the supply of nutrients available to the fetus and inhibit normal growth.

Nutrient transfer in the placenta is a complex process. It employs all the mechanisms used for the absorption of nutrients from the gastrointestinal tract: simple diffusion, facilitated diffusion, active transport, and pinocytosis. The difference, how-

ever, is that in the placenta two completely separate blood supplies are maintained. The maternal circulation remains in the intervillous space. The fetal capillaries are separated from the maternal blood by two layers of cells. Their thickness is approximately 5.5 μm.

Although the same nutrient may be simultaneously transferred by more than one mechanism, the major means of transport can be determined by comparing nutrient concentrations in maternal and cord blood. If the concentrations are equal, the transfer has most likely occurred by simple or facilitated diffusion. In these two processes nutrients move from high concentrations in the maternal blood to lower concentrations in the fetal capillaries until equilibrium is reached. Facilitated diffusion requires the assistance of a carrier protein to increase the solubility of the nutrient and its rate of transport. Water and the fat-soluble vitamins A, D, E, and K pass to the fetus by diffusion. Their transport becomes more rapid in the latter part of pregnancy, when the villi decrease in thickness and assume a larger surface area.

A higher concentration of nutrients in cord blood indicates that active transport against an electrochemical gradient is involved. Active transport also requires a carrier protein, but for it to be "pumped" against a concentration gradient, metabolic energy in the form of adenosine triphosphate (ATP) must be used. Amino acids, glucose, ascorbic acid, and the B vitamins as well as minerals such as calcium, sodium, and iron are all transported by active means.

Proteins do not cross the placenta, since their molecular size is too big to allow penetration through the cells of the villi. This protects the fetus from acquiring harmful agents of high molecular weight, but it also means that the fetus must synthesize all of its own proteins from its supply of amino acids. An exception is the maternal immunoglobulin IgG. It is not known why this particular protein crosses the placenta, but it appears that the selectivity is related to the structure and not to the size of the molecule. IgG is probably transported by pinocytosis. The benefits to the fetus are that it has the same resistance to infectious diseases as the mother. This resistance lasts from six to nine months after birth, until the infant can manufacture his own antibodies.

The placenta also acts to assure that once nutrients are transported to the fetus, they do not "slide back down" the concentration gradient into the mother's blood. Ascorbic acid, for example, crosses the placenta in its reduced form as dehydroascorbic acid. Once inside the fetus, it is converted back to active L-ascorbic acid, which is impermeable to the placenta. Calcium transport is subject to similar protection through the mediation of hormones. Active transport of calcium makes the mother hypocalcemic compared with the fetus. Her response is to secrete parathyroid hormone (PTH) to favor bone resorption and increase serum calcium levels. If PTH reached the fetus, the effect would be to reverse the normal process of bone development. The relative impermeability of the placenta to PTH prevents this from happening. Instead, the fetus responds to its own high blood calcium levels by secreting endogenous calcitonin —the hormone that enhances the deposition of calcium in bone. Meanwhile, the placenta is freely permeable to vitamin D, favoring calcium retention in both the mother and the fetus.[26]

These mechanisms of placental transport have implications for the nutritional management of pregnant women. Since vitamins A and D are both transported by simple diffusion, they will continue to accumulate in the fetus as long as maternal blood levels are high. Both vitamins A and D are toxic in excessive amounts. Administration of high doses of vitamin A to pregnant animals has produced cleft palate, abnormalities of the urinary tract, and malformations in other organs of the fetus arising from the mesoderm. The effects in humans are not as well documented, but Gal and co-workers[7] discovered high maternal blood levels and fetal liver concentrations of vitamin A with fetuses having malformations. It is reported that a mother who took high doses of vitamin A early in pregnancy had a child with urinary anomalies similar to those produced in experimental animals.[8]

Excessive doses of vitamin D can result in fetal hypercalcemia. Friedman and Mills[6] have induced aortic stenosis and abnormal skull development in rabbits by feeding their mothers high levels of vitamin D during pregnancy. Premature closure of the fontanel from excessive vitamin D has been reported in newborn humans as well.[8]

Megadoses of water-soluble vitamins are not toxic, since the fetus can excrete unneeded amounts, but high doses given to the mother may have other undesirable consequences. Malone[19] suggests that the physiological competition for transport carriers may become pathological when certain nutrients are in excess. If essential amino acids are forced to compete with unnecessarily large quantities of vitamin C or the B vitamins, the results could be impaired or defective growth. Malone therefore advises that the use of megavitamin therapy during pregnancy is not only unwarranted but potentially dangerous.

Respiratory and excretory exchange

Beside serving as a lifeline for nutrients, the placenta also functions in the exchange of respiratory gases and waste products between the mother and fetus.

The delivery of oxygen to the fetus is just as important to proper metabolism as an adequate supply of nutrients. The mother herself makes adjustments in her breathing to meet fetal oxygen needs, but the amount ultimately depends on the blood flow through the uterus to the placental villi. Near term the rate of flow through the intervillous space is 375 to 560 ml/min. Exchange is made between maternal red cells, which characteristically have a lower affinity for oxygen during pregnancy, and fetal red cells, which have a high affinity.

Maternal nutrition can influence oxygen exchange through the production of hemoglobin. Each gram of hemoglobin carries 1.34 ml of oxygen. In normal concentrations it can deliver up to 16 ml of oxygen per 100 ml of blood to the placenta. If maternal hemoglobin levels are depressed from iron deficiency, the supply of oxygen per 100 ml of blood is reduced. Since the fetus can tolerate little variation in the rate at which oxygen is supplied, the mother must compensate by increasing her cardiac output.

To rid the fetus of metabolic waste, the placenta is freely permeable to carbon dioxide, water, urea, creatinine, and uric acid. Hyperventilation on the part of the mother reduces her Pco_2 so that carbon dioxide exchange from the fetus is accomplished by simple diffusion. Urea, creatinine, and uric acid, which are the wastes of fetal amino acid metabolism, move through the placenta by diffusion and active transport.[20]

Placental hormones

During pregnancy, the placenta assumes a major role in the production of hormones. It becomes the primary source of progesterone and estrogen. The placenta also synthesizes several hormones that are unique to gestation. These include human chorionic gonadotrophin (HCG), human placental lactogen (HPL), human chorionic somatomammotrophin (HCS), and human chorionic thyrotrophin (HCT). As their names imply, these hormones stimulate many of the processes concerned with maternal development. They also have effects on metabolism and nutrition. Production of placental hormones depends on precursors from the fetus as well as the mother.

ROLE OF HORMONES

The pregnant woman secretes more than thirty different hormones throughout gestation. Some, like those just mentioned, are only present in pregnancy, whereas others that are normally present have altered rates of secretion that are modified by the pregnant state.

Most hormones are proteins or steroids that are synthesized from precursors like amino acids and cholesterol in endocrine glands throughout the body. Their production is influenced by the mother's general health and nutritional status. Under normal circumstances they are controlling factors in a complex feedback system that maintains homeostasis between cellular and extracellular constituents and metabolism. During pregnancy, many of these homeostatic mechanisms are "reset" so that changes occur in the retention, utilization, and excretion of nutrients. Some of the hormones that exert important effects on nutrient metabolism are summarized in Table 3-1. Only those which have more general implications for nutritional management are singled out for discussion here.

Progesterone and estrogen

Progesterone and estrogen are two hormones that have major effects on maternal physiology during pregnancy. The chief action of progesterone is to cause a relaxation of the smooth muscles of the uterus so that it can expand as the fetus grows, but it also has a relaxing effect on other smooth muscles in the body. Relaxation of the muscles of the gastrointestinal tract reduces motility in the gut, allowing more time for the nutrients to be absorbed. The slower movement is also a cause of the con-

Table 3-1. Hormonal effects on nutrient metabolism in pregnancy

Hormone	Primary source of secretion	Principal effects
Progesterone	Placenta	Reduces gastric motility; favors maternal fat deposition; increases sodium excretion; reduces alveolar and arterial Pco_2; interferes with folic acid metabolism
Estrogen	Placenta	Reduces serum proteins; increases hydroscopic properties of connective tissue; affects thyroid function; interferes with folic acid metabolism
Human placental lactogen (HPL)	Placenta	Elevates blood glucose from breakdown of glycogen
Human chorionic thyrotrophin (HCT)	Placenta	Stimulates production of thyroid hormones
Human growth hormone (HGH)	Anterior pituitary	Elevates blood glucose; stimulates growth of long bones; promotes nitrogen retention
Thyroid stimulating hormone (TSH)	Anterior pituitary	Stimulates secretion of thyroxine; increases uptake of iodine by thyroid gland
Thyroxine	Thyroid	Regulates rate of cellular oxidation (basal metabolism)
Parathyroid hormone (PTH)	Parathyroid	Promotes calcium resorption from bone; increases calcium absorption; promotes urinary excretion of phosphate
Calcitonin (CT)	Thyroid	Inhibits calcium resorption from bone
Insulin	Beta cells of pancreas	Reduces blood glucose levels to promote energy production and synthesis of fat
Glucagon	Alpha cells of pancreas	Elevates blood glucose levels from glycogen breakdown
Aldosterone	Adrenal cortex	Promotes sodium retention and potassium excretion
Cortisone	Adrenal cortex	Elevates blood glucose from protein breakdown
Renin-angiotensin	Kidneys	Stimulates aldosterone secretion; promotes sodium and water retention; increases thirst

stipation commonly experienced by pregnant women. General metabolic effects of progesterone are to induce maternal fat deposition, reduce alveolar and arterial Pco_2, and increase renal sodium excretion.

The secretion of estrogen is lower than that of progesterone during the early months of pregnancy, but it rises sharply near term. Its role is to promote the growth and control the function of the uterus, but it too has generalized effects on nutrition. One effect that has caused some difficulties for clinicians is the alteration of the structure of mucopolysaccharides in connective tissue. This alteration is beneficial because it makes the tissue more flexible and therefore assists in dilating the uterus at birth, but it also increases the affinity of connective tissue to water. The hydroscopic effects of estrogen and the sodium-losing effect of progesterone produce a confusing clinical picture of the pregnant woman's fluid and electrolyte balance. Because of estrogen, many pregnant women complain of excess fluid retention in the skin. Their faces and fingers become puffy, and there are other indications of generalized edema. In addition, changes in cardiovascular dynamics cause extracellular fluid to accumulate in the feet and legs.

Since excess fluid retention is one of the hallmarks of preeclampsia, some clinicians view these changes with alarm. Rather rigorous treatment with diuretics and a sodium-restricted diet is frequently initiated to promote water loss. The evidence, however, weighs against this practice. Thomson and associates[29] report that whereas the incidence of generalized and peripheral (ankle) edema is high, it is not associated with an increase in perinatal mortality when the two other symptoms of preeclampsia—hypertension and proteinuria—are absent. In fact, women with mild edema have slightly larger babies and a lower rate of prematurity.

The propensity of women to lose sodium from the action of progesterone is compensated by an increased secretion of aldosterone from the adrenal glands and renin from the juxtaglomerular gland of the kidneys. If sodium restriction is imposed, this system must work harder to maintain normal sodium concentrations in the body. Pushed beyond the stress naturally induced by pregnancy, the system could become exhausted so that, in the long run, less aldosterone and renin are produced. The sodium and water depletion that would result is more dangerous than the mild degrees of edema that the treatment is supposed to prevent. Pike and associates[25] have demonstrated this in pregnant rats that are placed on sodium-restricted diets that would be equivalent to a 1-gram sodium or "no added salt" diet in humans.

Although hormonal effects on fluid and electrolyte balance need more research, the mechanisms which are understood to date suggest that a mild degree of edema is physiological in pregnancy and that the measures commonly used to prevent it impose an unnecessary risk.

Thyroxine

The iodine-containing hormone thyroxine is secreted by the thyroid gland. Circulating levels of thyroxine regulate the rate of oxidation reactions that are involved in the production of energy. The hormone therefore has a major role in metabolism and influences caloric requirements.

The secretion of thyroxine is a good example of how hormonal interactions control homeostatic mechanisms during pregnancy. Normally, the manufacture and release of thyroxine are under the influence of thyroid-stimulating hormone (TSH)—a pituitary hormone which in turn is regulated by the hypothalamus. The hypothalamus appears to be sensitive to changing rates of nutrient utilization in the tissues. High rates of utilization send two kinds of messages through the hypothalamus. One stimulates appetite and the desire to eat; the other stimulates TSH and thyroxine release so that the nutrients in food can be used.

In pregnancy, progesterone and estrogen enter into this feedback and control system. Progesterone increases the sensitivity of the respiratory centers and causes the pregnant woman to "overbreathe." The reduction in Pco_2 that results depresses the circulating levels of thyroxine. Ordinarily this would excite the pituitary to secrete TSH so that levels of thyroxine can increase, but estrogen acts as a break to prevent overtaxation of the thyroid and keeps the process under control. The net effect is an overall rise in thyroxine with TSH maintained in the nonpregnant range (Fig. 3-2).

Although the picture is complex, it has implications for clinical management. The adaptive mechanisms under hormonal control are set to respond to increased rates of oxygen and nutrient utilization during pregnancy. These have an effect on oxygen requirements and caloric needs. Hyperventilation occurs spontaneously so that sufficient oxygen is available for the production of energy. When a pregnant woman is allowed to "eat to appetite," an adequate intake of the raw materials for energy production found in food is also ensured.

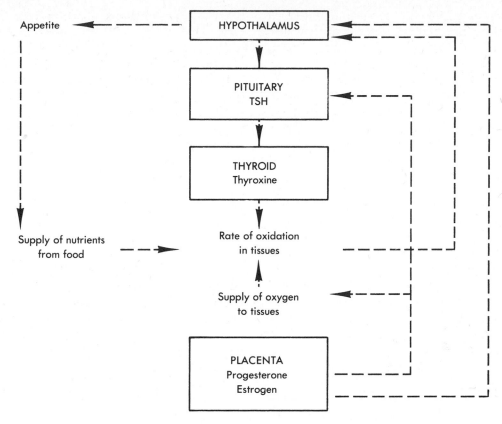

Fig. 3-2. Hormonal regulation of energy metabolism in pregnancy.

Insulin

There are a number of hormones concerned with maintaining the concentration of nutrients in the blood. Insulin affects blood glucose levels, and its action is critical in normal pregnancy. The fetus can use only glucose to meet its energy needs. Maternal metabolism is therefore keyed to make sure that adequate amounts of glucose are supplied.

The specific mechanisms of insulin secretion and glucose regulation in pregnancy are not fully understood. Normally, insulin is secreted by the beta cells of the pancreas when blood glucose levels are high. Insulin facilitates the transport of glucose to the cells, where it is used to produce energy or synthesize fat. The adequacy of insulin secretion is measured by the rate at which glucose disappears from the blood after an oral load.

Pregnant women have normal insulin responses to glucose in early pregnancy, but in the later months it takes more insulin to remove the same amount of glucose from the blood. Reasons for this are speculative. One explanation is simply that the increased needs for glucose by the growing fetus put a considerable strain on the system so that by the end of pregnancy the action of insulin becomes less efficient. But there are indications that other hormones of pregnancy are also involved. Those known to have an antagonistic relationship to insulin include human placental lactogen (HPL), human growth hormone (HGH), and cortisone.

HPL and HGH antagonize insulin by

continuing to feed glucose into the blood from the breakdown of glycogen. It is also possible that HPL increases the rate of insulin destruction in the placenta.

Cortisone also favors the elevation of blood glucose levels by stimulating its synthesis from amino acids that come from the breakdown of protein tissues. Cortisone levels are usually at or below normal in early pregnancy, but they rise steeply at term. This rise is induced by estrogen to help the mother through labor. High cortisone levels may increase the destruction of insulin in the liver.

Whatever specific mechanisms are involved, the effects of altered insulin efficiency in the face of other hormonal antagonists place a stress on the beta cells of the pancreas. Prediabetic women may show frank indications of impaired glucose tolerance. If diabetes exists prior to pregnancy, the condition may become worse. The diet of pregnant women must be managed to minimize this stress. As will be shown, there is a danger to both the mother and the fetus if impaired glucose metabolism results in ketoacidosis.

CHANGES IN BLOOD VOLUME AND COMPOSITION

Plasma is the fluid component of blood, whereas serum is the part of plasma that remains after its coagulation factors have been removed. Total plasma volume in a nonpregnant woman averages 2600 ml. Near the end of the first trimester of pregnancy, plasma volume begins to increase, and by thirty-four weeks it is about 50% greater than it was at conception.

There is considerable variation from these averages. Women who have small volumes to begin with usually have a greater increase, as do multigravidas and mothers with multiple births.

Hytten and Paintin[14] have shown that the increase in plasma volume is correlated with obstetrical performance. They found that women who have a small increase when compared with the average are more likely to have stillbirths, abortions, and low birth weight babies. Clearly, the restriction of a normal expansion of plasma volume is an undesirable condition in pregnancy.

If the availability of nutrients or the synthesis of normal blood constituents does not keep pace with the expansion of plasma volume, their concentrations per 100 ml of blood will decrease, even though the total amounts may rise. This is apparently what happens with red blood cells, serum proteins, minerals, and the water-soluble vitamins.

Red cell production is stimulated during pregnancy so that their numbers gradually rise, but the increase is not as large as the expansion of plasma volume. The hematocrit, which is normally around 35% in women, may be as low as 29% to 31% during pregnancy. The amount of hemoglobin in each red blood cell does not change, but because there are fewer red blood cells per 100 ml of blood, hemodilution occurs. Nonpregnant values of 13 to 14 gm/100 ml can drop as low as 10 or 11 gm/100 ml in the early months. In a nonpregnant woman this level of hemoglobin would indicate anemia, but in pregnancy the red blood cells are normochromic and normocytic.

Serum levels of the major nutrients typical for pregnant and nonpregnant women are compared in Table 3-2. Most of the reduction in serum proteins is due to a sharp decline in the albumin fraction. Alpha and beta globulins show a progressive increase. The reduction in serum albumin changes colloidal osmotic pressure of the blood. This, in conjunction with the expanded plasma volume, is another factor responsible for the tendency of pregnant women to accumulate extracellular fluid.

In contrast to the water-soluble nutrients, those which are fat soluble show increased serum concentrations during pregnancy. There are progressive increases in serum triglycerides, cholesterol, free fatty acids, and vitamin A. These higher lipid levels are what maintain the concentrations of alpha and beta globulins, since in

Table 3-2. Serum nutrient levels in pregnant and nonpregnant women*

Nutrient	Normal nonpregnancy range	Values in pregnancy
Total protein	6.5-8.5 gm/100 ml	6.0-8.0
Albumin	3.5-5.0 gm/100 ml	3.0-4.5
Glucose	<110 mg/100 ml	<120
Cholesterol	120-190 mg/100 ml	200-325
Vitamin A	20-60 μg/100 ml	20-60
Carotene	50-300 μg/100 ml	80-325
Ascorbic acid	0.2-2.0 mg/100 ml	0.2-1.5
Folic acid	5-21 ng/100 ml	3-15
Calcium	4.6-5.5 mEq/L	4.2-5.2
Iron/iron-binding capacity	>50/250-400 μg/100 ml	>40/300-450

*Modified from Aubry, R. H., Roberts, A., and Cuenca, V.: The assessment of maternal nutrition, Clin. Perinatol. **2**:207, 1975.

order to circulate, triglycerides and cholesterol must be protein bound. The mechanisms which support high lipid concentrations in pregnancy have not been fully elaborated, but it is probable that the steroid hormones are involved Cholesterol is a precursor for the synthesis of progesterone and estrogen in the placenta.

CHANGES IN RENAL FUNCTION

To facilitate the clearance of creatinine, urea, and other waste products of fetal and maternal metabolism, blood flow through the kidneys and the glomerular filtration rate are increased during pregnancy. The change in glomerular filtration is partially due to the lower osmotic pressure, which results from the fall in serum albumin. This is one adaptation that appears to be purely mechanical, since no effects of hormones on this aspect of kidney function have been shown. But there are consequences for nutrition.

In the words of Hytten and Thomson,[15] "The kidney during pregnancy shows an astonishing profligacy with nutrients." Normally, most of the glucose, amino acids, and water-soluble vitamins that are filtered by the kidneys are reabsorbed in the tubules to preserve the body's balance. But in pregnancy substantial quantities of these nutrients appear in the urine. The most satisfactory explanation at present is that the high glomerular filtration rate offers the tubules greater quantities of nutrients than they can feasibly reabsorb. Because the change in filtration rate is largely mechanical, there may not be an accompanying mechanism by which the tubules can readjust.

PROBLEMS IN DETERMINING NUTRIENT NEEDS

The low serum values of nutrients commonly seen during pregnancy and the tendency of the kidneys to excrete greater amounts have posed problems for setting nutrient requirements and making dietary recommendations. Some of the blood values typical in pregnancy would be judged borderline or deficient if they were seen in a nonpregnant woman. The picture is further complicated by the fact that most of the blood levels can be increased if oral supplements are given.

If no physical symptoms of deficiency or consequences to the course or outcome of pregnancy are observed when serum values differ from the norm, their clinical significance is difficult to determine. It is not presently known whether the total amounts of nutrients in the blood or their concentrations per 100 ml are most important for the mother and her growing child. Although the values may indicate increased needs, their nearly universal occurrence in pregnant women makes it hard to believe that they are all the result of dietary deficiencies.

Hytten and Leitch,[13] who have made extensive studies on the physiology of pregnancy, maintain that the profound changes which occur in maternal metabolism indicate that the pregnant woman cannot be judged by nonpregnant standards. To them the alterations in nutrient levels that are so typical in pregnancy suggest a common purpose. They see no reason to assume that vitamins and minerals such as folic acid, vitamin B$_6$, or iron require special attention, whereas other nutrients that are equally low (and usually less readily available as commercial supplements) are ignored.

On the other hand, more cautious clinicians have interpreted the lower serum values and altered rates of urinary excretion as indications of increased risk. They maintain that since intakes of nutrients necessary to achieve normal serum concentrations cannot be obtained without an inordinate increase in total calories, oral supplements should be used. Even though detrimental effects of the low serum values may not be apparent, these clinicians credit supplementation with the ability to prevent outright deficiencies that may be induced if women enter pregnancy with poor nutrient reserves.

This controversy cannot be resolved without further research. Because pregnancy is a time of growth, the need for nutrients is increased. It stands to reason that women who enter pregnancy in poor nutritional status run a risk of developing deficiencies that will have unfavorable effects on obstetrical performance. But for healthy women who enter pregnancy in good nutritional status, the picture is more obscure. Current standards used to evaluate the nutrition of pregnant women cannot be viewed as absolute until more about maternal metabolism and its effects on nutrient requirements is known.

RECOMMENDED DIETARY ALLOWANCES (RDA)

The Food and Nutrition Board of the National Research Council is well aware of the problems of determining nutrient requirements during pregnancy and takes them into consideration when setting dietary allowances and making recommendations about the need for supplementation. Recommended Dietary Allowances (RDA) are based on the best available evidence

from metabolic balance studies and from indirect estimates. Requirements for most nutrients are set at levels that prevent signs of deficiency and maintain intake in balance with urinary excretion. When making dietary recommendations, the requirements are adjusted upward to assure that the amounts derived from experimental subjects will cover individual variations in digestion, absorption, and utilization in the general population. As new evidence concerning requirements becomes available, the allowances are revised.

The 1974 edition of the Recommended Dietary Allowances for pregnant and nonpregnant adult women is presented in Table 3-3. The special needs of adolescent mothers will be discussed in Chapter 6.

Table 3-3. Recommended Dietary Allowances for adult women (ages 23 to 50 years)*

	Nonpregnant	Pregnant
Energy (kcal)	2000	2300
Protein (gm)	46	76
Vitamin A (RE)†	800	1000
(IU)	4000	5000
Vitamin D (IU)		400
Vitamin E (IU)	12	15
Vitamin C (ascorbic acid) (mg)	45	60
Folic acid (μg)	400	800
Niacin (mg)	13	15
Riboflavin (mg)	1.2	1.5
Thiamin (mg)	1.0	1.4
Vitamin B$_6$ (mg)	2.0	2.5
Vitamin B$_{12}$ (μg)	3.0	4.0
Calcium (mg)	800	1200
Phosphorus (mg)	800	1200
Iodine (μg)	100	125
Iron (mg)	18	18+
Magnesium (mg)	300	450
Zinc (mg)	15	20

*From Food and Nutrition Board, National Research Council, National Academy of Sciences: Recommended dietary allowances, ed. 8, Washington, D.C., 1974, Government Printing Office.
†RE (retinol equivalent) replaces IU (international unit) as the standard measure of vitamin A activity.

The figures in the table indicate the needs of a "reference" woman who is 64 inches tall and weighs 128 pounds at conception. Women may need more or less of the amounts listed for calories and protein depending on body size, activity, and health status. The allowances for vitamins and minerals provide sufficient room for individual variation so that they can be applied to all healthy women. They may not be adequate for women who enter pregnancy in poor nutritional status or who suffer from chronic diseases or other complicating conditions.

RDA have been set for only eighteen of the forty or so nutrients that are known to be needed to promote growth and maintain health. Strict attention to only those nutrients listed in the table without regard for the general quality and variety of foods in the diet can lead to a false sense of security. Intakes can be inadequate when highly fortified foods or vitamin pills are relied on as the primary source of nutrition, even though they contain 100% of the RDA. Daily consumption of foods from all of the food groups is necessary to make sure that nutrient needs, including those for which there is presently no RDA, are met.

NUTRIENT FUNCTIONS AND NEEDS

The nutrients enter into all of the major metabolic processes involving the production of energy, synthesis of cells, maintenance of their structure and function, and regulation of body processes. In considering each of these functions, emphasis will be given to those nutrients that have major roles, why their requirements during pregnancy increase, and where they can be found in foods. It should be kept in mind throughout that each of the nutrients has many interrelated functions in the body and that not all of the functions are known.

PRODUCTION OF ENERGY

Supplying sufficient energy to maintain life is the principal task of the body's metabolism. All other metabolic processes are subservient to this aim. During pregnancy, two factors that determine energy requirements are the mother's physical activity and the increase in her basal metabolism to support the work required for growth of the fetus and the accessory tissues. The cumulative energy cost of this extra work has been estimated at 80,000 calories, an amount derived from the caloric equivalents of protein and fat stored in the products of conception and from increased oxygen consumption of the mother. The total 80,000 calories break down to an addition of only 300 extra calories to the daily allowance of the nonpregnant reference woman. This is not a large increase when compared with the needs for extra protein, vitamins, and minerals. A portion of the energy increment may even be offset by the tendency of women to reduce their physical activity in the last trimester. The pregnant woman does not require a lot of additional food, but the quality of it must be high.

Since women differ in body size, individual needs can be calculated by allowing approximately 40 cal/kg of pregnant body weight, or about 18 cal/lb. *In no case* should the allowance drop below 36 cal/lb. It has been shown that energy intakes below this level impair adequate protein utilization in pregnancy.[23] Appetite and weight gain are the best indications that caloric needs are being met.

Sources of energy

The body produces energy by oxidizing carbohydrate, fat, or protein. Metabolites from all three of these nutrients can enter the citric acid (Krebs) cycle in the cells. Theoretically, the body can derive all of its energy from dietary or stored protein and fat. Carbohydrates are used preferentially by some cells and are required for intermediaries of the citric acid cycle, but they can be synthesized from protein. The exclusion of carbohydrate from the diet, however, has harmful effects. Since energy production is of primary importance, the body will use protein to manufacture citric acid cycle intermediaries and glucose if no preformed sources are available. This can impair growth. If the body must depend solely on dietary or stored fat for energy, metabolic products of fat oxidation accumulate in excess. These products, known as ketone bodies, cannot be metabolized when their concentrations reach high levels. Since they are acidic in nature, ketones disrupt the body's acid-base balance and can eventually lead to coma and death.

Ketoacidosis is the immediate consequence of uncontrolled diabetes mellitus. It is also produced in women who are on starvation diets. Even a mild condition can be dangerous in pregnancy. Maternal acetonuria from ketoacidosis is reported to be associated with neuropsychological defects in the infant. There is also evidence that maternal glucose levels influence the rate of fetal growth.[5] These are further reasons why weight reduction diets in general and low carbohydrate diets in particular must not be used in pregnancy.

For optimum protein utilization and to prevent ketosis, *at least* 5 grams of carbohydrate should be provided for every 100 calories of food. This would amount to 20% of total calories or 115 gm/day for the pregnant reference woman. To make the diet palatable and to meet vitamin and mineral needs, it is usual that 45% to 50% of total calories come from carbohydrate foods. Foods that supply carbohydrates as starch and contain other nutrients are preferable to foods containing mainly sugar. About 20% of dietary calories should be derived from protein foods of either animal or vegetable origin, and the remaining calories (30% to 35%) from fat.

Thiamin, riboflavin, and niacin

The process of energy production involves several other nutrients in addition to those which yield calories. The oxidation of carbohydrate proceeds in a series of reactions that convert glucose to pyruvic acid and then to acetylcoenzyme A (acetyl-CoA). This last step depends on a coenzyme, thiamin pyrophosphate (TPP). As its name implies, TPP contains the B vitamin thiamin and its availability can limit the rate at which energy from glucose is produced.

Riboflavin and niacin are also concerned with energy production. These two B vitamins are parts of the coenzymes flavin adenine dinucleotide (FAD) and niacin adenine dinucleotide (NAD), which assist in transferring hydrogen atoms through the respiratory chain in the cells. If protein must be used for energy, riboflavin is also needed as part of the coenzyme that helps to remove nitrogen from the amino acids.

Since thiamin, riboflavin, and niacin are all part of the reactions that produce energy in the body, requirements are related to caloric intake. The adult RDAs are 0.5, 0.6, and 6.6 mg/1000 cal for thiamin, riboflavin, and niacin, respectively. Since caloric allowances increase during pregnancy, the allowances for thiamin, riboflavin, and niacin automatically increase too. In addition, evidence from urinary excretion studies indicate that pregnant women have higher requirements for thiamin and riboflavin than nonpregnant women. The RDA for these two nutrients therefore contain additional adjustments.

Thiamin, riboflavin, and niacin are found in almost all foods but only a few are exceptionally good sources. Whole grains, legumes, organ meats, and pork are high in thiamin, whereas riboflavin is more plentiful in milk, cheese, lean meats, and leafy green vegetables. Foods that are high in thiamin and riboflavin are also good sources of niacin. Niacin is not only found preformed in food but it can also be made in the body from the amino acid tryptophan. For every 60 mg of tryptophan in the diet, 1 mg of niacin will be formed. Foods that are sources of good-quality protein are therefore good sources of niacin as well. Foods that contain only fat or sugar have no thiamin, riboflavin, or niacin.

In animals, severe deficiencies of thiamine, riboflavin, or niacin during pregnancy have resulted in fetal death, reduced growth, and congenital malformations. The skeleton and organs that arise from the ectoderm appear to be especially susceptible to riboflavin deficiency. Lack of riboflavin in the mother's diet was once thought to be a cause of prematurity in humans, but recent studies have failed to find a correlation.[10]

Heller and co-workers[11] have evaluated the thiamine status of pregnant women at various stages of gestation and have found that 25% to 30% have values which would be considered deficient by nonpregnant standards. Although there have been some reported cases of congenital beriberi from maternal thiamine deficiency, there is no evidence of impairment at the levels described by Heller and co-workers.

The niacin status of pregnant women has been inadequately investigated; however, there are no cases which indicate that niacin deficiency in humans produces the malformations noted in experimental animals.

Except in unusual circumstances, it appears that the primary nutritional problem to be anticipated in the energy metabolism of pregnant women is calorie imbalance, which is the result of socioeconomic conditions or ill-advised weight loss regimens which limit the quantity or quality of the diet.

SYNTHESIS OF NEW TISSUE

The promotion of optimum growth during pregnancy requires adequate supplies of energy and raw materials. Protein is essential because it forms the structural basis for all new cells and tissues in the mother and fetus. Other key nutrients are vitamins and minerals, which participate in the biochemical reactions that build amino acids into new protein molecules and maintain the structural and functional properties of the cells.

Protein

Nitrogen is the key element in protein that makes it different from carbohydrate and fat. Protein requirements therefore are usually determined by measuring the amount of nitrogen retained in the body for metabolic use. One gram of nitrogen is equivalent to 6.25 grams of protein.

In the factorial method, protein needs are estimated by totaling all the ways that nitrogen can be lost from the body. This gives an indication of how much protein nitrogen must be replaced each day. Urinary excretion when subjects are consuming a protein-free diet is used to estimate basic endogenous needs. Loss in feces during protein restriction shows how much is sloughed from cells of the gastrointestinal tract. Integumental loss indicates replacement needs for nitrogen in sweat and desquamated cells of the skin, hair, and nails. When these losses are calculated for the average reference woman, requirements are 2.84 grams of nitrogen or 18 grams of protein per day.

Requirements for protein during pregnancy are based on the needs of the nonpregnant reference woman plus the extra amounts needed for growth. The easiest way to determine how much extra protein is needed daily to support the synthesis of new tissue is to divide the amounts contained in the products of conception by the average length of gestation. About 925 grams of protein are deposited in a normal-weight fetus and in the maternal accessory tissues. When this is divided by the 280 days of pregnancy, the average is 3.3 grams of protein that must be added to normal daily requirements. The rate at which new tissue is synthesized, however, is not constant throughout gestation. Maternal and fetal growth do not accelerate until the second month, and the rate progressively increases until just before term. The need for protein follows this growth rate. Only about 0.6 extra grams of protein are used each day for synthesis in the first month of pregnancy, but by thirty weeks' gestation protein is being used at the rate of 6.1 gm/day. If this is added to the normal maintenance needs of the reference woman, one finds that 18.6 to 24.1 gm/day of protein are required during pregnancy.

These calculations would equal dietary allowances if 100% of the protein eaten could be used in the body. In actuality the efficiency of protein utilization depends on its digestibility and amino acid composition. Proteins which do not contain all of the eight essential amino acids in amounts proportional to human requirements are utilized less efficiently, but the utilization of even a high-quality protein, such as that from eggs, is only about 70%. Utilization from a mixed diet or from one in which protein is supplied totally from vegetable sources is less efficient.

Protein utilization also depends on caloric intake. Calloway[2] has shown that an extra 100 calories during pregnancy will have the same effect on nitrogen retention as an additional 0.28 gram of nitrogen itself. This means that calories from nonprotein sources (i.e., carbohydrate and fat) have a sparing effect. If these calories are inadequate, protein requirements would increase.

Finally, the trials that measure nitrogen loss are conducted on a limited number of subjects. There is much variation from the averages obtained. Since a dietary allowance must cover the needs of all healthy women, room for individual differences must be built in.

Because of these considerations, Recommended Dietary Allowances (RDA) for protein are set much higher than calculated requirements. The National Research Council allows 46 gm/day of protein for the nonpregnant reference woman with an extra 30 gm/day starting in the second month of pregnancy. If individual allowances are calculated on the basis of body weight, daily need would be 1.3 gm/kg of pregnant body weight or about 0.6 gm/lb. The RDA is based on a mixed diet in which at least one third of the protein comes from high-quality animal foods. Vegetarian diets which exclude all animal products can be made adequate when more total protein is consumed or when foods are selected so that those low in a particular amino acid are complemented by foods in which that amino acid is high.

Most people in the United States eat 100 grams of protein or more each day—well above the allowance for pregnant women. Since protein is one of the most expensive components of the diet, the food bill could be cut considerably by reducing protein intakes to the RDA. Calloway[2] and King,[17] however, have reasons for believing that typical intakes rather than recommended ones are more desirable for pregnant women. They have studied protein requirements using the nitrogen balance technique. This technique differs from the factorial method in that it measures the minimum amount of dietary protein which will maintain subjects in nitrogen equilibrium. Equilibrium is usually defined as an intake that exceeds excretion by 0.5 gm/day of nitrogen.[9]

When nitrogen balance is used on pregnant subjects, retentions that are two times greater than those estimated by the factorial method are obtained at all stages of gestation. King[17] hypothesizes that this discrepancy may be due to an underestimation of nitrogen storage by the factorial method. When the combined weights of the components of pregnancy are compared with the usual weight gain of pregnant women, there is a difference of approximately 3.3 kg. This extra weight has traditionally been thought to come from stored fat. The data of King suggest, however, that at least part of this weight may be fat-free tissue. The amount of lean tissue King estimates to be contained in this extra 3.3 kg is approximately equal to the higher nitrogen retention obtained from nitrogen balance. It is possible that nitrogen is stored throughout gestation as a reserve for increased fetal needs in the later months and for milk production during lactation.

This paradox of nitrogen retention illustrates the rationale for considering the RDA as general guidelines, not rigid standards. Pregnant women need at least 76 gm/day of protein, but until more is known about nitrogen needs in pregnancy, they should not be discouraged from intakes that exceed the RDA. This can be justified for reasons in addition to nitrogen balance. The practical aspects of menu planning are not taken into account when the National Research Council sets allowances. Furthermore, foods that are good sources of protein are also good sources of B vitamins and trace minerals. It may be difficult for women to meet their allowances for these nutrients if protein in the diet is curtailed.

Folic acid and vitamin B_{12}

The central place that protein occupies in the synthesis of new tissue sometimes obscures the emphasis which should be given to other nutrients. Growth, however, is a complex process that requires more than an adequate supply of protein and energy. To make new cells, DNA must replicate and transmit its genetic information to ribonucleic acid (RNA) intermediaries. RNA acts as templates for every new protein synthesized in the body.

Both DNA and RNA are composed of purines and pyrimidines. These ringlike substances are synthesized in the body from one-carbon (methyl) fragments and nitrogen. Derivatives of the B vitamin folic acid accept the carbon fragments from their biochemical donors and transfer them to their sites in the purine and pyrimidine rings. Folic acid also acts as a coenzyme in the synthesis of a nonessential amino acid, glycine. Glycine, in its turn, is a carbon and nitrogen donor in the synthesis of purines. Thus folic acid is involved in almost all aspects of DNA and RNA synthesis. If it is lacking, cell division cannot proceed normally. The effects are most detrimental in cells that have high turnover rates in the body.

One of the first signs of folic acid deficiency is anemia, which is due to the production of abnormal red blood cells. These cells are arrested in their development so that bone marrow contains a large number of immature megaloblasts and hemoglobin levels are reduced.

Megaloblastic anemia can also be produced by a deficiency of vitamin B_{12}, which indicates that the two vitamins somehow interact in the process of cell division. The exact nature of this interaction is still uncertain, but at least one reaction involving both folic acid and vitamin B_{12} as cofactors has been identified.

Chronic vitamin B_{12} deficiency is serious because in addition to the anemia it causes irreparable damage to the nervous system. A dietary-induced deficiency of vitamin B_{12} is rare, however, since it is present in all foods of animal origin. It is also manufactured by microorganisms in the gastrointestinal tract. The most common cause of a deficiency in humans comes from the inherited or acquired absence of intrinsic factor needed for the absorption of vitamin B_{12}, but long-term antibiotic therapy that destroys gastrointestinal flora or prolonged adherence to a vegetarian diet that eliminates all animal foods can lead to difficulties.

The dietary availability of folic acid is more limited than that of vitamin B_{12}. Leafy green vegetables are among the best sources, but as much as 80% of the vitamin's activity can be destroyed during storage and cooking. Liver, yeast, other green vegetables, legumes, nuts, and whole grains also supply folic acid, but the amount in most animal foods, fruits, other vegetables, and refined grains is poor.

The consequences of folic acid deficiency during pregnancy are controversial. Low serum folate levels have been reported in as many as 60% of patients in some clinical studies, but only a few of these women exhibit signs of megaloblastic anemia.

The low serum values of folic acid are believed to result from a number of factors. Problems with food selection, storage, and cooking losses, which place non-pregnant women in marginal status, are compounded in pregnancy by increased needs for folate to expand the maternal blood volume and for growth of the fetus. In addition, defects in the utilization of folic acid may be inherent in pregnancy because of the effects of steroid hormones.[18] The folic acid absorbed from food is converted by a series of reduction reactions to its active coenzyme form in the liver. High steroid levels may interfere with this process, since the liver is also the site where progesterone and estrogen are deactivated prior to excretion. The reactions for both the activation of folic acid and the deactivation of steroids involve similar biochemical mechanisms. A relationship is suspected because women taking oral steroid contraceptives are also likely to develop folic acid deficiencies.[27] In the case of contraceptives, the steroids are believed to inhibit gastrointestinal absorption of folate as well as interfere with its metabolism. A woman who plans her family by using oral contraceptives and later becomes pregnant would have sustained high steroid levels over quite some time. If steroids do interfere with folate absorption and metabolism, this woman would be extremely likely to show low serum levels during pregnancy.

Whether the low serum folate levels so common in pregnancy have any adverse effects on the course or outcome of pregnancy is unknown. Some investigators have been able to show highly significant associations between folic acid deficiencies with and without anemia and the incidence of fetal malformations, abruptio placentae, and abortion in human subjects, but others have failed to substantiate these relationships. Since the consequences of folic acid deficiency are potentially severe, the RDA during pregnancy is twice that of a nonpregnant woman. This amount is believed to protect most pregnant women from megaloblastic anemia and maintain serum levels in an acceptable range.

The question of oral supplementation is still a debatable issue. Average dietary intakes of folic acid range from 0.5 to 6 mg/day in the United States, but these values are unreliable because of limitations of methods for assaying the vitamin and its instability in foods. To be sure that women obtain enough folic acid, the National Research Council recommends that an oral supplement of 200 to 400 μg/day be given in the last half of pregnancy.

Vitamin B$_6$

Vitamin B$_6$, or pyridoxine, is another important nutrient concerned with amino acid metabolism and protein synthesis. In its active form as pyridoxal phosphate, the vitamin is a cofactor in reactions involving a group of enzymes known as transaminases. These enzymes work in the body to transfer the nitrogen-containing portion of certain amino acids to keto acid intermediaries from the Krebs cycle to synthesize some of the nonessential amino acids. Vitamin B$_6$ also functions in the reactions that convert tryptophan to niacin. Niacin, in turn, works as nicotinamide adenine dinucleotide (NAD) along with pyridoxal phosphate in some of the transamination reactions. This is another example of how interdependent the nutrients are in normal metabolism. Vitamin B$_6$ requirements increase in pregnancy not only because of the greater need for nonessential amino acids in growth but also because the body is making more niacin from tryptophan.

Urinary excretion of vitamin B$_6$ metabolites during pregnancy is ten to fifteen times higher than in nonpregnant women, whereas blood values are typically reduced. Investigators are not sure what the clinical significance of this is. For some time there have been efforts to link vitamin B$_6$ to preeclampsia because urinary excretion is even higher in preeclamptic patients than it is in normal pregnant women. It is far more likely that the observed values are the result of preeclampsia rather than a cause of it.

There is evidence that the placenta concentrates vitamin B_6 and that levels in cord blood are much higher than in the maternal circulation. This could mean that the reduced maternal blood levels are simply the result of physiological adjustments. On the other hand, there is also evidence that the fetus takes up more vitamin B_6 and that maternal levels increase when oral supplements are given.[3] The dietary allowance of 2.5 mg/day recommended in pregnancy is less than the amounts used by clinical investigators to bring blood levels up to nonpregnant standards, but since no clinically significant conditions can be attributed to the levels of vitamin B_6 that are commonly observed, the National Research Council does not believe that oral supplements are justified.

Even though the RDA is only 0.5 mg higher than normal, pregnant women will need some guidance in selecting foods to meet their allowance. Cereals and grains are good sources of vitamin B_6, but up to 75% of it is removed in processing. Unlike thiamin, riboflavin, and niacin, the vitamin B_6 content of cereals and grains is not restored by enrichment. Whole grains, wheat germ, bran, nuts, seeds, legumes, and some meats and fish supply vitamin B_6 in comparatively high amounts.

FORMATION OF HEMOGLOBIN

The importance of folic acid and vitamin B_{12} in the production of red blood cells has been discussed. These two nutrients must be accompanied by adequate amounts of protein and other vitamins and minerals for normal erythropoiesis. Adequacy of these supplies is indicated by the concentration of hemoglobin in the blood. Hemoglobin is responsible for carrying oxygen to the body's cells. One of its chief components is iron.

During pregnancy, iron is needed for the manufacture of hemoglobin in both maternal and fetal red blood cells. The fetus accumulates most of its iron during the last trimester. At term, a normal-weight infant has about 246 mg of iron in his blood and body stores. An additional 134 mg are stored in the placenta, and about 290 mg are used to expand the volume of the mother's blood.

Maintenance of erythropoiesis is one of the few instances during pregnancy when the fetus acts as a true parasite. It assures its own production of hemoglobin by drawing iron from the mother. Maternal iron deficiency therefore does not usually result in an infant who is anemic at birth. The most common cause of iron deficiency anemia in the infant is prematurity. The infant who has a short gestation does not have time to accumulate sufficient iron during the last trimester.

Iron deficiency in the mother does have adverse effects on her obstetrical performance. As has been previously noted, a reduction in hemoglobin concentration means that the mother must increase her cardiac output to maintain adequate oxygen consumption by placental and fetal cells. This extra work fatigues the mother and makes her more susceptible to other sources of physiological stress. A very low hemoglobin level places the mother at risk of cardiac arrest and leads to a poor prognosis for survival should she hemorrhage on delivery.[21]

Setting requirements for iron during pregnancy is complicated by changes in the erythropoietic system. Even when women are in adequate iron status at conception, the plasma volume increases faster than the number of red blood cells so that hemodilution occurs. But erythropoiesis is stimulated in the last half of pregnancy, and the rate of hemoglobin production is increased. If sufficient iron is available, hemoglobin levels should rise to at least 12 mg/100 ml by term.

It is generally conceded that the initial drop in hemoglobin is a normal physiological phenomenon, but there is concern that the usual iron intakes of pregnant women cannot support increased erythropoiesis and fetal demands in the last half of pregnancy. Iron absorption from the gastrointestinal tract increases during pregnancy, possibly to as much as 30% compared with the usual 10% absorption from the diet. Also working in the mother's favor are the 120 mg or so that she saves over the course of gestation because she is not menstruating. But even when these adjustments are taken into account, the pregnant woman still needs between 18 and 21 mg of iron in her diet each day. This could be supplied if large servings of iron-rich foods are eaten, but unfortunately, such foods are limited to organ meats, oysters, clams, and prune juice. These are not foods that people typically consume. From an average mixed diet, approximately 6 mg of iron are obtained from each 1000 calories of food. At this rate a pregnant woman would have to eat 3000 to 3500 cal/day to meet her iron needs. Furthermore, studies have shown that most women enter pregnancy with low iron stores so they have little to draw on to maintain normal hemoglobin concentrations in the later months. For these reasons the National Research Council recommends that pregnant women receive an oral iron supplement of 30 to 60 mg/day. This amount should maintain hemoglobin levels in normal pregnant women, but those who are anemic when they enter pregnancy will need a larger dose. Simple ferrous salts should be used. There are no advantages gained by using compounds purported to have unique properties that increase absorption or enhance erythropoiesis.

SKELETAL GROWTH AND DEVELOPMENT

Although ionic calcium and phosphorus both have important regulatory functions in the cells and blood, about 99% of the body's calcium and over 80% of its phosphorus are bound as hydroxyapatite, the primary structural component of bones and teeth. The importance of calcium and phosphorus during pregnancy is to promote adequate mineralization of the fetal skeleton and deciduous teeth.

The fetus acquires most of its calcium in the last trimester, when skeletal growth is maximum and teeth are being formed. Widdowson[30] has calculated that the fetus draws 13 mg/hr of calcium from the maternal blood supply, or 250 to 300 mg/day. At birth the infant has accumulated approximately 25 grams. Additional calcium is stored in the maternal skeleton as a reserve for lactation.

The levels of calcium maintained in the mother's blood and the amounts deposited in bones and teeth are regulated by the interactions of parathyroid hormone (PTH), calcitonin, and vitamin D. During pregnancy, these actions are mediated by human chorionic somatomammotropin (HCS) and estrogen so that, overall, there is a progressive increase in calcium retention. Exact amounts of dietary calcium needed to favor maximum retention are difficult to establish, since absorption and excretion are influenced by previous intake and other components of the diet. Ohlson and Stearns[22] maintain that most people eating diets that are typical in the United States cannot maintain calcium balance when intakes are less than 500 mg/day. To support fetal growth, a mother who consumes less than this amount would have to withdraw calcium from her own bones. Consistently low calcium intakes throughout the childbearing years could contribute to osteoporosis in later life.

The Recommended Dietary Allowance (RDA) for calcium is set well above the minimum level at 800 mg/day, with an additional 400 mg in the second and third trimesters of pregnancy. This allowance is based on average daily losses of 320 mg and an absorption of 40% of dietary intake.

Milk and milk products constitute the most important sources of calcium in the diet, but additional amounts are supplied by legumes, nuts, and dried fruits. Dark leafy green vegetables such as kale, cabbage, collards, and turnip greens contain calcium in high amounts that can be well absorbed, but some of the calcium in spinach, chard, and beet greens is bound with oxalic acid, which makes it unavailable to the body.

The fairly common occurrence of dental caries during pregnancy has led to a widely held belief that calcium deficiency causes demineralization of the teeth. A number of chemical analyses have been performed on animal and human teeth during pregnancy, but none has confirmed that demineralization occurs. James[16] quotes an interesting experiment in which a dog was maintained on a calcium-poor diet throughout pregnancy. The bones of the dog became so decalcified that they could hardly be seen on x-ray film, but its teeth showed no change. The dental caries that often accompany pregnancy are more likely to be due to a slight decrease in salivary pH. Good oral hygiene and the avoidance of cariogenic foods can counter this effect.

The RDA for phosphorus is the same as that for calcium—800 mg with an extra 400 mg during pregnancy. It is so widely available in foods that a dietary deficiency is rare. In fact, there is a possibility that the problem may be too much phosphorus rather than too little.

Calcium and phosphorus exist in a constant ratio in the blood. This ratio can be disturbed by the amounts of calcium and phosphorus in foods. If, for example, phosphorus is in excess, it will bind calcium in the gastrointestinal tract and limit the amount of calcium absorbed. A higher phosphorus-to-calcium ratio in the blood causes more calcium to be excreted in the urine.

The American diet is high in phosphorus. In addition to the naturally high levels in most animal protein foods, even greater amounts are found in processed meats, snack foods, and cola drinks. With the exception of dairy products, foods that are high in phosphorus contain only small amounts of calcium.

Several years ago, Page and Page[24] suggested that a calcium-phosphorus imbalance in the blood could be a cause of muscle spasms and leg cramps commonly experienced by pregnant women during the twenty-fourth to thirty-sixth weeks of gestation. Their remedy for treatment and prevention was to reduce milk intake to a cup per day (because of its high phosphorus content) and supply calcium with oral tablets.

Most adults can tolerate relatively wide variations in dietary calcium-phosphorus ratios when vitamin D is adequate. To protect the pregnant woman, a dietary intake of 400 IU/day is advised. But pregnancy is a time when calcium reserves are severely stressed. Lowered serum calcium concentrations and the mild alkalosis from the mother's reduced Pco_2 tend to increase muscular irritability. When this is compounded by exceptionally high phosphorus intakes, a disturbance of the calcium-phosphorus ratio in the body could result.

The fact that leg cramps can usually be relieved with aluminum hydroxide gels lends support to the idea that the calcium-phosphorus ratio may be involved. These gels bind phosphorus in the gastrointestinal tract and prevent it from interfering with calcium absorption. However, recent investigations have failed to show that too much milk is the cause of the imbalance or that leg cramps can be prevented if milk is curtailed.[1] A more reasonable approach is to limit high phosphorus foods such as processed snacks and soda pop rather than milk, which not only supplies calcium but vitamin D and other needed nutrients as well.

MAINTENANCE OF THE PROPERTIES OF CELLS

Vitamins A, C, and E have a number of specific functions in the body, but a role common to all three is to preserve the structural and functional properties of cells.

Vitamin A is essential to the welfare of epithelial tissues. These include the skin and the membranes that line glandless ducts and passages of the gastrointestinal, urinary, and respiratory tracts.

Vitamin C functions in reactions that oxidize proline, a nonessential amino acid, to hydroxyproline. Hydroxyproline is used to form the collagen matrix in connective tissue, skin, tendons, and bones.

The principal function of vitamin E is to prevent the oxidation of polyunsaturated fatty acids, which make up the structure of cell membranes. Vitamin E also prevents the oxidation of vitamin A in the gastrointestinal tract so that more vitamin A in the diet can be absorbed.

Although the need for these vitamins is increased during pregnancy, symptoms of deficiencies are seldom seen. The Recommended Dietary Allowances (RDA) can readily be met if a variety of foods is consumed. Preformed vitamin A is found in egg yolk, liver, butter, and fortified milk. It can also be formed in the body from its dietary precursor carotene, which is present in dark green and yellow vegetables and fortified margarine. Citrus fruits, berries, and green vegetables supply vitamin C, whereas vitamin E is present in vegetable oils, nuts, seeds, and whole grains.

Health enthusiasts frequently advocate intakes of vitamins A, C, and E in amounts that are many times greater than the RDA. This should be discouraged during pregnancy. Some of the dangers of too much vitamin A and vitamin D have already been discussed. There are other hazards that can be cited as well.

Two cases of infantile scurvy have been reported when mothers have taken megadoses of vitamin C during pregnancy.[4] The theory which explains this is that high levels during gestation may condition a higher than normal need for vitamin C in the infant. When he is born and begins to consume breast milk or formula, the levels are much lower than those which he has been getting in utero. Symptoms of vitamin C deficiency are temporarily induced until his body adjusts to a more natural intake. Since there are presently no scientifically

confirmed advantages for the mother, the risk of conditioning a need in the infant should outweigh any recommendation for taking large doses of vitamin C during pregnancy.

Similarly, there is no evidence that mothers or their infants can benefit from increased amounts of vitamin E. Numerous attempts have been made to demonstrate a relationship between vitamin E and a host of reproductive casualties, but none has proved significant for humans.

REGULATION OF BODY FUNCTIONS

The rate at which chemical reactions take place in the body is vital to health and well-being. If the reactions are too fast or too slow, normal body functions are impaired. Hormones and enzymes are responsible for maintaining proper balance, but so that they may do their work, mineral elements must accompany them in small amounts. Iodine, calcium, and phosphorus have long been known to be essential. The thyroid hormone is ineffective as a regulator of basal metabolism if iodine is unavailable. The calcium and phosphorus not bound in bones and teeth have a variety of regulatory roles. Calcium is needed for rhythmic muscular contractions and the activation of several enzyme systems. Among other things, phosphorus activates glucose and glycogen so that they can be metabolized for energy. Many of the B vitamins work as cofactors only after they are combined with phosphate (e.g., pyridoxal phosphate).

One of the more recent advances in nutrition research is the discovery that many other mineral elements are necessary for human reproduction, growth, and general health. Chromium, manganese, fluorine, cobalt, copper, zinc, magnesium, selenium, molybdenum, vanadium, tin, nickel, and silicon have all been shown to be needed by the body. Like iodine, calcium, and phosphorus, these elements (and likely others as well) participate in reactions that control body processes. Studies in animals have revealed that deficiencies produce widespread and serious metabolic defects. Limited knowledge of requirements in humans makes it impossible to establish RDA for the majority of these minerals. At the present time sufficient information is available only for magnesium and zinc.

Magnesium is much like calcium and phosphorus in that most of it is stored in bones. The amounts that are biochemically active are concentrated in nerve and muscle cells. Deficiencies of magnesium produce neuromuscular dysfunctions characterized by tremors and convulsions.

Not a great deal is known about the need for magnesium during pregnancy. The RDA is based on estimates of the amounts accumulated by the mother and the fetus. Green vegetables are good sources of magnesium because the element is part of the green pigment chlorophyll, but the best sources are nuts, wheat bran, soybeans, and wheat germ. Animal products and fruits are relatively poor sources of magnesium.

Zinc has an active role in metabolism because it is a component of insulin. It also is part of the carbonic anhydrase enzyme system that helps to maintain acid-base balance in the tissues. The action of zinc in the synthesis of DNA and RNA makes it a highly important element in reproduction. When zinc-free diets are fed to pregnant animals, growth is impaired and numerous malformations are produced. The skeleton and nervous system are most susceptible.

One of the more important implications of the animal work on zinc for humans is that a deficiency can come about in a very short time. Hurley and associates[12] have shown that maternal zinc restriction will produce fetal malformations almost immediately. This suggests that the mother is unable to mobilize her own zinc reserves to protect the fetus as she can in the case of calcium and iron. It is therefore essential that small amounts of zinc be supplied in the diet every day.

The 15 mg of zinc recommended as a dietary allowance during pregnancy are at the upper end of the range of intakes typically supplied by the American diet. It is difficult to meet the allowance if the diet does not contain some animal protein foods. Meat, liver, eggs, and seafood (especially oysters) are the best sources of zinc.

WEIGHT GAIN

The studies that were reviewed in Chapter 2 point to the importance of maintaining an adequate weight gain during pregnancy. By this time it should be apparent that much of the weight gained in a normal pregnancy is the result of physiological processes designed to foster fetal and maternal growth. Much of the weight gain can be accounted for by the products of gestation.

The total number of pounds gained in pregnancy will vary among individual women. Young mothers and primigravidas usually gain more than older mothers and multigravidas. A normal range for most healthy women is 26 to 30 pounds. Those who are underweight at conception may need to gain more. A gain of 40 pounds during pregnancy would not be unusual for these mothers.

Components of weight gain

Much of the past confusion about weight gain during pregnancy and the misguided attempts to restrict it are because of the failure to appreciate that the components and rate of weight gain are more important than the actual number of pounds a woman puts on. Pregnancy should be a positive period of growth in which most of the gain is in lean body (protein) tissue. A gain from too much fluid or too much fat is not conducive to good health.

Table 3-4 shows how weight gain is normally apportioned from conception to term. Almost 16 pounds (7.3 kg) of a typical weight gain comes from the fetus, placenta, amniotic fluid, and growth of the uterus and breasts. Another 11 pounds is

Table 3-4. Components of the average weight gained in normal pregnancy*

Component	10 weeks	Amount (gm) gained at 20 weeks	30 weeks	40 weeks
A. Total gain of body weight	650	4,000	8,500	12,500
Fetus	5	300	1,500	3,300
Placenta	20	170	430	650
Amniotic fluid	30	250	600	800
Increase of				
Uterus	135	585	819	900
Mammary gland	34	180	360	405
Maternal blood	100	600	1,300	1,250
B. Total (rounded)	320	2,100	5,000	7,300
C. Weight not accounted for (A-B)	330	1,900	3,500	5,200

*From Committee on Maternal Nutrition, Food and Nutrition Board, National Research Council, National Academy of Sciences: Maternal nutrition and the course of pregnancy, Washington, D.C., 1970, Government Printing Office.

from general growth of the mother's body and storage of nutrient reserves.

What should be noted is that weight gain in the first ten weeks is small and that much of it is due to growth of the uterus and expansion of the mother's blood. At this time the fetus weighs only about 5 grams, but toward the end of pregnancy growth of the fetus accounts for the largest portion of the weight increment. This pattern explains why many of the Recommended Dietary Allowances do not increase until the second trimester. The mother's rate of weight gain should parallel these trends. If she eats to appetite, the mother should gain a total of 2 to 4 pounds by the end of the first trimester and about 1 pound each week thereafter. If pounds gained are plotted over the weeks of gestation, the curve would resemble that shown in Fig. 3-3.

A sudden weight gain that greatly exceeds this rate is likely to be due to excess fluid retention. It has been repeatedly stated throughout this chapter that mild generalized edema and some accumulation of fluid in the lower limbs is not unphysiological. Women with edema can gain as much as 9 liters of fluid and still have clinically normal pregnancies.[29] But it should be emphasized that this accumulation is

gradual. A large shift in water balance reflected by a sudden increase in weight is usually an indication of toxemia, particularly if it occurs after the twentieth week.

Because of the action of progesterone, pregnant women have a tendency to lay down extra fat. Fat storage is commonly believed to be responsible for part of the weight unaccounted for in Table 3-4. Skinfold thicknesses that measure subcutaneous fat have been shown to increase at the abdomen, back, and upper thighs of pregnant women from ten to thirty weeks' gestation.[28] This fat storage at midpregnancy is insurance against the high energy costs of fetal growth in the last ten weeks and of labor and birth. Although the increased adiposity may be of concern to figure-conscious mothers, most will lose it in the postpartum period, especially if they breastfeed.

Recommendations for weight management

The goal of weight management during pregnancy should be to promote optimum nutrition for the mother and child. There is no good evidence that caloric restriction or weight loss will prevent toxemia or any other complicating condition, but there are clear indications that a 26- to 30-pound

PRENATAL WEIGHT GAIN GRID

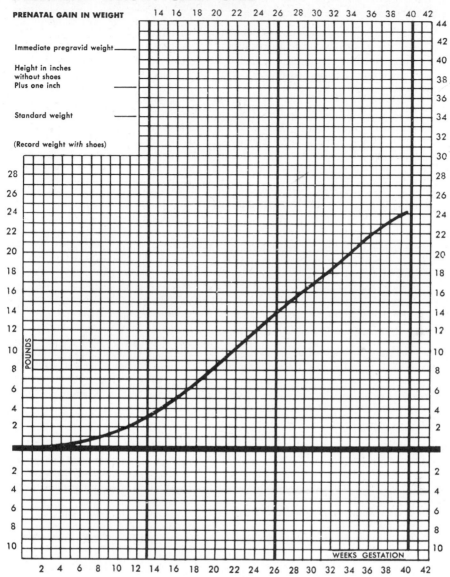

Fig. 3-3. Pattern of normal prenatal weight gain. (From Committee on Maternal Nutrition, Food and Nutrition Board, National Research Council, National Academy of Sciences: Maternal nutrition and the course of pregnancy, Washington, D.C., 1970, Government Printing Office.)

gain produces the most favorable outcome. This gain cannot be achieved if deliberate efforts are made to restrict food intake. At the same time obesity is *not* one of the outcomes of pregnancy that health professionals should seek to promote. The recommendation that pregnant women should

"eat to appetite" must not be taken as a license to overindulge in empty-calorie foods. To achieve the optimum balance, guidance should be given in the selection of foods that are nutritious, appealing, and conducive to weight gain within the normal range. Since each woman is an individual with her own history, preferences, and needs, management should be flexible and personalized. Every woman should have an evaluation of her weight status at conception along with' her usual dietary and activity patterns to determine the weight gain that is best for her.

REFERENCES

1. Abrams, J., and Aponte, G. E.: The leg cramp syndrome during pregnancy: the relationship to calcium and phosphorus metabolism, Am. J. Obstet. Gynecol. **76:**32, 1958.
2. Calloway, D. H.: Nitrogen balance during pregnancy. In Winick, M. E., editor: Nutrition and fetal development, vol. 2, New York, 1974, John Wiley & Sons, Inc.
3. Cleary, R. E., Lumeng, L., and Li, T.: Maternal and fetal plasma levels of pyridoxal phosphate at term: adequacy of vitamin B-6 supplementation during pregnancy, Am. J. Obstet. Gynecol. **121:**25, 1975.
4. Cochrane, W. A.: Overnutrition in prenatal and neonatal life: a problem? Can. Med. Assoc. J. **93:**893, 1965.
5. Committee on Maternal Nutrition, Food and Nutrition Board, National Research Council, National Academy of Sciences: Maternal nutrition and the course of pregnancy, Washington, D.C., 1970, Government Printing Office.
6. Friedman, W. F., and Mills, L. F.: The relationship between vitamin D and the craniofacial and dental anomalies of the supravalvular aortic stenosis syndrome, Pediatrics **43:**12, 1969.
7. Gal, I., Sharman, I. M., and Press-Davies, J.: Vitamin A in relation to human malformations. In Woolam, D. H. M., editor: Advances in teratology, vol. 5, New York, 1972, Academic Press, Inc.
8. Giroud, A.: The nutrition of the embryo, Springfield, Ill., 1970, Charles C Thomas, Publisher.
9. Hegsted, D. M.: Variation in requirements of nutrients—amino acids, Fed. Proc. **22:**1424, 1963.
10. Heller, S., Salkeld, R. M., and Korner, W. F.: Riboflavin status in pregnancy, Am. J. Clin. Nutr. **27:**1225, 1974.
11. Heller, S., Salkeld, R. M., and Korner, W. F.: Vitamin B-1 status in pregnancy, Am. J. Clin. Nutr. **27:**1221, 1974.
12. Hurley, L. S., Dreosti, I. E., Swenerton, H., and Gowan, J.: The movement of zinc in maternal and fetal rat tissues in teratogenic zinc deficiency, Teratology **1:**216, 1968.
13. Hytten, F. E., and Leitch, I.: The physiology of human pregnancy, ed. 2, Oxford, 1971, Blackwell Scientific Publications, Ltd.
14. Hytten, F. E., and Paintin, D. B.: Increase in plasma volume during normal pregnancy, J. Obstet. Gynaecol. Br. Commonw. **70:**402, 1963.
15. Hytten, F. E., and Thomson, A. M.: Maternal physiological adjustments. In Committee on Maternal Nutrition, Food and Nutrition Board, National Research Council, National Academy of Sciences: Maternal nutrition and the course of pregnancy, Washington, D.C., 1970, Government Printing Office.
16. James, J. D.: Dental caries in pregnancy, J. Am. Dent. Assoc. **28:**1857, 1941.
17. King, J. C.: Protein metabolism during pregnancy, Clin. Perinatol. **2:**243, 1975.
18. Kitay, D. Z., and Harbort, R. A.: Iron and folic acid deficiency in pregnancy, Clin. Perinatol. **2:**255, 1975.
19. Malone, J. I.: Vitamin passage across the placenta, Clin. Perinatol. **2:**295, 1975.
20. MacRae, D. J., and Palavradje, D.: Maternal acid-base changes in pregnancy, J. Obstet. Gynaecol. Br. Commonw. **74:**11, 1967.
21. McFee, J. G.: Anemia: a high-risk complication of pregnancy, Clin. Obstet. Gynecol. **16:**153, 1973.
22. Ohlson, M. A., and Stearns, G.: Calcium intake of children and adults, Fed. Proc. **18:**1076, 1959.
23. Oldham, H., and Sheft, B. B.: Effect of caloric intake on nitrogen utilization during pregnancy, J. Am. Diet. Assoc. **27:**847, 1951.
24. Page, E. W., and Page, E. P.: Leg cramps in pregnancy: etiology and treatment, Obstet. Gynecol. **1:**94, 1953.
25. Pike, R. L., Miles, J. E., Wardlaw, J. M.: Juxtaglomerular degranulation and zona glomerulosa exhaustion in pregnant rats induced by low sodium intakes and reversed by sodium load, Am. J. Obstet. Gynecol. **95:**604, 1966.
26. Pitkin, R. M.: Calcium metabolism in pregnancy: a review, Am. J. Obstet. Gynecol. **121:**724, 1975.
27. Shojania, A. M., Hornaday, G. J., and Barnes, P. H.: The effect of oral contraceptives on folate metabolism, Am. J. Obstet. Gynecol. **111:**782, 1971.
28. Taggart, N. R., Holliday, R. M., Billewicz, W. Z., Hytten, F. E., and Thomson, A. M.: Changes in skinfolds during pregnancy, Br. J. Nutr. **21:**439, 1967.
29. Thomson, A. M., Hytten, F. E., and Billewicz, W. Z.: The epidemiology of oedema during pregnancy, J. Obstet. Gynaecol. Br. Commonw. **74:**1, 1967.
30. Widdowson, E. M.: Growth and composition of the fetus and newborn. In Assali, N. S., editor: Biology of gestation, vol. 2, New York, 1968, Academic Press, Inc.
31. Watchstein, M., and Gudiatis, A.: Disturbance of vitamin B-6 metabolism in pregnancy, J. Lab. Clin. Med. **40:**550, 1952.

4

Nutritional guidance in prenatal care

Sue Rodwell Williams

RELATION OF NUTRITION AND PREGNANCY

From the discussion presented in the preceding chapters, it is clear that much of the counsel given to pregnant women over the past few decades has been based more on tradition than on scientific fact. Increasing evidence indicates that positive nutritional support of pregnancy, rather than past restrictions born of limited knowledge and false assumptions, builds for a positive outcome of pregnancy and increased health and vigor of mothers and infants alike.

False assumptions and folklore

As is true in all cultures, over time a great body of folklore has grown up around pregnancy. This is understandable, since reproduction and childbirth form a profound core of human life experience. As a result, many traditional practices and diets have developed and been followed from time to time, most of which have had little basis in fact. Especially through the ups and downs of the past decades, beginning with roots in European medicine and spreading to American medical practice, maternal nutrition has suffered from ignorance and neglect. For example, as we have seen, early in the 1900s the pronouncement of the German obstetrician, Ludwig Prochownick, that, "Semi-starvation of the mother is really a blessing in disguise because curtailment of food would produce a small light-weight baby easier to deliver," gained recognition. He repeated this dictum during the strict food rationing of World War I, proposing a diet low in calories, low in carbohydrate and protein, and restricted in water and salt. Incredible as it now seems in retrospect, in the light of present advanced knowledge and research, despite any scientific evidence to support such ideas, this general view became implanted in obstetrical textbooks and practice, passed from one generation of physicians to the next.

Until recently, much of the clinical advice given to pregnant women in American obstetrical practice has been based on such unfounded tradition and supposition. As a result, two false assumptions have grown and formed the basis for wrong advice over the years: (1) the *"parasite" theory*—whatever the fetus needs, it will draw from the stores of the mother despite the maternal diet; and (2) the *"maternal instinct" theory*—whatever the fetus needs, the mother will instinctively crave and consume. Both of these theories are obviously false. On the contrary, as we have seen from research to date, the scientific evidence for positive nutritional demands of pregnancy is increasingly apparent.

Positive physiological demands of pregnancy

Therefore, in the past few years, several factors have led to reconsideration of practices in maternal care, especially nutritional counsel. The first factor has been a growing awareness of the poor American statistics for maternal and infant morbidity rates, particularly in "reproductive casualties" among infants (Chapter 1). In these worldwide statistics, the United States has ranked thirteenth among the nations of the world in infant mortality rates, despite its relative position of wealth, medical knowledge, and skill, and even lower—seventeenth—in the broader, perhaps more significant statistics of low birth weight babies. Such premature or poorly formed infants suffer a higher death rate or incidence of defects than do well-formed infants.

A second factor that has influenced the positive changes that are taking place in American maternal care practices is twofold: (1) the increasing knowledge of nutritional science and its relation to the outcome of pregnancy, as indicated in the previous chapters; and (2) the increasing number of studies reporting the effective reduction of morbidity and mortality rates by applying this knowledge of optimum nutrition in sound education programs during pregnancy. Data gathered from clinic populations in the United States, Europe, and Canada, for example, have demonstrated a remarkable reduction in these "reproductive casualties" with vigorous programs of sound nutrition that include (1) adequate protein of high biological value, (2) sufficient calories to spare protein for tissue synthesis, and (3) enough salt and other regulatory agents of vitamins and minerals, rather than the traditional erroneous priority given to weight control and salt restriction.

National Research Council report

These concerns led a few years ago to the formation of a subcommittee of the National Research Council, the Committee on Maternal Nutrition. After a three-year study of the research up to that time, the committee issued a definitive report entitled *Maternal Nutrition and the Course of Pregnancy*. This report clearly showed the need for change in traditional practices of care, toward a positive approach to the dietary management of pregnancy.

From the large amount of evidence involved in the committee's deliberations and report, reinforced further by subsequent increased research, several important considerations emerge as individual determinants of specific nutritional requirements during pregnancy. Thus there are four basic principles on which to base individual assessment and guidance.

Age and parity of the mother. Higher risk is involved at both ends of the age cycle in reproduction. The teenage mother adds to her own growth needs those introduced by her pregnancy. At the other end of the reproductive span, hazards increase with age. Also parity, the number of pregnancies, and the time intervals between them have a strong influence on the needs of the mother and the outcome of the pregnancy.

Preconception nutrition. The mother brings to her pregnancy all of her previous life experiences, including her diet, her food habits, her attitudes. Her general health and fitness and the state of her nutrition at her infant's conception are products of her lifelong habits and possibly those of generations before her.

Complex metabolic interactions of pregnancy. Three distinct biological entities are involved in pregnancy—the mother, the fetus, and the placenta. Together they form a unique biological *synergism*. Constant metabolic interactions are going on among them all the while. Their functions, although unique, are at the same time interdependent. Any number of variables therefore may combine at any point in time to determine individual needs and events

Individual needs and adaptations. Thus individual nutritional needs may vary with time and circumstance. Homeostatic mechanisms appear to operate with special efficiency during pregnancy, but special conditions of stress increase nutrient requirements above those needed for usual circumstances.

Changing concepts in maternal nutrition

As a result of this background study and the clear, definitive report and recommendations of the National Research Council, there has been a growing awareness of the vital importance to the outcome of pregnancy of meeting the nutritional demands during this period. Two concepts, the perinatal and synergism concepts, form a basis for understanding these needs and developing a relevant program of nutritional counseling.

Perinatal concept. The prefix "peri" comes from a Greek root meaning "about, around, surrounding." As nutritional knowledge and understanding has increased, health professionals realize that the whole of the individual woman's life experiences surrounding her pregnancy must be considered. Her nutritional status developed over previous years of living and the degree to which nutritional reserves have been established and maintained are important factors. Throughout her life a woman is providing for the ongoing continuum of life through the food she eats. It is thus that she provides nourishment for her unborn child. Moreover, in the broader sense she carries over the same nutritional principles and beliefs in her feeding and teaching to her growing child, who in turn in the next generation passes on this heritage to her child. All of these factors surrounding the total reproductive cycle must be considered, not merely the nine months of an individual pregnancy.

Synergism concept. The word *synergism* comes from two Greek roots, "syn" meaning "with" or "together" and "ergon" meaning "work." Thus synergism is used to describe biological systems in which two or more factors *work together* to produce a total effect greater than and *different* from the sum of their parts. In short, a new *whole* is created by the unified joint effort of the blending of the parts, in which each part strengthens and makes possible the actions of the others.

Of the many biological and physiological interactions providing examples of synergism, pregnancy is a prime example in point. Here there are three distinct biological entities involved—the mother, the fetus, and the placenta. However, during this unique period, no one of them exists as a separate whole. All parts combine to create a *new whole,* which did not exist before and will never exist again. Together they produce a total effect greater than, and different from, the sum of their parts, all for the specific purpose of sustaining and nurturing the pregnancy and its offspring. Measures of physiological health change therefore during this synergistic response to the pregnancy. For example, the total body water and circulating blood volume increase 50% or more, the cardiac output increases, the ventilation rate and tidal volume of air increase. Thus physiological norms of the nonpregnant woman do not apply, nor can normal physiological adjustment to the pregnancy be viewed as abnormal or pathological with the application of treatment procedures for that same type of response in an abnormal state. For example, the physiological generalized edema of pregnancy is a normal protective response. It should not be confused with or treated as abnormal edema in pathological states such as heart failure. This specific protective response of benign edema is associated with improved reproductive performance, and in the well-nourished woman it is a healthy phenomenon.

Implications for prenatal care and counseling

As a result of increased knowledge of pregnancy and nutrition from basic and applied research, some of which has been discussed in this book, former negative priorities and practices in prenatal care are giving way to improved current positive nutritional priorities and practices. Earlier misplaced priorities have centered on strict weight control and sodium restriction, whereas current sound priorities focus on increased nutritional requirements and individual assessment and counseling.

Former negative priorities and practices

Weight control in pregnancy—quantity versus quality. The former concept of severe caloric restrictions to avoid large total weight gains and hence complications of pregnancy is without foundation. Weight gain *alone* gives an incomplete measure of health status during pregnancy; it provides only one parameter and must be interpreted on an individual basis in terms of weight history, nutritional-medical-obstetrical histories, current nutritional status and reserves, and overall weight pattern during the pregnancy. Thus the primary consideration lies not in the quantity of the weight gain so much as it does in the *quality* of the weight gain. Optimum weight gain of the mother during pregnancy makes an important contribution to successful course and outcome. Evidence has mounted, as we have indicated, from many sources that healthy women produce healthy babies over a wide range of total weight gains. Depending on a woman's weight and nutritional reserves at conception, her range of weight change in pregnancy may vary from very little to a gain of about 60 pounds. A normal outcome may be found anywhere in that range. Thus, when we say that an *average* weight gain during pregnancy is about 25 to 30 pounds, we mean just that—an *average* around which many variations on an individual basis may occur, not a rigid norm or restriction to which all women must be held, regardless of individual needs. Therefore each pregnant woman must be carefully assessed in terms of her individual health status and life situation, and care and guid-

Table 4-1. Average weight of the products of pregnancy

Products	Weight (pounds)
Fetus	7.5
Placenta	1.0
Amniotic fluid	2.0
Uterus (weight increase)	2.5
Breast tissue (weight increase)	3.0
Blood volume (weight increase)	4.0 (1500 ml)
Maternal stores	4.0 to 8.0
Totals	24 to 28 pounds

ance must be provided accordingly. To act otherwise would be simplistic, invalid, and unscientific maternity care practice.

As an initial basis for evaluation, the average weight of the products of pregnancy may be considered (Table 4-1).

In addition to the components of growth and development usually attributed to a pregnancy, an important item is listed here—maternal stores. This laying down of extra adipose fat tissue is necessary to provide maternal reserves for energy to sustain fetal growth during the latter part of pregnancy and energy for labor and birth and maintaining lactation after birth. About 4 to 8 pounds of adipose tissue are commonly deposited for these needs, presumably as a result of stimulus by progesterone, acting centrally to reset the "lipostat"—a fat-producing mechanism in the hypothalamus. When the pregnancy is completed, the lipostat reverts to its usual nonpregnant state and the added fat not used is lost. Sometimes there has been a failure by some practitioners to distinguish between weight gained as the result of edema and that due to deposition of these fat stores. The important factor therefore is the nature or *quality* of the weight gain and the *foods consumed to bring it about*, rather than a routine restriction on the quantity of weight gain alone. Clearly, severe caloric restriction is an unphysiological and potentially harmful practice, both for the developing fetus and for the mother. Usually it is accompanied by restriction of vitally needed nutrients essential to the growth process during pregnancy. Therefore weight reduction should *never* be undertaken during pregnancy. To the contrary, adequate weight gains should be encouraged with the use of a nourishing, well-balanced diet as outlined in Tools D and E (pp. 76-78, 86, 87).

Rate of weight gain. A more useful index is the rate of weight gain during pregnancy. On the whole, about 2 to 4 pounds comprise an average gain during the first trimester. Thereafter, about a pound a week, more or less, during the remainder of pregnancy is usual. There is no scientific justification for routinely limiting weight gain to lesser amounts. It is only unusual patterns of gain, such as a sharp sudden increase in weight about the twentieth week of pregnancy, which may indicate abnormal water retention, that should be watched.

Sodium restriction in pregnancy. Routine restriction of sodium during pregnancy, just as restriction of calories, is unphysiological and unfounded. Physicians who prescribe diets low in calories and low in sodium are placing pregnant women and their offspring at particular disadvantage and unnecessary risk. A number of studies have indicated the need for sodium during pregnancy and the harm to maternal-fetal health by restricting salt. Combined with the added injury of routine use of diuretics, such a program places the pregnant woman and her child in double jeopardy. The National Research Council report on maternal nutrition labels such routine use of salt-free diets and diuretics as potentially dangerous.

Current positive nutritional priorities and practices

Increased nutritional requirements. In the preceding chapters extensive foundation has been laid for the increased nutritional demands of pregnancy. These demands focus on nutrient needs basic to human growth and development, increased protein, vitamins, and minerals to sustain the necessary building process, as well as sufficient energy input from calories to do the work. The basic concept provides a logical framework for nutrition education and guidance in prenatal care.

Individual nutritional assessment and guidance. The second positive nutritional priority—individual assessment and guidance—follows from the first priority of increased nutrient demands of pregnancy. As indicated, a number of variables may combine to produce individual needs. These needs may be physiological, psychological, situational, cultural, economic, or other personal needs. Thus individual nutrition assessment should be an integral part of every obstetrical workup, and nutritional guidance and education based on that assessment should be a continuing part of the individual ongoing plan of prenatal care. Some basic tools and approaches for planning and carrying such an individualized program of nutritional care during pregnancy are suggested here.

NUTRITION ASSESSMENT IN PRENATAL CARE

It is clearly evident that nutrition—*optimum* nutrition, vigorously supported—is an integral part of sound maternity care, basic to the successful outcome of a woman's pregnancy. To ensure that this fundamental requirement for successful pregnancy is met, an initial individual assessment of nutritional status and need must be made at the beginning of prenatal care and supported by continuing evaluation throughout the pregnancy.

Methods of assessment

In planning health care in any field, the three following basic methods of assessment provide the data necessary to determine needs: (1) clinical observations and physical examination, (2) laboratory tests, and (3) history.

Clinical observations

In making nutritional assessment from clinical observations, the following two basic problems exist: (1) there is generally considerable variation among observers in interpretation of physical signs, partly because of differences in expertise and experience of the observers, problems in standardization of definition of a particular sign, or the low general prevalence and nonspecificity of clinical signs of malnutrition in developed areas except in high-risk groups; and (2) there is sometimes confusion in specific interpretation of signs during pregnancy; for example, gingival hypertrophy may sometimes occur normally in pregnancy and is not necessarily a sign of ascorbic acid deficiency.

Nonetheless, together with more definitive data from laboratory studies of hematological and biochemical analysis and from careful medical-obstetrical-social-nutritional histories and their evaluation, much valuable information may be gained from good clinical observation by trained observers. In general, three areas of observation are useful.

Weight-height evaluations. Important clinical parameters predictive of the birth weight of the child are the mother's prepregnancy weight and her pattern of gain or loss during her pregnancy. Prepregnancy weight is the result of her genetic pattern, her previous nutrition history, and her environment, given no other coexisting serious illnesses. Extremes of underweight or overweight should be investigated for underlying poor eating habits, environmental or social factors, or illness so that the mother may be counseled appropriately.

Dental examination. General screening for dental health status signs provides helpful data on nutritional health or disease. Areas observed should include obvious dental caries; periodontal disease with signs such as hyperemia, edema, ease of bleeding, or retraction; calculus deposits; and soft materia alba. Trained dental observers may further quantify these findings using standardized calculations of decayed-missing-filled index (DMF), periodontal disease index (PDI), and oral hygiene index (OHI). Persons found to have dental disease related to eating habits can be counseled about improvement in their dietary patterns or, according to need, referred for specific preventive measures of dental treatment.

General physical inspection. General examination of skin, mucous membranes, tongue, eyes, and hair condition provide useful information for assessing nutritional status during pregnancy. These signs must, of course, be evaluated in relation to other data from laboratory procedures and histories, recognizing that various signs have different degrees of reliability. However, they present useful clues for further investigation or monitoring. General reference may be made to definition of physical signs of nutritional status as reviewed in Table 4-2.

Table 4-2. Clinical signs of nutritional status

Body area	Signs of good nutrition	Signs of poor nutrition
General appearance	Alert, responsive	Listless, apathetic, cachexic
Weight	Normal for height, age, body build	Overweight or underweight (special concern for underweight)
Posture	Erect, arms and legs straight	Sagging shoulders, sunken chest, humped back
Muscles	Well developed, firm, good tone, some fat under skin	Flaccid, poor tone, undeveloped, tender, "wasted" appearance, cannot walk properly
Nervous control	Good attention span, not irritable or restless, normal re-	Inattentive, irritable, confused, burning and tingling of hands and feet (paresthesia),

Table 4-2. Clinical signs of nutritional status—cont'd

Body area	Signs of good nutrition	Signs of poor nutrition
Nervous control—cont'd	flexes, psychological stability	loss of position and vibratory sense, weakness and tenderness of muscles (may result in inability to walk), decrease or loss of ankle and knee reflexes
Gastrointestinal function	Good appetite and digestion, normal regular elimination, no palpable organs or masses	Anorexia, indigestion, constipation or diarrhea, liver or spleen enlargement
Cardiovascular function	Normal heart rate and rhythm, no murmurs, normal blood pressure for age	Rapid heart rate (above 100 beats/min tachycardia), enlarged heart, abnormal rhythm, elevated blood pressure
General vitality	Endurance, energetic, sleeps well, vigorous	Easily fatigued, no energy, falls asleep easily, looks tired, apathetic
Hair	Shiny, lustrous, firm, not easily plucked, healthy scalp	Stringy, dull, brittle, dry, thin and sparse, depigmented, can be easily plucked
Skin (general)	Smooth, slightly moist, good color	Rough, dry, scaly, pale, pigmented, irritated, bruises, petechiae
Face and neck	Skin color uniform, smooth, pink, healthy appearance, not swollen	Greasy, discolored, scaly, swollen, skin dark over cheeks and under eyes, lumpiness or flakiness of skin around nose and mouth
Lips	Smooth, good color, moist, not chapped or swollen	Dry, scaly, swollen, redness and swelling (cheilosis), or angular lesions at corners of the mouth or fissures or scars (stomatitis)
Mouth, oral membranes	Reddish pink mucous membranes in oral cavity	Swollen, boggy oral mucous membranes
Gums	Good pink color, healthy, red, no swelling or bleeding	Spongy, bleed easily, marginal redness, inflamed, gums receding
Tongue	Good pink color or deep reddish in appearance, not swollen or smooth, surface papillae present, no lesion	Swelling, scarlet and raw, magenta color, beefy (glossitis), hyperemic and hypertrophic papillae, atrophic papillae
Teeth	No cavities, no pain, bright, straight, no crowding, well-shaped jaw, clean, no discoloration	Unfilled caries, absent teeth, worn surfaces, mottled (fluorosis), malpositioned
Eyes	Bright, clear, shiny, no sores at corner of eyelids, membranes moist and healthy pink color, no prominent blood vessels or mound of tissue or sclera, no fatigue circles beneath	Eye membranes pale (pale conjunctivas), redness of membrane (conjunctival injection), dryness, signs of infection, Bitot's spots, redness and fissuring of eyelid corners (angular palpebritis), dryness of eye membrane (conjunctival xerosis) dull appearance of cornea (corneal xerosis), soft cornea (keratomalacia)
Neck (glands)	No enlargement	Thyroid enlarged
Nails	Firm, pink	Spoon shape (koilonychia), brittle, ridged
Legs, feet	No tenderness, weakness, or swelling; good color	Edema, tender calf, tingling, weakness
Skeleton	No malformations	Bowlegs, knock-knees, chest deformity at diaphragm, beaded ribs, prominent scapulas

Laboratory tests

More objective and precise data concerning nutritional status may be obtained by laboratory methods. However, for assessment during pregnancy, some problems in interpretation exist here also, including (1) a lack in many instances of established norms for pregnant women for some of the tests and (2) a need for more knowledge of the relation of certain nutrients to prepregnant and pregnant states. For example, the use of steroid contraceptives have been implicated in alterations in serum folate, vitamin B_6, vitamin B_{12}, and ascorbic acid, which may be important in developing chronic depletion in maternal stores. Evidence has been found for some progressive decrease in plasma ascorbic acid levels during pregnancy. Also, more knowledge is needed of the effects of maternal distribution of plasma proteins, serum cholesterol, and triglycerides on the future health of the infant.

Despite these limitations, however, laboratory data provide vital baseline information for nutritional assessment at the beginning of pregnancy as well as ongoing monitoring of its course throughout gestation. In general, laboratory tests may determine deficiencies or needs in several nutrient areas.

Blood-forming nutrients. Measures of the blood-forming nutrients—iron, folacin, pyridoxine (vitamin B_6), and cobalamin (vitamin B_{12})—are important guides for use in preventing and treating anemias often associated with pregnancy or with depletion of prepregnant stores of these hematological agents. Along with protein, these agents are necessary to combat anemia, the most common nutritional complication of pregnancy and the interconceptual period, by providing materials for the synthesis of hemoglobin, the oxygen-carrying protein of blood. Other differential causes of anemia are discussed in Chapter 6. Basic routine tests during pregnancy include measures of hemoglobin and hematocrit levels: hemoglobin less than 11 gm/100 ml (or

hematocrit less than 33%) late in pregnancy is suspect for anemia, and hemoglobin less than 10 gm/100 ml is a certainty. Further examination of a stained erythrocyte smear will help to determine the specific cause of the anemia. Also, measures of serum iron and total iron-binding capacity (TIBC) help to evaluate iron-deficiency anemia more specifically.

Serum protein. Of special interest during pregnancy is the serum albumin level because of its function in helping to maintain normal flow of tissue fluids from the circulating blood through the tissues for nourishment of cells and back into circulation by means of the capillary fluid shift mechanism. The operation of this mechanism depends on a normal balance between two pressures: the blood pressure and the colloidal osmotic pressure of plasma albumin. Thus a protein deficit would contribute to a lowered plasma albumin level and in turn to an imbalance in the fluid shift mechanism with resulting edema. An acceptable level during pregnancy of serum albumin is 3.5 gm/100 ml or above.

Other minerals and vitamins. According to individual indication, tests of other vitamin and mineral levels may be performed, including determinations of the water-soluble vitamins thiamine, riboflavin, niacin, and vitamin C; the fat-soluble vitamins A, D, E, and K; and iodine and other trace minerals.

Blood lipids, glucose, and enzymes. Routine testing for urine sugar and ketone bodies will screen for latent diabetes or gestational glycosuria. More extensive care and monitoring can then be provided for those mothers indicated. Other tests may be indicated in chronic diseases such as heart disease, renal disease, or tuberculosis (Chapter 5).

Historical information

The third and most important method of nutritional assessment in pregnancy is that of history taking. These data must include basic information from carefully taken medical, obstetrical, nutritional, family, and social histories, all of which have a bearing on nutritional status. Primary factors in historical data that should be included are age; previous obstetrical history; and medical, social, personal, and nutrition histories.

Age. Increased risk accompanies pregnancy in adolescents and older women.

Previous obstetrical history. Poor reproductive history may indicate nutritional deficiencies. Data should be obtained about (1) *parity and outcome*—sequential listing of total previous pregnancies and their result, including stillbirths, premature infants, and abortions (spontaneous and therapeutic); (2) *birth weights of previous infants*—low birth weights, which may be suggestive of nutritional problems, or larger birth weights, which may be correlated with latent diabetes; (3) *maternal weight changes in previous pregnancies*—amount and pattern of weight gain as a potential indicator of possible high-risk mothers; and (4) *interconceptual period*—repeated pregnancies or lactation within one-year intervals with depletion of nutritional reserves; use of steroid contraceptives, which may affect nutritional status through inhibition of folic acid absorption; intercurrent illnesses of a metabolic nature such as diabetes, which pregnancy intensifies; or infections or neoplastic disease.

Medical history. In addition to the incidence of intercurrent illnesses just listed, chronic illnesses such as renal disease or heart disease and family history of diabetes as well as overt signs provide relevant information for nutritional assessment in pregnancy. Any prior incidence of hypertension, syphilis, tuberculosis, or other infections will be needed. Previous nutritional deficiencies with conditions such as anemia should be described fully.

Social history. Family situation, number in family, housing, economic status with family income available for food, the need and accessibility and use of food assistance programs are prime factors of concern in nutritional assessment in pregnancy. Also important is a knowledge of the occupation and physical activity of the mother. Food habits are closely related to ethnic patterns so that data concerning cultural background are needed.

Personal history. Additional personal data should include cigarette smoking and use of drugs or alcohol. An increased incidence of low birth weight babies occurs among women who smoke. Drug addiction and alcoholism create special problems of nutritional deficiencies. Also, a general review of all medications used should be made, exploring possible nutrient-drug interactions and avoiding all drugs during pregnancy that are not specifically prescribed and administered under medical supervision.

Nutrition history. In addition to data concerning food habits, many additional items such as allergies, tolerances, dieting experiences, and others will need to be explored in detail. Because this aspect of historical information is most basic to nutritional assessment in pregnancy, the following separate section discusses needs and approaches in this area of dietary evaluation.

Nutrition assessment

In all patient care and education the initial principle is to begin where persons are. Thus in nutrition assessment in pregnancy, which is a time in the human life cycle when nutrition is of special importance, it is particularly necessary to learn who the mother is, where she is, what her needs are, and how they can best be met. Only in this context of individual life situations and need can realistic guidance be provided. Nutrition assessment in pregnancy therefore involves three basic areas: background data, diet history, and diet analysis.

Personal background data

The life situation and values, as well as physical and emotional factors, are closely related to food habits and attitudes. Thus, if nutritional counseling is to be valid, it must be based on an individually adapted plan of care. Information about the following items will provide helpful background data on which the nutritionist can develop such a personalized plan.

Living situation. As her nutrition counselor, ask the mother to help you see her in her living situation to plan together a food guide to meet her particular needs during pregnancy. This information will include any contingencies or influences on food use and eating behavior, such as home setting, housing, life-style, family members, occupations, general socioeconomic status, food assistance needs, and family roles and attitudes concerning food, especially food practices in pregnancy.

Cultural-ethnic food practices. Any culturally related food patterns will be explored, including types of food, ethnic dishes, methods of cooking, and taboos associated with pregnancy. From many sources in her community and family, the pregnant woman receives much culturally based advice concerning what she should eat.

Special diet practices. Any personal diet beliefs, values, practices, and experiences will also be explored. These areas that may bring out special nutritional needs include any recent weight reduction "dieting" the mother may have experienced that reduced her nutritional reserves, any faddist or unusual patterns that may be nutritionally unsound such as "macrobiotic" or other restricted diets, pica patterns such as cravings for clay or laundry starch, severe vegetarian regimens such as fruitarianism, and any other arbitrarily adopted pattern harmful to her pregnancy.

Food allergies or intolerances. Any particular food allergies, milk or lactose intolerance, or any other indications for omission of certain foods need to be explored. It may be a true allergy or intolerance, and modified forms of the food will need to be sought such as cultured forms of milk or lactose-free substitutes. In other cases it may be a simple dislike or unpleasant association with the food, and discussion about the cause or alternative ways of using it may be the solution for acceptance.

Medications or supplements. The use of all medications or supplements needs to be explored. Medications may need to be used with caution, certainly only under medical supervision, and nutritional supplements should be discussed. Specific nutrient supplements of iron and folic acid are recommended by the National Research Council report, and routine comprehensive supplementation with vitamins and minerals may not be needed with careful diet planning. Certainly the counsel that such routine supplementation does not remove the need for increased dietary intake is important. The increased demand for protein and energy, for example, is not met by such broad vitamin and mineral supplementation.

Diet history

Depending on the time available in the clinic or the skills of the practitioner, a diet history may be obtained in several different ways. The two most commonly used methods are the food record and the nutrition interview.

Food record. To obtain as valid a record as possible, the nutritionist should make the request in an open and supportive manner, explaining the reasons for the record, giving assurances concerning the use that will be made of it, and providing clear directions for keeping the record. For example, the nutritionist's conversation with the mother may go something like this:

"One of the most important things you can do for yourself during your pregnancy is to eat the best foods for your own health and the health of your baby."

"Why does it matter what I eat?"

"Because the foods you eat supply the building materials for the baby to grow, and certain foods supply more of these building materials than others. Also, these foods will keep you healthy, too, and give you the energy you need. One way you can see if you are eating the foods you need is to keep a record of the foods you eat.

Name _____

Medical record no. _____

Date _____

TOOL A
Food record: diet history*

TOTAL FOOD INTAKE

Meals and snacks		Description of food items			With whom eaten?	COMMENTS
Time	Place	Food	Amount	Type or preparation		Any related factors?—associated activity, place, persons, money, feelings, hunger, etc.

*From Williams, S.: Handbook of maternal and infant nutrition, Berkeley, Calif., 1976, SRW Productions, Inc.

Then we can go over it together on your next visit and help you plan your diet."

"Well, what kind of a record should I keep?"

"Here is a record form you might use if you like." (Show the mother a copy of *Tool A—Food Record: Diet History,* and give her assurances that it is not a "test" but only a means of helping her and can only be helpful if it is accurate and complete.)

"I know a lot of things influence what we eat, and we usually don't eat the same foods each day—there's no 'perfect' eating every day. This record is just to help you see where you are and what your food needs are. There's a space here, you see, not only for the foods you eat but also the time that you eat them, who you are with, and any comments you might have about the situation or things that may have influenced your food choices or just how you felt at the time."

"Should I put everything down or just my regular meals?"

"Everything—be sure to include everything you eat or drink at any time, with the amount you had. Try to write them down right after eating so you won't forget anything."

"When should I start?"

"Right now, if you like. I can help you start today's page, for example." (Take a record sheet and write in the mother's responses as she gives them.)

"What did you have to eat this morning?" (After a few entries are made to give examples and to clarify directions, give the required number of record sheets to the mother for her to complete during the coming week.)

"Here are enough sheets for you to write down everything you eat or drink for one week. Bring these sheets with you after you fill them out, when you come to your next clinic visit. Then we can look at your record together, and you can see if you are getting what you need for your pregnancy. Then whatever we find your needs are, you and I can plan a good food guide for you that will meet your needs during your pregnancy as well as being one that you will like and enjoy."

On the mother's next clinic visit, the nutritionist uses the food record the mother brings in as a general basis for analyzing and discussing her diet, according to her food and nutrient needs for her pregnancy.

A guide such as *Tool C—Nutrition Analysis Sheet* may be helpful in leading the mother to make her own analysis of her food intake record.

Nutrition interview. An alternative method of obtaining a diet history is the nutrition interview, which is a basic history-taking type of interview. Perhaps one of the simplest and most helpful means of conducting such an interview is the *activity-associated general day's food intake pattern* (AADFP). Since for most people eating is related to usual activity pattern or work throughout the day, making use of the two provides a structure. People usually eat according to where they are and what they are doing. Thus this type of an interview schedule gives both the interviewer and the client a structure—a beginning, a middle, and an ending—and provides a series of "memory jogs" on which to bring out the greater detail of food habits that will aid constructive diet counseling.

Using a form such as *Tool B—Nutrition Interview: Diet History,* the interview has three basic stages.

Stage I—Beginning introductions and background. A few introductory statements, introductions, and questions help to establish the purpose of the interview and build a rapport that allows mutual trust and exchange of information. It helps to draw a profile of the individual as a person of worth and integrity. It gives a picture of her living situation and other personal factors that she may wish to discuss and that may impinge on her food availability and choice. In this beginning you are trying to get a clear picture of who the client is as a person and where she is in terms of life situation and her general understanding of her health needs during her pregnancy. You will refer to such items as those given earlier under personal background data (p. 63).

Stage II—General pattern of the day's activities and food intake. In the main body of the interview, lead the client through her usual day's routine activities, from the time she

TOOL B

Nutrition interview: diet history*

Activity-Associated General Day's Food Intake Pattern

Age _____ Height _____ Prepregnant weight _____

Gravida _____ EDC _____ Present weight _____

Living situation

Housing _____

Members of household _____

Culture _____

Occupation: Husband _____

Self _____

Recreation, physical activity _____

Present food habits	Place	Time
Morning		
Noon		
Evening		
Snacks		
Comments		

Checklist

Protein foods
Milk   Fish
Cheese   Poultry
Meat   Eggs
Breads, cereals, legumes
Breads (whole-grain, enriched)
Cereals
Pastas
Dried beans, peas, lentils
Vegetables
Dark yellow   Potato
Deep green   Others
Fruits   Fats and oils
Citrus   Butter
Others   Margarine
               Others

Desserts, sweets
Soft drinks, candy
Alcohol
Vitamin, mineral supplements
Medications, drugs

*From Williams, S.: Handbook of maternal and infant nutrition, Berkeley, Calif., 1976, SRW Productions, Inc.

TOOL C
Nutritional analysis sheet*

Food groups	Major nutrient contributions	Recommended daily intake (number of servings)	Patient intake	Analysis of food needs
Protein-rich foods Milk-cheese	Protein (complete, high biological value); Ca, P, Mg; vitamin D; ribo-flavin	1 qt milk 2 oz cheese or ½ cup cottage cheese		
Egg-meat	Protein (complete, high biological value); B complex vitamins; folic acid (liver); vitamin A (liver); iron (liver especially)	2 eggs 2 servings meat (3-4 oz each) Liver once a week at least		
Vitamin- and mineral-rich foods Grains, whole or enriched, breads or cereals, legumes	Protein (incomplete, supplementary); B complex vitamins; iron, Ca, P, Mg; energy (protein sparing)	4 or more servings		
Green and yellow vegetables	Vitamin A; folic acid	1-2 servings		
Citrus fruits and other vitamin C–rich fruits and vegetables	Vitamin C	2 servings		
Potatoes and other vegetables and fruits	Energy (protein sparing); added vitamins and minerals	1 serving or as needed for calories		
Fats—margarine, butter, and oils	Vitamin A (butter, fortified margarine); vitamin E (vegetable oils); energy (protein sparing)	1-2 tbsp as needed for calories		
Iodized salt	Iodine	Use with food to taste		

*From Williams, S.: Handbook of maternal and infant nutrition, Berkeley, Calif., 1976, SRW Productions, Inc.

arises in the morning until she retires at night, all the while relating these activities to her food intake. Omit labels for informal meals so that she will remember to mention food which she eats but does not consider a meal. Since the family dinner is usually the only fairly structured meal, however, review it carefully one item at a time from the main dish through starch accompaniment, vegetables, salad, dessert, bread, and beverage. In the case of each item, ask questions in terms of general habit—food item form, frequency, preparation, portion, seasoning, likes and dislikes —not in terms of any one specific day's food intake. Sometimes pictures or models of portion sizes may be helpful in arriving at a clear picture of this family's general habits of food use.

Stage III—Cross check by nutrient food groups. The final stage of the diet history interview is designed to reflect back to the client her original responses concerning the use of foods according to groupings by main nutrient contribution. This review helps her to validate or correct her original statements. It also helps to tally the day's use of given types of foods as a beginning aid to the nutritional analysis to follow. By referring to a cross list of food items that have been categorized according to nutrient groups, the general intake of basic nutrients is analyzed:

1. *Protein foods*—meat, milk, fish, poultry, egg, cheese
2. *Cereal grains, bread*—whole grain or enriched, forms used, frequency
3. *Fruits and vegetables*—vitamin A and C sources, citrus and substitutes, deep green and yellow fruits and vegetables, how cooked
4. *Desserts*—form and frequency, milk base
5. *Beverages*—coffee, tea, soft drinks, alcohol
6. *Snack items*—candy, chips, nuts, cookies
7. *Nutrient supplements*—vitamins and minerals
8. *Other drugs used*—prescribed medications and "over-the-counter" drugs such as aspirin, laxatives, antacids

Instead of the foregoing cross-check method, at this point you may wish to use *Tool C—Nutritional Analysis Sheet,* entering food items used in a day in the respective food groupings indicated. Another method of cross check is to ask for a 24-hour recall of specific foods eaten in the previous day for comparison with the responses given during the interview.

Throughout the interview weighted phrases such as "only one" or "plenty of", approving or disapproving tones or facial expressions, or other "body language" should be avoided because these tend to imply judgments and prevent realistic responses. Important clues to food attitudes and values are being communicated, and you do not want to miss any of them. Note these carefully and store them in your mind for later thought and possible exploration. If your manner throughout has been warm, interested, and accepting, the information the client gives should be valid and straightforward. If you are judgmental or authoritarian at this point, she will probably tell you only what she thinks you want to hear or what will make you think well of her, not what her true situation may be.

Example of a nutrition history interview. For example, such a nutrition interview may go as follows:

"Good morning, Mrs. Morton. I'm Dale Johnson, the nutritionist here in our prenatal clinic. Why don't you sit over here? I think this chair is more comfortable. I see by your chart that this is your first baby. How are you feeling?"

"Oh, I'm fine, so far—just a little 'queasy' in the morning, but it doesn't last long."

"Queasy? Are you having any trouble with your food?"

"Not really, I guess. I just don't have much appetite."

"Well, it's important that you do eat certain foods during your pregnancy, so perhaps we can plan some way to help your appetite so you can eat and enjoy your food. Why do you think it's so important how you eat now during your pregnancy?"

"I know I must need more food for my baby to grow."

"That's right. One of the most important things you can do during your pregnancy to keep yourself and your baby healthy and to help the baby grow is to eat a good diet—foods to feed both you and your baby. So this is our main purpose at this first visit here at the beginning of your pregnancy—to review your food habits and see what your nutritional needs are and to help you plan your diet. So we want to go over anything that influences your needs and the way you eat. Let's see, what age are you?"

"Nineteen."

"And you're how tall?"

"Five feet four."

"Let's check your weight before we go on." (The mother steps on the scale, and the nutritionist adjusts the balances. They return to their seats beside each other.)

"One hundred thirty pounds. Is that your usual weight?"

"Yes, it's been that for the past few years."

"Well, let's see. Is there anything about your living situation that might affect your eating? For example, what is your living arrangement? How many persons in your household?"

"Only two, my husband and I. We have an apartment near the campus."

"Do you both work? Or go to school at the university?"

"Well, both. My husband works evenings driving a taxi and has classes at the university mornings. I work at the courthouse as a clerk during the day. I hope some day to study law."

"Well, that's a pretty full schedule. It sounds to me like you two could do just about anything you set your minds to. Do you eat most of your meals at home?"

"Yes, we can't afford to go out. Most Sundays we have dinner at my mother-in-law's house."

"Well, let's see what a usual day's food pattern is for you. Take me through your usual day's activities, and let's see what you usually eat. When does your day begin? When do you usually get up?"

"About 6:30. I have to be at work by 8:30 and Mike has 8:00 o'clock classes most mornings."

"After you get up, do you usually have something to eat? Can you give me some examples of what you might have?"

"I rarely have time for anything. I just have some coffee."

"Black or cream and sugar?"

"Just black coffee."

"Then you get to work about 8:30. Through the morning at work do you have a break? Would you get something to eat then?"

"My break is at 10:15. But we only have vend-

ing machines, so I usually get a candy bar or a Coke."

"Then, what about your next break at noon. What do you do about your lunch?"

"I usually carry it from home. I can't afford to buy my lunch every day."

"What do you bring?"

"A sandwich and some cookies."

"What kind of a sandwich?"

"Oh, it varies, usually cold cuts and cheese or tuna. And I usually get another Coke from the machine."

"Anything else?"

"No, that's about all."

"Then you go back to work. Is there also an afternoon break? Do you have something to eat then?"

"No, I usually don't take a break so I can leave earlier."

"What time do you get off?"

"At 4:45. I'm usually home by 5:30."

"Then what do you do?"

"Well, Mike usually comes in for his dinner break at 7:00 o'clock so I start getting it ready for him."

"I know dinners vary, but give me some examples of what you might have. For example, do you usually have some kind of meat? How do you cook it?"

"We can't afford much meat, but I usually try to have something like hamburger or chicken or fish. I usually fry it."

"What do you have with it? Do you usually have some sort of starch, such as potatoes, rice, corn, beans, pastas such as macaroni or noodles or spaghetti?"

"Yes, Mike and I both like french fried potatoes. And we have dumplings often."

"What about vegetables? Do you usually have some sort of vegetable—cooked, or raw in a salad?"

"Not very often. Mike doesn't eat many vegetables, and I'm not very good at cooking them. But we sometimes have some mixed tossed salad, once or twice a week, I guess."

"What about bread with your dinner?"

"We each have about one or two slices of bread or hot biscuits."

"Do you usually have a dessert of some kind?"

"No, only on weekends or special occasions."

"And what do you usually drink with your dinner?"

"Coffee, black."

"Then after dinner what do you usually do?"

"Well, Mike goes back to work, and I watch TV or catch up on some of the housework."

"Later on in the evening, before you go to bed, do you usually have something to eat?"

"Yes, I usually get something from the kitchen, like a dish of ice cream. But usually, since I have to get up so early, I'm in bed as a rule by midnight."

"Well, you do have quite a busy, long day, don't you. Let's see now if this is right as to the general food you eat. You didn't mention drinking milk at all. Would you say you don't use it at all? Do you not like it or are you just not in the habit of using it?"

"Oh, I don't dislike it. I use it occasionally, about once a week, I guess. I just don't think about it."

"You mentioned cheese in your lunch sandwich. How often would you say you eat cheese?"

"Oh, just about every day. I like cheese of any kind, and we have potatoes almost every day."

"You spoke of some kind of meat at dinner and a cold cut or tuna in your sandwich. Would you say you usually have two servings of meat every day?"

"Yes, I guess that's about right."

"You didn't mention eggs. Do you eat eggs at all?"

"Yes, I guess I have about one or two a week. I like them. I just don't think to fix them."

"What about the amount of bread you eat? You said you have a sandwich at lunch—that's two slices. But you didn't mention cereal or other forms. Oh, yes, your bread or biscuits at dinner. Would you say, then, that you have about four pieces or servings of bread a day?"

"Yes, that's about right."

"You said you didn't have many vegetables. What are some you like? Would you say you have about three servings a week?"

"Yes, I guess that's about right. I like vegetables, but I just haven't been fixing them."

"You didn't mention fruit. Do you usually eat any?"

"Oh, yes, I forgot. I usually drink some orange juice in the mornings. But that's about it."

"You mentioned coffee at breakfast and at dinner and a Coke midmorning and at lunch. Are those the only beverages you have?"

"Yes, except for some wine occasionally at dinner at Mike's house."

"Have you been taking any vitamins or minerals?"

"No."

"Thank you. You've given me some very helpful information. Now let's look back over what you've told me about your food habits and the foods you like, and compare this with your nutritional requirements during your pregnancy. Then we can see what your needs are and help you with a food plan you can use. Then you'll be assured that you are giving your baby what he needs to grow on and what you need to keep healthy."

Diet analysis

After obtaining the client's diet history, either by food record or by nutrition interview, analyze your findings in terms of the increased nutritional demands of pregnancy. The two methods of analysis that may be used are nutrient calculation and nutrient check by food groups.

Nutrient calculation. Sometimes, when specific nutrient intake data are needed, you may need to tally foods for calculation of protein, calories, and key vitamins and minerals. Food value tables in standard references[2,4,12] or in textbook appendices may be used; then totals of each nutrient may be compared with the Recommended Dietary Allowances for pregnancy stated by the National Research Council[5] or as given here (pp. 76-78). Any areas of deficiency can then be discussed with the mother and emphasized in her food plan.

Nutrient check by food groups. In most cases the adequacy of the mother's food pattern can be checked with her using basic groupings of foods according to major nutrient contributions. Effort is made to determine amounts of food from each group given to meet the increased needs for key nutrients during pregnancy. *Tool C—Nutritional Analysis Sheet* provides such a guide.

First, the mother should be familiarized with the food groups and the basis of the groupings—the major nutrients each contains. Second, the mother should be asked to name some foods that would be included in each group. This will provide a basis for reviewing the basic nutrients needed during pregnancy and why each is needed.

Emphasis, in turn, will be given to protein, calories, and key vitamins and minerals, with basic core foods emerging that fill these needs. Third, the nutritionist should review her own food record or the findings of her nutrition interview with the mother. Taking one food group at a time, ask the mother to list all the food items she can find in her own diet that go in that food group, with the amount of each food that she usually eats. Continue in this way with each of the food groups. This activity will fill in the column under *My intake* on Tool C.

Finally, taking one group at a time, the nutritionist should ask the mother to compare her food intake with the recommended increased amount listed on the sheet for each food group to meet the needs of her pregnancy. As a result of this comparison, the mother should be asked to state her dietary needs in each food group. Then, on the basis of this analysis, the nutritionist develops with her a food plan to meet her nutritional needs for her pregnancy as well as her personal needs as discovered in the nutrition interview.

NUTRITION EDUCATION AND GUIDANCE IN PRENATAL CARE

What is the nutritionist going to do at this point with the findings from diet surveys in the prenatal clinic? What kind of educational program and continuing guidance is needed to build and strengthen healthy food practices? When the diet histories of clients are analyzed, the nutritionist will find a variety of food practices. Some of these practices will be beneficial and need only encouragement. Some may be harmless and can be ignored. Other food practices, however, will be harmful because they produce deficiencies in specific nutrients that are needed in increased amounts during pregnancy, and hence these practices need to be overcome and corrected. All of these situations present an educational challenge. Because the successful outcome of the pregnancy of each woman in the nutritionist's care is of par-

ticular concern, and because nutrition plays such a primary role in determining that outcome, nutrition education becomes one of the major responsibilities of the nutritionist in prenatal care.

Principles of learning

The teaching-learning process, however, is not a simple matter. Essentially, learning means *change*. Often this involves change in deeply rooted habits, values, and beliefs, and such change seldom is easy. There is a vast difference between a person who has *learned* and a person who has only been *informed*. Thus, to guide her work at this point, the nutritionist should remember and apply three important principles of learning:

1. *Learning is very personal and individual.* It cannot be imposed on one from the outside. Rather, it takes place *inside* a person in response to his own felt *needs* and through interaction with his environment. Therefore valid learning must meet personal needs and involve the learner.

2. *Learning is associative or developmental.* It builds on prior learning and prior experience and knowledge. Therefore valid learning must blend the new with the familiar.

3. *Learning results in changed behavior.* In the last analysis therefore valid learning must be measured largely in terms of behavior change.

Learning framework: concept of building

The word *concept* comes from the Latin roots for the prefix "with" and the verb "to seize." Thus it carries a dynamic idea of learning by seizing on new thought and putting it together with other thought to form new knowledge. A concept, then, is a general notion or idea of something formed by mentally combining all its characteristics or particulars to make a concrete construct. The concept thus forms a framework, or "hook," on which to place various parts of the thing being learned to give it meaning and relationship and wholeness. Essentially, from a cognitive viewpoint, persons learn things in two basic interrelated ways. One way is to respond to collections of things or ideas by distinguishing among them, thus forming categories. Another way, even more important as a human capability, is to put things into an overall class and to respond to the class as a whole, to relate the parts to the whole. This learning that makes it possible for a person to respond to things or events as a whole or as a class is called *concept learning.*[6]

The concept of *building* provides a useful framework, or hook, for prenatal nutrition education. This idea is a concrete one with numerous illustrative associations from prior learning and experience. Applied to pregnancy, it gives a dynamic notion to the profound reality of building a new human life. Using this concept of building, the nutrition principles may be presented and interpreted and learned in relation to the basic idea of growth and development—building, with each component providing a necessary part for a successful outcome of the building process.

Building materials: protein

In the human building system the specific necessary building material is *protein* and its individual construction units the *amino acids.* During the period of pregnancy, the human life grows from a single fertilized egg cell (ovum) to a fully developed, specifically constructed infant weighing about 7 pounds—the most rapid building period of the entire human life span. It is evident therefore that the rapid growth period of pregnancy places primary demand on larger amounts of the growth-promoting material protein in the diet of the mother, who is the master builder. We shall consider the amount of the protein building material needed in the mother's diet, the reasons for this increased need, and ways she can be sure that she gets this needed protein in foods that she eats.

Amount of protein increase needed for building. The latest recommendations of the National Research Council for protein intake during pregnancy reflect this increased demand for building material. As mentioned previously, the council indicates a general required increase of 30 gm/day over the amount (45 to 50 grams) needed by a nonpregnant adult woman. This makes an increased need of about 60% more protein, or about 80 to 85 grams. Some high-risk or active women would need even more, nearer 100 grams, or about double their previous intake.

Reasons for the increased protein requirement. A number of reasons for increased protein building material reflect the tremendous growth period involved.

Rapid growth of the baby. A study of fetal tissue composition indicates that the amount of nitrogen, the unique distinguishing element of protein structure, stored by the embryo rises from 0.9 gram at conception to 55.9 grams at birth. The mere increase in size of the fetus during pregnancy indicates how much protein is required for building the baby's body during so brief a period of time.

Development of the placenta. The mature placenta at term has stored about 17 grams of nitrogen. Sufficient protein is required for its complete building and unique development during pregnancy as the necessary vital organ to sustain, support, and nourish the baby. It is literally the baby's "lifeline."

Enlargement of maternal tissue. Increased development of breast and uterine tissue is required to support pregnancy. An estimated 17 grams of nitrogen is incorporated in the developing maternal breast tissue and nearly 40 grams in the increased tissue of the uterus. In addition, a general maternal reserve tissue is required. About 200 to 350 grams of nitrogen is stored for the approaching losses during labor and birth. For example, 300 to 500 ml of blood (protein tissue) or more may be lost during childbirth. Also, increased tissue reserves are required in preparation for the physiological demand of lactation to follow.

Increased maternal circulating blood volume. A particular increase of protein building material is demanded by the increase in the mother's circulating blood volume, which is 50% or more above her normal blood volume. This increase is necessary to provide the transportation system required by the increased metabolic work load going on in the mother's body during pregnancy, to carry the increased "traffic" of nutrients back and forth to cells, and thus to nourish and support the mother's body and the baby's body as well as the bridging placenta between them. With this increased blood volume there is an independent need for increased synthesis of constituents of blood, especially hemoglobin and plasma protein, both of which are proteins vital to the support of the pregnancy. Increased hemoglobin is required to supply increased oxygen need for the growing cells and increased metabolic work load. One particular plasma protein needed in increased amount is albumin, which creates an osmotic force to keep the increased blood volume circulating. The albumin provides the necessary colloidal osmotic pressure (COP) to maintain operation of the *capillary fluid shift mechanism,* a fundamental homeostatic mechanism designed to maintain normal fluid and electrolyte balance in the body (p. 101). As the blood pressure constantly "pushes" body fluids and their nutrients out of capillaries into tissues to nourish cells, the COP exerted by plasma albumin molecules constantly "pulls" the tissue fluids and their products of cell metabolism back into circulation. Thus body fluids and their solutes are kept in constant circulation, thereby guarding the total vascular volume and preventing accumulation of fluid in the tissues (edema). Other binding proteins in the blood are also needed in increased amounts; for example, iron-binding protein is required to handle the increased metabolic need for iron during pregnancy, and thyroxine-binding protein is required to handle the increased need for this hormone controlling basal metabolic rate. In turn, to synthesize the needed thyroxine, more iodine is needed.

Formation of amniotic fluid. The fluid surrounding the infant in the uterus is designed to protect him from shock or trauma. It contains protein; hence, its formation requires more protein.

Storage reserves. Increased storage reserves are required in maternal tissue to prepare for labor, birth, the immediate postpartum period, and lactation. As indicated, about 200 to 350 grams of nitrogen are stored thus as a maternal reserve.

Food sources of protein building material. The prime quality building material, called *complete protein* because it supplies all eight essential construction units—amino acids—the body cannot manufacture and hence must come from food humans eat, is found only in four commonly used foods: milk, cheese, eggs, and meat. Therefore these "core foods" assume prime importance in the diet of a pregnant woman. Additional building material comes from some *incomplete proteins,* so called because they do not supply enough of one or more of the eight essential construction units (amino acids) that the diet must provide. Although less therefore in quality by comparison, these supplementary protein building materials found in plant foods such as legumes, grains, nuts, and seeds are also important additions to the mother's diet.

Energy for the building work: calories

The work of building tissue requires energy. Thus calories must be supplied by the mother's diet in sufficient amount to meet these increased energy needs and thereby spare protein for tissue building. The National Research Council indicates that at least an additional 300 calories is required during pregnancy, making a basic total of 2200 to 2400 cal/day for the pregnant woman, which is about a 15% increase over her usual intake. However, this amount may be insufficient still for many nutritionally deficient or active women, who may need as much as 2500 to 3000 calories. The emphasis therefore should be a positive one on sufficient calories to ensure *individual* nutrient and energy needs, not a negative idea of blanket restriction of calories.

Control agents for regulating the building process

Just as any building process must have specifications and control agents regulating the building process to bring about the specific construction guided by the plans, even so must the human building system have specific regulatory agents at each step of the process to control its orderly progress according to plan. These control agents in the human system are the vitamins and minerals. In their roles in regulating various parts of the building process, they function in two basic types of ways: (1) as construction material, they contribute needed units to build tissue; for example, calcium builds bones and tooth buds, iron builds hemoglobin, vitamins A and C participate in building tissue in general; and (2) as enzyme partners they regulate specific building and energy-producing processes; for example, vitamin D helps to regulate calcium use and hence bone-building activity, and the family of B vitamins act largely as coenzymes to regulate a large number of specific actions in the overall building and energy-producing processes.

In planning nutrition education and guidance for a prenatal care program using this conceptual approach to learning, the nutritionist can relate discussion about each of the key nutrients and their food sources to this basic concept of building. References using this approach may be consulted for background material and ideas.[13,14] Also, for a review of these nutrient demands of pregnancy, the increases recommended by the National Research Council, reasons for the increases, and food sources supplying these needs, a summary

table is provided in *Tool D—Nutrient Needs of Pregnancy.*

Positive approach to build motivation for learning

Perhaps at no other time in the human life cycle is a person more open to nutrition education, more motivated by a sense of responsibility for another human life, than during the period of pregnancy. A positive personalized approach can build on this feeling of responsibility and anticipation of parenthood to develop motivation for learning. Moreover, nutrition learning during this period will go far in carrying over to the young parents' attitudes toward feeding their children as they continue to grow to maturity, and in turn contribute to the health habits of another generation.

Personal motivation therefore is a prime requisite for learning. Without it any "educational program" remains on paper, an exercise in futility, wasted energy, and a "flailing at windmills." With it learning becomes the very human adventure it can be. In short, the whole business of motivation is tied up with sending your learners away from your instruction anxious to use what you have taught them—and eager to learn more.[8] A positive personalized approach in individual prenatal counseling can help to accomplish this aim.

How will you begin? Consider the two general types of food behavior you will discover in your prenatal clinic work with mothers: (1) good food intake that meets all of the recommended nutrient needs and ensures optimal nutritional intake for pregnancy, and (2) inadequate food intake that does not meet the recommended nutrient needs for pregnancy and creates deficiencies that may contribute to serious complications. In each case an analysis of individual food habits in terms of positive reinforcement of good habits and positive teaching to help correct deficiencies will be useful. Then, on this basis, a personal food plan may be developed.

TOOL D
Nutrient needs of pregnancy*

Nutrient	Amount (NRC)		Reasons for increased nutrient need in pregnancy	Food sources
	Nonpregnant adult need	Pregnancy need		

Protein	46 gm	76-100 gm	Rapid fetal tissue growth
			Amniotic fluid
			Placenta growth and development
			Maternal tissue growth: uterus, breasts
			Increased maternal circulating blood volume:
			  a. Hemoglobin increase
			  b. Plasma protein increase
			Maternal storage reserves for labor, delivery, and lactation
				Milk
				Cheese
				Egg
				Meat
				Grains
				Legumes
				Nuts

Calories	2100	2400	Increased BMR, energy needs Protein sparing	Carbohydrates Fats Proteins
Minerals Calcium	800 mg	1200 mg	Fetal skeleton formation Fetal tooth bud formation Increased maternal calcium metabolism	Milk Cheese Whole grains Leafy vegetables Egg yolk
Phosphorus	800 mg	1200 mg	Fetal skeletal formation Fetal tooth bud formation Increased maternal phosphorus metabolism	Milk Cheese Lean meats
Iron	18 mg	18+ mg (+30-60 mg supplement)	Increased maternal circulating blood volume, increased hemoglobin Fetal liver iron storage High iron cost of pregnancy	Liver Meats Egg Whole or enriched grain Leafy vegetables Nuts Legumes Dried fruits

*From Williams, S.: Handbook of maternal and infant nutrition, Berkeley, Calif., 1976, SRW Productions, Inc.

TOOL D
Nutrient needs of pregnancy—cont'd

Nutrient	Amount (NRC)		Reasons for increased nutrient need in pregnancy	Food sources
	Nonpregnant adult need	Pregnancy need		
Iodine	100 μg	125 μg	Increased BMR—increased thyroxine production	Iodized salt
Magnesium	300 mg	450 mg	Coenzyme in energy and protein metabolism Enzyme activator Tissue growth, cell metabolism Muscle action	Nuts Soybeans Cocoa Seafood Whole grains Dried beans and peas
Vitamins A	4000 IU	5000 IU	Essential for cell development, hence tissue growth Tooth bud formation (development of enamel-forming cells in gum tissue) Bone growth	Butter Cream Fortified margarine Green and yellow vegetables
D	0	400 IU	Absorption of calcium and phosphorus, mineralization of bone tissue, tooth buds	Fortified milk Fortified margarine
E	12 IU	15 IU	Tissue growth, cell wall integrity Red blood cell integrity	Vegetable oils Leafy vegetables Cereals Meat Egg Milk
C	45 mg	60 mg	Tissue formation and integrity Cement substance in connective and vascular tissues Increases iron absorption	Citrus fruits Berries Melons Tomatoes Chili peppers Green peppers Green leafy vegetables Broccoli Potatoes
Folic acid	400 μg	800 μg (+200-400 mcg supplement)	Increased metabolic demand in pregnancy Prevention of megaloblastic anemia in high-risk patients	Liver Green leafy vegetables

Continued.

TOOL D
Nutrient needs of pregnancy—cont'd

Nutrient	Amount (NRC)		Reasons for increased nutrient need in pregnancy	Food sources
	Nonpregnant adult need	Pregnancy need		
Folic acid— cont'd			Increased heme production for hemoglobin Production of cell nucleus material	
Niacin	13 mg	15 mg	Coenzyme in energy metabolism Coenzyme in protein metabolism	Meat Peanuts Beans and peas Enriched grains
Riboflavin	1.2 mg	1.5 mg	Coenzyme in energy metabolism and protein metabolism	Milk Liver Enriched grains
Thiamine	1.0 mg	1.3 mg	Coenzyme for energy metabolism	Pork, beef Liver Whole or enriched grains Legumes
B₆ (pyridoxine)	2.0 mg	2.5 mg	Coenzyme in protein metabolism Increased fetal growth requirement	Wheat, corn Liver Meat
B₁₂	3.0 μg	4.0 μg	Coenzyme in protein metabolism, especially vital cell proteins such as nucleic acid Formation of red blood cells	Milk Egg Meat Liver Cheese

Positive reinforcement of good food habits

To strengthen good food habits, give positive feedback immediately for those food behaviors you find in a mother's food records and interview responses when you analyze them together, that fulfill recommended food choices and amounts for pregnancy. You may provide positive reinforcement for this desired behavior by the following basic actions:

1. *Relate the mother's food practices to the nutritional needs of her pregnancy.* Guide her to identify for herself how her particular food practices are meeting the needs of her pregnancy. You may use Tool C to help her relate some specific key foods she is using to the nutrients needed.

2. *Review the reasons for these increased nutrient needs of pregnancy.* Further reinforce her good food habits by guiding her to see *why* it is important that she

get these increased nutrients during her pregnancy. Relate the functions of the key nutrients to the changes taking place in her own body and to the rapid growth of her baby and its protection. The summary of functions in Tool D may be useful here.

3. *Give verbal recognition for her efforts.* Commend her openly and warmly for her good food habits. Simple phrases, such as "Good work" or "You're doing a good job," are needed occasionally by everyone.

Positive teaching to correct nutrient deficiencies

To correct inadequate food practices, provide teaching rather than dire pronouncements to help the mother change those food habits that need improving. In a similar manner to your approach to reinforcing good habits, you may provide positive thinking and concern for habit change by four basic actions.

Helping the mother relate her food habits to unmet nutrient needs of her pregnancy. Guide the mother to identify for herself the instances in which her particular food intake fails to meet the nutritional demands of her pregnancy. Again, you may find Tool C useful here to help her see for herself some key nutrients she needs more of and some specific foods that supply them.

Discussing the reasons for these increased nutrient needs of pregnancy. Again, this is your previous approach, but here you are trying to build motivation for making the desired behavior change by helping the mother to see why it is important for her to do so. Point to the positive results for her baby's health, as well as for her own health, of such changed food behavior. Here, too, Tool D may be a useful guide for your discussion.

Identifying reasons for the mother's dietary deficiencies. What are her problems in obtaining appropriate foods? What limiting factors exist in her personal living situation? What personal reasons are there for her usual food choices? A variety of factors may be involved, and they are often interrelated. On the whole, problems hindering the mother from getting the food she needs relate to three basic areas: (1) the nature of the available food supply, (2) the physical status and personal characteristics of the woman herself, or (3) the nature of her personal environment. Some of these factors may be simple reasons of which the woman is aware and can readily change. Others, however, may be larger problems requiring team help from the nutritionist, the social worker, the nurse, and the physician. In any event, possible problem areas should be considered in your analysis of the individual client's needs.

The food supply. There may be a lack of food available because of poor marketing resources, insufficient funds for a large family, inadequate food storage facilities and food spoilage and waste, and lack of skills in general food management and preparation.

The person herself. Physical problems may be present, such as underlying disease, food intolerances or aversions, poor appetite or low energy level, and general low nutritional reserve. Personal problems may include ignorance of food needs or food values, special beliefs concerning food, lack of education, illiteracy, language barrier, carelessness, lack of concern or general apathy, and underlying psychological or emotional needs. In many of these situations there may be a pride that prevents disclosure of problems related to personal needs.

The environment. Too often problems attributed to personal factors, as just listed, are in reality the result of environmental factors that have overwhelmed the woman's coping resources, and she needs assistance. She may not be living in a home of her own and may have little control over food selection and preparation. Also, there may be cultural or family food customs, especially during pregnancy, that limit food choices. There may be, in addition, socioeconomic problems stemming from low income, unemployment, or frank poverty. Moreover, in some communities there may be attitudes or political influences that limit the availability of food assistance programs for pregnancy.

Exploring possible solutions to problems or alternative practices available. Whatever the situation discovered, identify any needs or limitations on the woman's ability to make the desired changes and explore with her possible solutions.

Low income. If lack of money sufficient for food needs is a problem, depending on degree of need, two areas of assistance may be discussed: (1) economy buying suggestions to help the woman spend her limited budget more wisely; and (2) possible food assistance programs available to her in the community, through government, church,

or lodge groups. Consultation with a social worker will provide guidance.

Food aversions or intolerances. The basis of the rejection should be reviewed as a means of securing acceptance of the food (or a reasonable alternative) or determining another form of the food in question.

Cultural food patterns. Nutrient needs should be related to a variety of acceptable food forms and preparations within the appropriate cultural food pattern. However, within one general cultural group, individual food habits may vary widely so that careful exploration of individual needs and desires is necessary. Several general cultural pattern guides are included here (Tables 4-3 to 4-7), and expanded references are available.[10,14]

Table 4-3. Characteristic Mexican-American food choices*

Protein foods	Milk and milk products	Grain products	Vegetables	Fruits	Other
Meat	Milk	Rice	Avocado	Apple	Salsa
Beef	Fluid	Tortillas	Cabbage	Apricots	(tomato-
Pork	Flavored	Corn	Carrots	Banana	pepper-
Lamb	Evaporated	Flour	Chilies	Guava	onion relish)
Tripe	Condensed	Oatmeal	Corn	Lemon	Chili sauce
Sausage	Cheese	Dry cereals	Green beans	Mango	Guacamole
(chorizo)	American	Cornflakes	Lettuce	Melons	Lard
Bologna	Monterey	Sugared	Onion	Orange	(manteca)
Bacon	Jack	Noodles	Peas	Peach	Pork cracklings
Poultry	Hoop	Spaghetti	Potato	Pear	Fruit drinks
Chicken	Ice cream	White bread	Prickly pear	Prickly pear	Kool-aid
Eggs		Sweet bread	cactus leaf	cactus fruit	Carbonated
Legumes		(pan dulce)	(nopales)	(tuna)	beverages
Pinto beans			Spinach	Zapote	Beer
Pink beans			Sweet potato	(sapote)	Coffee
Garbanzo beans			Tomato		
Lentils			Zucchini		
Nuts					
Peanuts					
Peanut butter					

*Modified from Nutrition during pregnancy and lactation, Sacramento, Calif., 1975, California Department of Health.

Table 4-4. Characteristic black food groups*

Protein foods	Milk and milk products	Grain products	Vegetables	Fruits	Other
Meat	Milk	Rice	Broccoli	Apple	Salt pork
Beef	Fluid	Cornbread	Cabbage	Banana	(fat back)
Pork, ham	Evaporated	Hominy grits	Carrots	Grapefruit	Carbonated
Sausage	in coffee	Biscuits	Corn	Grapes	beverages
Pig's feet,	Buttermilk	Muffins	Green beans	Nectarine	Fruit drinks
ears, etc.	Cheese	White bread	Greens	Orange	Gravies
Bacon	Cheddar	Dry cereal	Mustard	Plums	Coffee
Luncheon meats	Cottage	Cooked cereal	Collard	Tangerine	Iced tea
Organ meats	Ice cream	Macaroni	Kale	Watermelon	
Poultry		Spaghetti	Spinach		
Chicken		Crackers	Turnip		
Turkey			Lima beans		
Fish			Okra		
Catfish			Peas		
Perch			Potato		
Red snapper			Pumpkin		
Tuna			Sweet potato		
Salmon			Tomato		
Sardines			Yam		
Shrimp					
Eggs					
Legumes					
Kidney beans					
Red beans					
Pinto beans					
Black-eyed peas					
Nuts					
Peanuts					
Peanut butter					

*Modified from Nutrition during pregnancy and lactation, Sacramento, Calif., 1975, California Department of Health.

Table 4-5. Characteristic Chinese food choices*

Protein foods	Milk and milk products	Grain products	Vegetables	Fruits	Other
Meat	Milk	Rice	Bamboo shoots	Apple	Soy sauce
Pork	Flavored	Noodles	Beans	Banana	Sweet and sour
Beef	Whole milk	White bread	Green	Figs	sauce
Organ meats	(used in	Barley	Yellow	Grapes	Mustard sauce
Poultry	cooking)	Millet	Bean sprouts	Kumquats	Ginger
Chicken	Ice cream		Bok choy	Loquats	Plum sauce
Duck			Broccoli	Mango	Red bean paste
Fish			Cabbage	Melons	Black bean
White fish			Carrots	Orange	sauce
Shrimp			Celery	Peach	Oyster sauce
Lobster			Chinese	Pear	Tea
Oyster			cabbage	Persimmon	Coffee
Sardines			Corn	Pineapple	
Eggs			Cucumbers	Plums	
Legumes			Eggplant	Tangerine	
Soybeans			Greens		
Soybean			Collard		
curd (tofu)			Chinese		
Black beans			broccoli		
Nuts			Mustard		
Peanuts			Kale		
Almonds			Spinach		
Cashews			Leeks		
			Lettuce		
			Mushrooms		
			Peppers		
			Potato		
			Scallions		
			Snow peas		
			Sweet potato		
			Taro		
			Tomato		
			Water		
			chestnuts		
			White radish		
			White turnip		
			Winter melon		

*Modified from Nutrition during pregnancy and lactation, Sacramento, Calif., 1975, California Department of Health.

Table 4-6. Characteristic Japanese food choices*

Protein foods	Milk and milk products	Grain products	Vegetables	Fruits	Other
Meat	Milk	Rice	Bamboo shoots	Apple	Soy sauce
Beef	Cheese	Rice crackers	Bok choy	Apricot	Nori paste
Pork	Ice cream	Noodles	Broccoli	Banana	(seasoned
Poultry		(whole	Burdock root	Cherries	rice)
Chicken		wheat:	Cabbage	Grapefruit	Bean thread
Turkey		soba)	Carrots	Grapes	(konyaku)
Fish		Spaghetti	Cauliflower	Lemon	Ginger (shoga;
Tuna		White bread	Celery	Lime	dried form
Mackerel		Oatmeal	Cucumbers	Melons	called
Sardines		Dry cereal	Eggplant	Orange	denishoga)
(dried form:			Green beans	Peach	Tea
mezashi)			Gourd	Pear	Coffee
Sea bass			(kampyo)	Persimmon	
Shrimp			Mushrooms	Pineapple	
Abalone			Mustard	Pomegranate	
Squid			greens	Plums	
Octopus			Napa cabbage	(dried, pickled	
Eggs			Peas	plums called	
Legumes			Peppers	umeboshi)	
Soybean curd			Radishes	Strawberries	
(tofu)			(white rad-	Tangerine	
Soybean paste			ish: daikon;		
(miso)			pickled		
Soybeans			white:		
Red beans			takawan)		
(azuki)			Snow peas		
Lima beans			Spinach		
Nuts			Squash		
Chestnuts			Sweet potato		
(kuri)			Taro (Japanese		
			sweet potato)		
			Tomato		
			Turnips		
			Water		
			chestnuts		
			Yam		

*Modified from Nutrition during pregnancy and lactation, Sacramento, Calif., 1975, California Department of Health.

Table 4-7. Characteristic Filipino food choices*

Protein foods	Milk and milk products	Grain products	Vegetables	Fruits	Other
Meat	Milk	Rice	Bamboo shoots	Apple	Soy sauce
Pork	Flavored	Cooked cereals	Beets	Banana	Coffee
Beef	Evaporated	Farina	Cabbage	Grapes	Tea
Goat	Cheese	Oatmeal	Carrots	Guava	
Deer	Gouda	Dry cereals	Cauliflower	Lemon	
Rabbit	Cheddar	Pastas	Celery	Lime	
Variety meats		Rice noodles	Chinese celery	Mango	
Poultry		Wheat noodles	Eggplant	Melons	
Chicken		Macaroni	Endive	Orange	
Fish		Spaghetti	Green beans	Papaya	
Sole			Leeks	Pear	
Bonito			Lettuce	Pineapple	
Herring			Mushrooms	Plums	
Tuna			Okra	Pomegranate	
Mackerel			Onion	Rhubarb	
Crab			Peppers	Strawberries	
Mussels			Potato	Tangerine	
Shrimp			Pumpkin		
Squid			Radishes		
Eggs			Snow peas		
Legumes			Spinach		
Black beans			Squash		
Chick peas			Sweet potato		
Black-eyed peas			Tomato		
Lentils			Water chestnuts		
Mung beans			Watercress		
Lima beans			Yam		
White kidney beans					
Nuts					
Cashew					
Peanuts					
Pili nuts					

*Modified from Nutrition during pregnancy and lactation, Sacramento, Calif., 1975, California Department of Health.

Vegetarian food patterns. Exploration first must be made concerning the level or type of vegetarian pattern the woman may be following. Many vegetarian food plans exclude only meat, some even allowing fish. With these patterns ample protein may be obtained from dairy foods and eggs. However, if a strict vegetarian pattern is followed, extremely careful planning is necessary to obtain sufficient complete protein from mixtures of plant food sources. A vegetarian food guide is given in Table 4-8, and expanded references are available.[3,7]

Personal food plan

On the basis of individual findings, the nutritionist should plan with the client a personal food guide that she can enjoy. A diet consisting of a variety of foods can supply needed nutrients and make eating a pleasure. A core plan, such as that in *Tool E—Daily Food Plan For Pregnancy,* may

Table 4-8. Vegetarian food guide

General guidelines

1. Follow nutrition guide for regular food plan during pregnancy as outlined in Tools E and F.
2. Eat a wide variety of foods, including milk and milk products and eggs.
3. If no milk is allowed, use a supplement of 4 μg of vitamin B_{12} daily. If goat and soymilk are used, partial supplementation may be needed.
4. If no milk is taken, also use supplements of 12 mg of calcium and 400 IU of vitamin D daily. Partial supplementation will be necessary if less than four servings of milk and milk products are consumed.
5. Select a variety of plant foods (especially grains, legumes, nuts, and seeds) to obtain "complete" proteins by complementary combinations, as indicated in the list below.
6. Use iodized salt.

Complementary plant protein combinations*		
Food	Amino acids deficient	Complementary protein food combinations
Grains	Isoleucine Lysine	Rice + legumes Corn + legumes Wheat + legumes Wheat + peanut + milk Wheat + sesame + soybean Rice + Brewer's yeast
Legumes	Tryptophan Methionine	Legumes + rice Beans + wheat Beans + corn Soybeans + rice + wheat Soybeans + corn + milk Soybeans + wheat + sesame Soybeans + peanuts + sesame Soybeans + peanuts + wheat + rice Soybeans + sesame + wheat
Nuts and seeds	Isoleucine Lysine	Peanuts + sesame + soybeans Sesame + beans Sesame + soybeans + wheat Peanuts + sunflower seeds
Vegetables	Isoleucine Methionine	Lima beans Green beans Brussels sprouts } + Sesame seeds or Cauliflower Brazil nuts or Broccoli mushrooms Greens = millet or rice

*Modified from Lappé, F. M.: Diet for a small planet, New York, 1971, Friends of the Earth/Ballantine.

TOOL E
Daily food plan for pregnancy*

Foods	Daily amount	Suggested uses
Protein-rich foods		
Primary protein		
Dairy products	1 qt milk	Beverage, in cooking, or milk
Milk, cheese	2+ oz brick cheese or ½ cup+ cottage cheese	based desserts such as ice milk, custards, puddings, cream soups; cheese in cooked dishes, salads, or snacks throughout the day
Eggs	2	Breakfast use, chopped or sliced hard egg, in salads, custards, whole boiled eggs, deviled eggs, plain or in sandwiches
Meat	2 servings (total of 6 to 8 oz) liver frequently, 1-2 times per week	Main dish, sandwich, salad, snack
Supplementary protein		
Grains	4 to 5 slices or servings	Bread, plain or toast, sand-
Enriched or whole grains, breads, cereals, crackers	whole grain or enriched	wiches, with meals, snacks, cereal (breakfast or snack), cooked grain as meal ac- companiment (corn, rice, pasta, grits, hominy, hot breads: corn bread, biscuits, etc.)
Legumes, seeds, nuts	Occasional servings as meat or grain substitute	Cooked and served alone or in combination with grains,
Dried beans and peas	or in combination with meat or grains	cheese, or meat; soups, salads; nuts as snacks or in
Lentils		salads; peanut butter sand- wich
Mineral-rich foods		
Calcium-rich		
Dairy products	1 qt milk (as above)	As above
Grains, whole or enriched	4-5 slices or servings (as above)	As above
Green leafy vegetables	1 serving	Cooked or raw in salads
Iron-rich		
Organ meats, espe- cially liver	1-2 servings per week	
Grains, enriched	4-5 slices or servings	Breakfast cereals, main dish, or combination with meats, cheese, egg, cooked grain foods, enriched breads
Egg yolk	2	As above
Green, leafy vegeta- bles or dried fruits	1-2 servings	Cooked or stewed, raw in salads, snacks

*From Williams, S.: Handbook of maternal and infant nutrition, Berkeley, Calif., 1976, SRW Productions, Inc.

TOOL E
Daily food plan for pregnancy—cont'd

Foods	Daily amount	Suggested uses
Mineral-rich foods—cont'd		
Iodine-rich		
Iodized salt	Daily in cooking and on foods	On salads, in cooked food dishes, according to taste
Seafood	1-2 servings per week	Main dish, salad, sandwiches
Vitamin-rich foods		
Vitamin A		
Animal sources		
Butter fat (whole milk, cream, butter)	2 tbsp butter (or fortified margarine)	In cooking or on foods
Liver	1-2 servings per week	Main dish
Egg yolk	2 (as above)	As above
Plant sources		
Dark green or deep yellow vegetables or fruits	1-2 servings	Cooked dishes, salads, snacks
Fortified margarine	2 tbsp	In cooking and on foods
Vitamin C		
Fruits		
Citrus	1 or 2 servings	Snacks, salads, juices
Other fruits— papayas, strawberries, melons	Occasional serving to substitute for one citrus portion	Salads, snacks
Vegetables		
Broccoli, potatoes, tomato, cabbage, green or chili peppers	1 serving as a substitute for 1 citrus occasionally	Cooked, snacks, salads, juices
Folic acid		
Liver, dark green vegetables, dried beans, lentils, nuts (peanuts, walnuts, filberts)	1 serving	Cooked as main dish or soups, snacks, in salads

be used initially. Additional foods may be added or changed according to individual needs, cultural patterns, or personal lifestyles. Tool F provides a follow-up checklist of basic foods to be included in a daily food plan, and it may be used for reinforcement on a continuing basis.

However, in each case the food plan must be *realistic* to be useful. In a large number of cases, broad food habits exist with few if any limitations present. For these women basic guidance and encouragement will suffice to meet needs. However, for some women with real problems for whom risks exist for a successful pregnancy, extremely careful and supportive counseling is necessary and may well determine the outcome of their pregnancies.

TOOL F
Checklist of foods needed during pregnancy*

Foods	Daily amount
Milk	1 qt
Eggs	1-2
Meat	2 servings (liver often)
Cheese	1-2 servings, additional snacks
Grains (whole, enriched)	4-5 slices or servings
Legumes, nuts	1-2 servings a week
Green and yellow fruits, vegetables	1-2 servings
Citrus fruit	2
Additional vitamin C foods	Frequently, as desired
Other vegetables and fruits	1-2 servings
Butter, fortified margarine	2 tbsp (or as needed)
Other foods: grains, fruits, vegetables, other proteins	As needed for energy and added vitamins and minerals

*From Williams, S.: Handbook of maternal and infant nutrition, Berkeley, Calif., 1976, SRW Productions, Inc.

Some form of follow-up support and evaluation should be built into the continuing plan of care. Ongoing nutrition awareness and concern should be made an integral part of every clinic visit, and the nutritionist should show positive interest for continuance of the food plan, continue to look for any problems that may need adjustment, and use occasional food records for continuing evaluation of nutritional needs. It is often of great encouragement to the mother to see visible means whereby her food habit changes are indeed making actual increases in her nutrient intake and hence meeting her nutritional requirements.

Common functional gastrointestinal problems

General nutritional guidance may also be needed during pregnancy for common functional gastrointestinal difficulties encountered. These complaints are highly individual in form and extent. They will therefore require individual counseling and assurances for control. Usually these difficulties are relatively minor. However, if they persist or become extreme, they will need medical attention. In most cases general investigation of food practices will reveal some areas where diet counseling may help to relieve them. Some of the more common difficulties include nausea, constipation, hemorrhoids, or heartburn.

Nausea and vomiting. Difficulty with nausea and vomiting is usually mild and limited to early pregnancy. It is commonly called "morning sickness" because it occurs more often on arising than later in the day. A number of factors may contribute to the condition. Some are physiological based on hormonal changes that occur early in pregnancy. Other factors may be psychological, various situational tensions or anxieties concerning the pregnancy itself. Additional contributory causes may be poor diet habits.

Simple treatment generally improves food toleration. Small frequent meals, fairly dry and consisting chiefly of easily digested energy foods such as carbohydrates, are more readily tolerated. Liquids are best taken between meals instead of with the food. If the condition persists and develops into *hyperemesis* (severe, prolonged, persistent vomiting), the physician will probably hospitalize the patient and feed her intravenously to prevent complications and dehydration. However, such an increase in the symptoms is usually rare. Most conditions pass early in the pregnancy and respond to the simple dietary remedies given here.

Constipation. The condition of constipation is seldom more than minor. Hormonal changes in pregnancy tend to increase relaxation of the gastrointestinal muscles. Also, the pressure of the enlarging uterus on the lower portion of the intestine, especially during the latter part of pregnancy, may make elimination somewhat difficult. Increased fluid intake, use of naturally laxative foods such as whole grains with added bran, dried fruits (especially prunes and figs), and other fruits and juices generally induce regularity. Laxatives should be avoided. They should only be used in special situations under medical supervision.

Hemorrhoids. A fairly common complaint during the latter part of pregnancy is that of hemorrhoids. These are enlarged veins in the anus, often protruding through the anal sphincter. This vein enlargement is usually due to the increased weight of the fetus and the downward pressure it causes. The hemorrhoids may cause considerable discomfort, burning and itching. Occasionally they may rupture and bleed under pressure of a bowel movement during constipation, therefore causing more anxiety for the patient. The difficulty is usually remedied by dietary suggestions given earlier to control constipation. Also, observing general hygiene recommendations concerning sufficient rest during the latter part of the day may help to relieve the pressure of the uterus on the lower intestine.

Heartburn or full feeling. The related complaints of "heartburn" or a "full feeling" are sometimes voiced by pregnant women. These discomforts may occur especially after meals, usually caused by the pressure of the enlarging uterus crowding the adjacent digestive organ, the stomach, thereby causing some difficulty after eating. Food mixtures may be pushed back into the lower part of the esophagus, causing a "burning" sensation due to the acid mixed with the food mass. This burning sensation is commonly called heartburn because of the proximity of the lower esophagus to the heart. Obviously, however, it has nothing to do with the heart and its action. A full feeling usually refers to general gastric pressure, due to lack of normal space in the area, and is accentuated by a large meal or gas formation. These complaints are generally remedied by dividing the day's food intake into a number of small meals during the day, rather than large meals at one time. Attention may also be given to relaxation, adequate chewing, eating slowly, and avoiding tensions during meals.

PLACES AND PROVIDERS OF PRENATAL CARE

Nutrition services in prenatal care are assuming an increasing variety in the nature of the places and persons providing care. In the changing society and overall changing health care delivery system in the United States, there is an increasing awareness of the relation of social issues and problems to health and disease, and an increasing sense of responsibility for reaching high-risk population groups and for involving the people more in decisions concerning their own care. More programs of care are developing around these principles of positive health maintenance, in which sound nutrition is fundamental, and use of more health-oriented, nonphysician practitioners along with physicians for providing care. As a result of these trends, prenatal care is taking place in a variety of settings with a variety of professional participants.

Settings of prenatal care

Over the past years, modern American obstetrical-medical practice has moved from the home into the hospital, removing the woman from family and familiar surroundings and assigning her a patient role in a clinically oriented setting. As more and more women, husbands, and families are voicing a sense of loss in this transition of personal and human needs involved in the profound human experience of childbirth, more alternatives of care are being provided according to individual needs and situations. These alternatives involve both private and community facilities.

Private settings. Although the line of distinction between the private and public sectors of medical and health care are becoming increasingly blurred, private facilities may be distinguished in general use from public programs of care. Individuals may seek out and employ the services of a private medical specialist, an obstetrician-gynecologist, receive care in his or her private office and be delivered at a private hospital used by the specialist. This has been the medical model. However, with rising costs of such care, this model is becoming diffused to involve group practice and third party payment systems of health insurance.

Community settings. With increasing social awareness and government legislated funding, a number of community-based programs of care have developed. Various Health Maintenance Organizations (HMO) provide care through community health centers and clinics, seeking to reach underserved and economically depressed areas. Special projects such as Women and Infant Care (WIC), Maternal-Infant-Child (MIC), and others provide additional outreach services. The new comprehensive health care legislation, Public Law 93-641: Health Planning and Resources Development Act of 1974, signed into law in 1975 and presently being developed and administered, will seek to coordinate health care services in a better manner.

Other community settings of care may stem from various community action groups. Innovative health projects and food advocacy programs have resulted, often reaching out to meet needs outside the mainstream of medical care. Resources developed by some of these groups for use by their community workers are available.[1,9]

Providers of care: role of the health team

Concept of the health team. As scientific knowledge has expanded with its attendant proliferating technology, and increasing population-socioeconomic pressures have brought rapid social change, the concept of a team of health care workers has grown to meet needs. In this framework various skilled persons with expertise in related areas of health care can work as an efficient group to identify health problems and plan comprehensive care to meet these problems. Such health care teams may include not only health professionals but also assistants and community workers. This broader application of the team concept helps to bridge the provider-consumer gap that exists in many areas and to bring the clients in need of special services more into the planning process concerning their care, thus restoring some of the humanistic aspects of care sought by many providers and consumers alike.

Primary care providers. Recognizing this need for a more coordinated, comprehensive, and personalized program of health care, groups of primary care providers have begun to develop. The term *primary care* has come into general usage in relation to levels of care: primary care—immediate, face-to-face, coordinated care for individuals and families; secondary care—resource specialists used by the primary care providers according to problem or need; tertiary care—long-term problems of care for chronic illness or trauma requiring specialized treatment, as in rehabilitation facilities.

These providers of primary care involve a number of health professionals with broad education and training, particularly problem oriented, and experienced in family and community health care. This primary care team includes physicians with backgrounds in family and community medicine, nurses with expanded training as nurse-practitioners, and nutritionists with community, family, and clinical skills.

In the area of prenatal care, as well as infant and early childhood care, other members of the primary care team may include specialized professionals such as OB-GYN nurse-clinicians or pediatric nurse-practitioners, as well as specially trained and certified practicing midwives. Such assistants bring particular skills and personal strengths to a family-centered maternity care program.

COMMUNITY RESOURCES

In any community setting of prenatal care, a number of possible community resources for nutritional needs may exist. These should be explored, constantly updated, and used for consultation, referral, or sources of materials or services. Some of these resources may include those from government, professional, private centers, industry, volunteer groups, education, and other groups.

Government agencies

Public health departments and services. Local, state, and federal health agencies conduct many services and educational activities. Skilled public health nutritionists provide consultation and direct services to help assess nutritional needs in community situations, to plan nutrition components for health care programs and individual care, to assist in solving family-related problems, and to educate co-professionals and clients in nutritional care.

Welfare departments. Local and state welfare departments also supply resources in assisting families in need of care. Through their social workers they can provide help in planning for food assistance such as food stamps or in securing financial aid as needed for medical care.

Agricultural Extension Service. Through state land-grant universities, the Agricultural Extension Service provides assistance to the community through nutrition specialists, home advisors, and consumer specialists. These persons are particularly able to give resources in wise food buying, especially for those with low incomes.

Professional groups

Local professional organizations—medical, nursing, dietetics—provide general health education resources in a number of ways. Nutrition resources may be found through two main groups: (1) the American Dietetic Association, local district as well as state and national organizations; and (2) the Society for Nutrition Education. The latter group, through its national office in Berkeley, California, provides a large collection of nutrition education materials in its National Nutrition Education Clearing House (NNECH), as well as evaluated and annotated lists of available resources in a variety of media.[11]

Community hospitals and medical centers

Dietitians employed by local community hospitals work in inpatient and outpatient services. They may be consulted as needed concerning special prenatal care problems or to procure nutrition education materials. Most community centers providing prenatal care services also employ a nutritionist to counsel staff and clinic patients concerning nutritional care.

Food industry groups

A number of food industry–related organizations, such as the Dairy Council, the National Livestock and Meat Board, and the Cereal Institute, sponsor research and community workshops, produce nutrition education materials, and sometimes underwrite special community nutrition projects. For example, local Dairy Council nutritionists may be available for consultation concerning nutrition education materials for maternity care.

County and state interagency nutrition councils

Nutrition councils have been organized in many areas to help coordinate nutrition services and education. They plan community health activities, including maternity nutrition conferences and prenatal care resource materials.

Volunteer health agencies

Community resources may also be available for special needs of pregnant women with diabetes or heart disease through the local, state, or national diabetes or heart associations. They provide special resource materials and conduct group teaching for patients and conferences for professionals.

REFERENCES
Specific

1. Children's Defense Fund: Doctors and dollars are not enough, 1520 New Hampshire Ave., N.W., Washington, D.C. 20036.
2. Church, C. F., and Church, H. N.: Food values of portions commonly used, Philadelphia, 1976, J. B. Lippincott Co.
3. Clamp, B. A.: Cooking with low-cost proteins, New York, 1976, Arco Publishing Co., Inc.
4. Consumer and Food Economics Research Division, Agricultural Research Service: Nutritive value of foods, Home and Garden Bull. No. 72, Washington, D.C., 1970, United States Department of Agriculture.
5. Food and Nutrition Board, National Research Council, National Academy of Sciences, Recommended dietary allowances, ed. 8, Washington, D.C., 1974, Government Printing Office.
6. Gagne, R. M.: The conditions of learning, ed. 2, New York, 1970, Holt, Rinehart & Winston, Inc.
7. Lappé, F. M.: Diet for a small planet, New York, 1971, Friends of the Earth/Ballantine Books, Inc.
8. Mager, R. F.: Developing attitude toward learning, Palo Alto, Calif., 1968, Fearon Publishers, Inc.
9. National Child Nutrition Project: Federal food program workbook, 303 George St., New Brunswick, N.J. 08901.
10. Nutrition during pregnancy and lactation, Sacramento, 1975, California Department of Health.
11. Society for Nutrition Education: Resource list for maternal and infant nutrition, 2140 Shattuck Ave., Suite 1110, Berkeley, Calif. 94704.
12. Watt, B. K., and Merrill, A. L.: Composition of foods: raw, processed, prepared, Agriculture Handbook No. 8, Washington, D.C., 1976, United States Department of Agriculture.
13. Williams, S. R.: Essentials of nutrition and diet therapy, St. Louis, 1974, The C. V. Mosby Co.
14. Williams, S. R.: Nutrition and diet therapy, ed. 3, St. Louis, 1977, The C. V. Mosby Co.

General

Aubry, R. H., et al.: Assessment of maternal nutrition, Clin. Perinatol. **2:**207, 1975.
Christakis, G., ed.: Nutritional assessment in health programs, Am. J. Public Health **63**(supp.):1, Nov., 1973.
Committee on Maternal Nutrition, Food and Nutrition Board, National Research Council, National Academy of Sciences: Maternal nutrition and the course of pregnancy, Washington, D.C., 1970, Government Printing Office.
Committee on Maternal Nutrition, Food and Nutrition Board, National Research Council, National Academy of Sciences: Nutritional supplementation and the outcome of pregnancy, Washington, D.C., 1973, Government Printing Office.
Grieve, J. F.: Prevention of gestational failure by high protein diet, J. Reprod. Med. **13:**170, 1974.
Grieve, J. F.: A comment on the relation between protein and weight gain in pregnancy, J. Reprod. Med. **14:**55, 1975.
Guyton, A. C.: Textbook of medical physiology, ed. 5, Philadelphia, 1976, W. B. Saunders Co.
Hytten, F. E., and Leitch, I.: The physiology of human pregnancy, ed. 2, Oxford, 1971, Blackwell Scientific Publications, Ltd.
Jacobson, H. N.: Weight and weight gain in pregnancy, Clin. Perinatol. **2:**233, 1975.
King, J. C.: Protein metabolism, Clin. Perinatol. **2:**243, 1975.
Lowe, C. U.: Research in infant nutrition: the untapped well, Am. J. Clin. Nutr. **25:**245, 1972.
Pike, R.: Further evidence of deleterious effects produced by sodium restriction during pregnancy, Am. J. Clin. Nutr. **23:**883, 1970.
Pitkin, R. M., chairman: Nutrition in maternal health care, Chicago, 1974, Committee on Nutrition, American College of Obstetricians and Gynecologists.
Pitkin, R. M.: Calcium metabolism in pregnancy: a review, Am. J. Obstet. Gynecol. **121:**724, 1975.
Pitkin, R. M.: Vitamins and minerals in pregnancy, Clin. Perinatol. **2:**221, 1975.
Pitkin, R. M., Kaminetzky, H. A., Newton, M., and Pritchard, J. A.: Maternal nutrition: a selective review of clinical topics, Obstet. Gynecol. **40:**773, 1972.
Primrose, T., and Higgins, A.: A study in human antepartum nutrition, J. Reprod. Med. **7:**257, 1972.
Shank, R. E.: A chink in our armor, Nutr. Today **5:**2, Summer, 1970.
United States Department of Health, Education, and Welfare: Health Planning and Resources Development Act of 1974, DHEW Pub. No. (HRA) 76-14015, Washington, D.C., 1975, Government Printing Office.

5
Nutritional therapy in special conditions of pregnancy

Sue Rodwell Williams

NUTRITIONAL COMPLICATIONS OF PREGNANCY

The condition of pregnancy may induce complications of two general types, the anemias and the toxemias of pregnancy, both of which have nutritional relationships. Anemia is by far the most common complication encountered in pregnancy. The incidence of toxemia varies, apparently, with socioeconomic situation and prenatal care. Both conditions require nutritional care, with prevention being the basic objective.

Anemias of pregnancy

A general "physiological anemia" is commonly related to the normal adaptations in maternal physiology that support and sustain the pregnancy. This tendency may be compounded, however, by deficiencies in key nutrients having specific roles in red blood cell (RBC) division or hemoglobin synthesis for RBC maturation. In addition to the basic protein requirement, the two main nutrients needed are iron and folic acid, both of which are required in increased amounts during pregnancy.

Definition of anemia

The term *anemia* stems from a Greek root meaning "want of blood." It is generally defined as a significant reduction in hemoglobin and red blood cells, as measured by (1) concentration of hemoglobin per 100 ml of blood, (2) volume of packed red blood cells per 100 ml of blood (hematocrit), or (3) number of mature red blood cells (erythrocytes) per cubic millimeter of blood. Repeated measures of these indices of hematological values indicate that the hemoglobin concentration as a base value for healthy young women averages 13.7 gm/100 ml with a range of 12 to 15.4 gm/100 ml.[44]

The life-sustaining feature of the hemoglobin molecule is its ability to form a loose and reversible combination with oxygen, thus providing the necessary oxygen for cell metabolism. Oxygen binds with the iron of the heme part of the hemoglobin molecule; thus iron is an exceedingly important element of the hemoglobin structure. In the lungs oxygen binds easily with the iron but separates from the iron just as easily in the tissue capillaries to supply the

93

tissue cells with needed oxygen. Because of this vital function of hemoglobin, the signs and symptoms common to anemia include pallor, fatigue, anorexia, weakness, lassitude, dyspnea, and edema.

In addition to iron, a number of other nutrients are involved in hemoglobin synthesis. Protein must supply the necessary amino acids. It can be calculated from the known composition of hemoglobin, for example, that the globin (the protein moiety of hemoglobin) portion contains a total of 574 amino acids. Other minerals needed include copper, cobalt, and nickel. Special vitamins necessary for hemoglobin synthesis are vitamin B_{12} and folic acid. The lack of these essential coenzyme factors causes the delayed and disordered maturation of red blood cells that characterizes megaloblastic anemias. An additional B vitamin, pyridoxine, is also involved in hemoglobin synthesis.

Normal hematological alterations in pregnancy

In pregnancy, normal physiological changes occur in the blood for the purpose of supporting the synergistic metabolism of the maternal organism, the fetus, and the placenta necessary to sustain the pregnancy. First, the blood volume increases by about 50% to meet increased circulatory needs, especially to the highly vascular placenta and to other increased tissue, maternal and fetal. This plasma volume increase starts at about three months' gestation, reaches its maximum level in the third trimester especially the ninth month, decreases slightly at term, and returns to normal by about three weeks' post partum. This expanded volume amounts to about 1000 ml for a single fetus pregnancy, more for multiple pregnancy. The probable stimulus for the increased blood volume may be placental lactogen, which in turn causes increased aldosterone secretion.[36,41]

Second, the total red blood cell volume and hemoglobin mass increases by 25% during pregnancy, beginning at six months, peaking at term, and returning to normal about six weeks' postpartum. This increase in total red blood cell mass amounts to about 300 to 350 ml. The probable stimulus for this increase may be the interrelationship between maternal hormones and the increased levels of erythropoietin found during pregnancy.[36]

By comparison of these two changes therefore, it becomes evident that the increase in red blood cell mass is not sufficient to compensate for the marked increase in plasma volume. Thus, by dilution, a "physiological anemia" ensues with development of decreased values for hemoglobin and hematocrit. These values begin to decrease at three to five months' gestation, reach their powest point at five to eight months' gestation, rise slightly at term, and return to normal at six weeks post partum.[20]

Types of anemias in pregnancy

Anemia occurs frequently in pregnancy.[59] Compounded by socioeconomic status, as many as 56% of pregnant women are anemic.[14] The majority of these cases are nutritional in origin, with iron-deficiency anemia being by far the most common. A second related cause is acute blood loss from hemorrhage. A third less common nutritional anemia is that caused by a deficiency of folic acid—specific megaloblastic anemia. The following summarizes the acquired and hereditary causes, in general order of incidence, of the anemias of pregnancy in the United States.* Because of their greater nutritional significance, the two anemias related to deficiency of iron and of folic acid are discussed here.

Acquired
  Iron-deficiency anemia
  Anemia due to acute blood loss
  Megaloblastic anemia due to folate deficiency

---

*From Committee on Maternal Nutrition, Food and Nutrition Board, National Research Council, National Academy of Sciences: Maternal nutrition and the course of pregnancy, Washington, D.C., 1970, Government Printing Office, p. 81.

Anemia caused by infection
Acquired hemolytic anemia
Aplastic or hypoplastic anemia

Hereditary
Thalassemia
Sickle cell anemia
Sickle cell–hemoglobin C disease
Other hemoglobinopathies
Hereditary hemolytic anemia without hemo-
    globinopathy

Iron-deficiency anemia. A characteristic microcytic hypochromic anemia is produced by a deficiency of iron, the major mineral element required for the synthesis of hemoglobin. Because of the widespread incidence of iron deficiency among females during the reproductive years of menstruation, women become highly vulnerable to iron-deficiency anemia when pregnancy places a greater physiological demand on their already tenuous iron balance. As indicated in Table 5-1, the "iron cost" of a pregnancy is high, and negative balances can easily occur. To counteract this tendency toward an iron-deficiency anemia in pregnancy, the National Research Council report on maternal nutrition and the course of pregnancy has recommended a daily supplement of 30 to 60 mg of iron.[18] Commonly used iron compounds are ferrous sulfate or ferrous fumarate, both of which contain about 33% elemental iron. Since the third compound available, ferrous gluconate, contains only about 11% elemental iron, a larger dosage is required.

Iron-deficiency anemia accounts for about 77% or more of the nonphysiological anemias in pregnancy. The increased demand for iron during pregnancy is caused by the increased need for hemoglobin synthesis as described and by the large fetal need for liver storage to meet iron needs of the infant during the first 3 to 6 months of life, since milk—the first food—contains little or no iron. Furthermore, up to two years of normal diet are required to replace

Table 5-1. Maternal and fetal iron balance*

Input		Output	
Stores		Increased requirement	
Normal adult female iron stores (total)	2 gm	Maternal red blood cell mass	450 mg
Red blood cells (60%-70%)	1.2-1.4 gm	Fetus (single), placenta, cord	360 mg
Liver, spleen, and bone marrow (10%-30%)	0.3 gm	Total	810 mg
Other cell compounds (remainder)		Lactation (daily)	0.5-1.0 mg
Diet		Losses	
Average absorption (280 days)	1.3-2.6 mg/day‡	Gastrointestinal, renal, sweat (280 days)	0.5-1.0 mg/day
Supplementation		Birth† (including placenta and lochia)	200-250 mg
Daily iron supplement 12%-25% absorption: ferrous sulfate, ferrous fumarate, 33% iron; ferrous gluconate, 11% iron	30-60 mg		

*Data from references 20, 31, 41, 56, 59.
†Cesarean section or birth of twins results in an additional loss of approximately 140 mg of iron.
‡Some investigators estimate that a pregnant woman requires more than 4 mg/day of iron, an amount which exceeds that absorbed from a normal diet, even if the woman is iron deficient.[20]

the iron lost during a pregnancy. Hence, if there is a shorter time interval between pregnancies, an even greater drain is placed on the mother's depleted iron stores.[31]

The diagnosis of iron-deficiency anemia is made on the basis of a hemoglobin concentration value of 10 gm/100 ml of blood or less, a hematocrit value of 30% or less, and the appearance of characteristic red blood cells on a stained erythrocyte smear. The cells are smaller than usual with a fading red color. In the development of iron-deficiency anemia, the first changes that occur are the depletion of iron stores in the liver, spleen, and bone marrow, followed by a decrease in serum iron and an increase in serum total iron-binding capacity (TIBC). Finally, the anemic state develops as hematocrit levels drop below normal, and the change in red blood cell development follows. Usually the microcytosis (production of smaller cells) precedes the hypochromia (the fading red color). A serum iron level below 50 to 60 μg/100 ml and less than 15% to 16% saturation of transferrin is usually indicative of iron-deficiency anemia, given the ruling out of other causes of decreased serum iron.[56]

Treatment of iron-deficiency anemia centers on the correction of the low hemoglobin concentration with medicinal iron, usually up to 200 mg/day of iron, depending on the severity of the anemia. Moreover, it can be prevented by appropriate iron supplementation and emphasis on food sources of iron in the daily diet. Such supplementation is particularly important to those women who are susceptible to deficiency states, that is, those with poor dietary intake, frequent pregnancies, or a history of prior iron depletion. A diet such as that outlined in Chapter 4 will help to prevent such a nutritional anemia.

Folic acid–deficiency anemia. A characteristic megaloblastic anemia is produced during pregnancy by a deficiency of folic acid, which can exist as a single deficiency state but is more commonly found in association with iron deficiency.[12] Folates have widespread physiological function, participating as they do in methionine, purine, and thymine biosynthesis. Hence, not only do they assist in hemoglobin synthesis but they also are necessary for deoxyribonucleic acid (DNA) synthesis; thus a deficiency has far-reaching consequences.

The nonpregnant adult woman is believed to require about 50 to 100 μg/day of folic acid. Thus the National Research Council recommends 400 μg/day to ensure the absorption of that quantity. In pregnancy the requirement for folic acid rises to 150 to 300 μg/day; hence the National Research Council's recommendation is 800 μg/day. This increased demand for folic acid in pregnancy is due to a somewhat decreased absorption during pregnancy and to increased maternal and fetal tissue synthesis needs.[43] In folic acid–deficiency ane-

Table 5-2. Guidelines for laboratory evaluation of anemia in pregnancy[*]

	Hemoglobin (gm/100 ml)	Hematocrit (packed cell vol %)	Serum iron (μg/ 100 ml)	Transferrin saturation (%)	Serum folacin (ng/ml)[†]	Serum B_{12} (pg/ml)[‡]
Pregnancy						
Deficient	<9.5	<30	<40	<15	<2.0	<100
Marginal	9.5-10.9	30-32	40	15	2.1-5.9	100
Acceptable	>11.0	>33	>40	>15	>6.0	>100
Nonpregnant woman						
Normal values	>12.0	36-50	>50	>15	6.0-25.0	>100

[*]Modified from U.S. Department of HEW: Ten State Nutrition Survey, 1968-1970, DHEW Pub (HSM) 72-8130 Atlanta, 1972, Center for Disease Control.
[†]Nanograms per milliliter.   [‡]Picograms per milliliter.

mia the characteristic red blood cell is larger than usual and immature; this hematologic condition is called megaloblastosis.

Since the requirement for folic acid is markedly increased during pregnancy, and because an inadequate dietary intake is frequent especially in lower socioeconomic groups, the National Research Council recommends a supplementation during pregnancy of 200 to 400 μg/day of folic acid. Food sources of folic acid should be assured in the diet. These include leafy vegetables, liver, and to some extent nuts, cheese, eggs, and milk. A food plan such as that described in Chapter 4 will help to prevent this nutritional anemia. Such a diet emphasis along with the folic acid supplementation indicated will help to prevent the 50% to 60% incidence of serum folate depletion found among pregnant women in the United States.[15]

Table 5-2 presents a summary of guidelines for laboratory evaluation of anemia in pregnancy.

Toxemias of pregnancy

The toxemias of pregnancy collectively represent varying degrees of a hypertensive syndrome seen in late pregnancy. This disease complex is still called by many "the disease of theories," and much has been written of the conflicting views concerning its origin and its treatment. However, as more knowledge has been gained concerning the physiology of pregnancy, of nutritional science, and of the relation of optimum nutrition to the outcome of pregnancy and to the prevention of complications, it seems to be increasingly evident that nutritional factors play a primary role. The basic physiological concept of pregnancy is that of *growth,* the initiation and sustaining of new life through two fundamental factors: (1) physiologic synergistic adaptation to facilitate the growth process, and (2) optimum increased nutrition to ensure adequate building materials necessary for growth. By applying this basic concept, perhaps a greater understanding can be achieved of this disease complex that complicates pregnancy. Problems in clarifying the nature, etiology, and treatment of toxemia have come in large measure from lack of widely accepted definitions of the disease process and of variance in accepted symptomatic criteria. Here, then, we will look at a definition of the disease and its symptoms, its related epidemiology and pathology, and hence its associated nutritional factors in prevention and treatment.

Definition of toxemia of pregnancy

The term *toxemia* is a misnomer here, in that its actual meaning, "blood toxins," does not apply. It is a general term given historically to degrees of the disorder of late pregnancy called *eclampsia,* which comes from a Greek word "eclampsis," meaning "a sudden flash," or "a sudden development." Thus more accurately the terms *preeclampsia* and *eclampsia* are used referring to the nature and degree of the symptoms involved. A definition of this disorder unique to pregnancy perhaps may be best understood by a review of its cardinal clinical symptoms: hypertension, proteinuria, and edema, usually occurring after the twentieth week of gestation.

Hypertension. Usually hypertension in pregnancy is defined as a systolic blood pressure of 140 mm Hg, or a diastolic pressure of 90 mm Hg, or both. These blood pressure levels must be observed on two or more occasions at least 6 hours or more apart. However, more definitive criteria are needed on an individual basis to identify abnormal disease states better, as indicated by the National Research Council's Committee on Maternal Nutrition and working group on nutrition and the toxemias of pregnancy.[18] National health survey data indicate that among females 18 to 34 years of age, fewer than 3% have a systolic pressure of 140 mm Hg or greater, and fewer than 4% have a diastolic pressure of 90 mm Hg or greater. Instead, 75% of these younger women have a blood pressure of less than 120/80 mm Hg.[55] The usual minimum diagnostic values of 140/90 mm Hg may thus miss hypertensive conditions in young women displaying lower values. Young teenagers, for example, have blood pressures of about 90/60 mm Hg, and it is in this group of young primiparas that the risk factor is greater. A more significant level for determining hypertension therefore would be based on usual individual blood pressure: a rise of 20 to 30 mm Hg in systolic pressure and/or of 10 to 15 mm Hg in diastolic pressure observed on two or more occasions at least 6 hours apart. Further confusion in the clinical identity of pregnancy toxemias lies in the common problem of lack of distinction between chronic hypertensive vascular disease complicated by the pregnancy and a true pregnancy toxemia state. In any event the use of blood pressure values of 140/90 mm Hg as the upper limit of normal appears to have little real meaning in pregnancy. Recent data from a collaborative study of the clinical criteria from toxemia have shown that blood pressures above 125/75 mm Hg prior to thirty-two weeks' gestation were associated with significant increases in fetal risk, as were pressures above 125/85 mm Hg at term.[27]

Proteinuria. Although the degree of proteinuria is variable in preeclampsia and eclampsia, it rarely exceeds 5 gm/day. Often it is fluctuating or transient and may be minimal even in more severe cases. These observations of proteinuria must be made on clean voided specimens, two or more taken at least 6 hours apart.

Edema. The normal physiological edema of pregnancy, manifested mainly in the extremities, is not to be confused with the pathological generalized edema associated with toxemia states, elevated blood pressure, and increased sensitivity to angiotensin.[28] Thus the accumulation of fluid in the legs alone is not significant in the diagnosis of preeclampsia. The majority of pregnant women develop edema in the last trimester.

In eclampsia characteristic convulsions may be a fourth symptom, viewed generally as an end result of preeclampsia and distinguishing the two states.

In preeclampsia additional common complaints of the patient include dizziness, headache, visual disturbances, upper abdominal pain, facial edema, anorexia, nausea, and vomiting. Further probing usually discloses a history of acute starvation or fasting due to the gastrointestinal problems, superimposed on an underlying chronic state of malnutrition, often related to socioeconomic, personal, or psychological problems.

Epidemiology of toxemia of pregnancy

A study of the incidence of toxemia, especially of its mortality rate, in the United States in recent years reveals a close association of high incidence rates with *low income and poverty*. General reports from hospitals in various parts of the country have indicated a higher incidence among clinic populations when compared with private populations and among women in the southern states compared with elsewhere. Moreover, more reliable data on the mortality rates from the acute toxemias of pregnancy show striking relationships to economic factors, as can be seen in Table 5-3.[18] Counting the District of Columbia as a state and dividing the states into three groups of seventeen states each, according to income per capita, we find the greatest mortality rate from toxemia in the lowest income group. This correlation supports the long-held view that standards of living, hence quality of prenatal care and nutritional status, are related to the incidence of toxemia.

The relation of toxemia to *race* has been suggested in the past, but the figures in Table 5-3 dispute this factor. Although there is a greater black population in the South (hence a greater proportion of nonwhite births than in any other region) and the toxemia mortality rate is greatest in southern states, this relation to nonwhite births does not hold in the District of Columbia.

The District has the highest percentage of nonwhite births among the states, but it also has the highest per capita income. Its

Table 5-3. Mortality rates from toxemia of pregnancy by states ranked according to per capita income*

States in rank order (1963-1965)	Rate per 100,000 live births
Group I: High income states (first 17 states)	3.8
Washington, D.C.	5.1
Nevada, Connecticut, Delaware, California, New York, New Jersey, Illinois, Alaska, Massachusetts, Maryland, Michigan, Hawaii, Washington, Rhode Island, Ohio, Indiana	
Group II: Middle income states (second 17 states)	5.9
Oregon, Pennsylvania, Colorado, Wisconsin, Kansas, Missouri, Minnesota, Wyoming, Iowa, New Hampshire, Nebraska, Montana, Arizona, Florida, Utah, Virginia, Texas	
Group III: Low income states (third 17 states)	11.9
Idaho, Vermont, Oklahoma, Maine, New Mexico, North Dakota, Georgia, South Dakota, Louisiana, Kentucky, North Carolina, West Virginia, Tennessee, Alabama, Arkansas	
South Carolina (nonwhite: 42.8)	21.0
Mississippi (nonwhite: 52.4)	30.2
United States—national rate	6.2

*Modified from Committee on Maternal Nutrition, National Research Council, National Academy of Sciences: Maternal nutrition and the course of pregnancy, Washington, D.C., 1970, Government Printing Office.

toxemia mortality rate is less than the national average, less than one sixth the rate for Mississippi (the lowest income state and the highest nonwhite percentage of births), and less than half the average for the low-income group of states. Thus it seems that the relation is not to race per se or any such intrinsic biological characteristic. Instead the cause appears to be deeply rooted in social issues and problems, including medical care and nutrition, associated with home and community and political environment. Additional support for this view is the fact that the other states with high toxemia mortality rates are those in which the nonwhite population is largely American Indian (Idaho, Nevada, Arizona, North Dakota, New Mexico, and South Dakota), as shown in Table 5-4. Thus the poverty cycle takes its toll.

A number of factors closely associated with poverty and having a bearing on the course and outcome of pregnancy are the availability and quality of prenatal care, general prevalence of poor health with chronic conditions such as cardiovascular-renal disease, general prevalence of poor nutrition from a lifetime of poor eating and health habits, ignorance of health factors, emotional stress, and general prevalence of younger age at first pregnancy with high parity—multiple pregnancies with shorter time intervals intervening.

Pathology of toxemia of pregnancy

Characteristic lesions have been found in postmortem tissue examination showing alterations in eclampsia in several organ systems. The main organ system involved appears to be the liver. The major finding is a hemorrhagic necrosis, patchy in places but predominantly in the right lobe and in the peripheral part of the hepatic lobule. The lesions appear grossly as irregularly shaped reddish areas, giving the liver a mottled look. Microscopical examination shows that the areas of hemorrhagic necrosis are usually associated with extensive thrombosis in the smallest blood vessels in the periportal connective tissue, followed by fibrin deposits. Although the main hepatic necrosis of eclampsia is periportal, the lesion may sometimes extend into the center of the hepatic lobule, as Acosta-Sison[1]

Table 5-4. States with highest mortality rates from the toxemias of pregnancy among nonwhite women*

State	Rate per 100,000 live births
Idaho	58.1
Mississippi	52.4
South Carolina	42.8
Alabama	36.8
Nevada	36.1
Kentucky	34.4
North Carolina	31.6
Tennessee	30.7
Arizona	30.0
North Dakota	29.2
New Mexico	29.1
Virginia	24.8
South Dakota	23.3
Texas	22.9
Arkansas	22.1
Florida	20.5
Iowa	19.8

*Data from U.S. Department of Health, Education, and Welfare, Social and Rehabilitation Service, Children's Bureau, Public Health Service, National Center for Health Statistics. In Committee on Maternal Nutrition, National Research Council, National Academy of Sciences: Maternal nutrition and the course of pregnancy, Washington, D.C., 1970, Government Printing Office.

described in her classical early study of 38 pregnant women in Manila who died from eclampsia and who had no prenatal care. Some investigators postulate that the hemorrhagic changes in the liver are due to intense vasospasm of the hepatic arterioles.[46] Others attribute the liver tissue changes to more fundamental metabolic malfunction due to underlying malnutrition.[6] Eastman and Hellman[21] conclude that important as vascular constriction is in rationalizing the pathology of acute toxemia, it may well be a secondary manifestation of the disease.

Similar changes occur in renal tissue. The glomeruli are enlarged by about 20%, often protruding into the neck of the renal tubule.[46] The endothelial cells of the glomeruli are swollen and lay down deposits of fibrinlike material, with resulting leakage of protein and secondary tubular lesions from the protein filtrate. Usually these renal changes regress rapidly after birth. Apparently, endothelial cells of glomerular capillaries possess reticuloendothelial properties and can phagocytize precipitated fibrin.[9] Other endothelial tissue becomes involved, and small hemorrhages are found in the adrenals, lungs, brain, and endothelial surfaces of the heart.

Nutritional factors in toxemia of pregnancy

As indicated here and in previous chapters, the condition of pregnancy presents the human organism with a profound physiological and metabolic challenge. It is small wonder therefore that the major metabolic organ of the body—the liver—should bear in large measure the heightened metabolic challenge and reflect in its function its increased capacity to process the varied nutrient materials and their myriad metabolites, thus supporting in turn fundamental physiological processes throughout the rest of the body as a synergistic *whole*. Hence, the health and integrity of liver tissue is basic to this increased functional demand during pregnancy and to the prevention of a disordered metabolism such as occurs in toxemias of pregnancy, and it is on optimum nutritional input that the integrity of liver tissue, indeed any body tissue, ultimately depends. Thus nutritional factors in toxemias of pregnancy include directly or indirectly all of the nutrients and their metabolites, with particular emphasis on certain members of each group.

Protein. Since protein provides the basic structural units for all human tissues—the amino acids—it holds a primary position in human metabolism in close interrelationship with other nutrients. Such is true in the fundamental *growth* process that characterizes pregnancy. Especially, however, in relation to toxemias of pregnancy, three functional roles of protein may be considered.

1. *Fluid and electrolyte balance.* The major homeostatic mechanism maintaining the vascular volume and keeping circulating fluids moving through the body tissues is the capillary fluid shift mechanism (p. 74). Normal fluid circulation allows for ongoing nourishment of cells along with maintenance of appropriate blood volume and prevention of edema. This fundamental water balance mechanism is controlled by the plasma protein, mainly albumin, and the colloidal osmotic pressure it exerts in balance with the constant hydrostatic pressure—blood pressure. Any situation in which the serum albumin is decreased, therefore, would alter this balance between osmotic and hydrostatic pressure and foster edema. Thus albumin is of major importance in maintaining serum osmotic balance. Each gram of albumin per 100 ml of serum exerts an osmotic pressure of 5.54 mm Hg, whereas the same quantity of serum globulin, for example, exerts a pressure of only 1.43 mm Hg. One gram of albumin will hold 18 ml of fluid in the blood. Albumin infusions of 25 grams in 100 ml of diluent are equivalent in osmotic effect to 500 ml of citrated plasma.[30] It is clear that this effect would be beneficial in the treatment of shock or in any situation where the clinical objective is to remove excess fluid from the tissues and to increase the blood volume.

The liver is the sole source of the plasma protein, albumin. The precursor building materials for albumin and other plasma proteins are the amino acids, which derive, in large part, from dietary proteins. Studies have shown that the most effective food proteins in supplying materials for the regeneration of plasma proteins are lactalbumin (a milk protein), egg white, beef muscle, liver, and casein. Thus the two factors necessary to the synthesis of plasma albumin, and hence the normal operation of the capillary fluid shift mechanism and water exchange throughout the body, are (1) a constant optimum dietary source of adequate protein to supply the essential amino acids and (2) a healthy functioning liver to do the metabolic work of plasma protein synthesis.

2. *Lipid transport.* Protein functions also as the major means of transporting lipids in a water medium—the bloodstream. The transport vehicles are protein-lipid compounds, the lipoproteins, formed mainly in the liver from endogenous circulating lipids and plasma proteins produced from dietary protein. To the degree that this process is hindered by lack of an adequate dietary protein supply or diseased liver tissue, this metabolic work of converting fats to lipoprotein transport forms cannot take place, with the result that fats tend to accumulate in the liver. Fatty infiltration of liver tissue is a pathological state that can ultimately depress normal cellular functions in this tissue.

3. *Tissue synthesis.* Protein through its constituent amino acids is the basic necessity for building and maintaining all tissue proteins. Especially here in these metabolic relationships described, the maintenance of a healthy functioning liver (as well as other organs), is dependent on optimum protein supply and utilization.

All of these basic protein functions have relationships to overall metabolism, especially to metabolic functions of the liver, and in turn to the toxemias of pregnancy. It has long been established by the classical work of Strauss[48] and Ross[42] and reinforced by subsequent investigators and clinicians[5,26] that characteristic clinical findings in conditions of preeclampsia and eclampsia are hypoalbuminemia and hypovolemia, with subsequent hemoconcentration often masking anemia and the lowered total plasma albumin. Blood volume may be reduced 35% to 50%, and serum albumin may be as low as 2.0 gm/100 ml, when it should be 3.5 gm/100 ml to be acceptable.

Calories. Always closely associated with protein functions in tissue synthesis is a sufficient supply of nonprotein calories to ensure energy needs and prevent protein breakdown to supply energy. This is true in

Table 5-5. Relation of excessive gain in weight during full-term pregnancy to incidence of preeclampsia*

	Number		Percent	
Women gaining more than 30 pounds	1,933		15.0	
With preeclampsia		172		8.9
Without preeclampsia		1,761		91.1
Women gaining less than 30 pounds	10,789		85.0	
With preeclampsia		639		5.9
Without preeclampsia		10,150		94.1

*Data from N. J. Eastman, Johns Hopkins Hospital. In Committee on Maternal Nutrition, National Research Council, National Academy of Sciences: Maternal nutrition and the course of pregnancy, Washington, D.C., 1970, Government Printing Office.

pregnancy. Especially in relation to the toxemias of pregnancy, the former practices of restricting calories to control weight and hence reduce risk of toxemic complications are unwarranted, unscientific, and dangerous. To the contrary, Tompkins and co-workers[51] found a greater incidence of toxemia among underweight women who failed to gain weight normally during pregnancy. Eastman's data (Table 5-5) also refutes the correlation of "excessive" weight gain with incidence of preeclampsia and eclampsia. The overwhelming evidence indicates that the total amount of weight gain per se is not the significant factor; rather, it is the *quality* of the gain as determined by the nutritional value of the diet and the pattern of that gain which are of vital importance.

Minerals. The full spectrum of major and trace minerals are required to support the enhanced metabolic and structural functions during pregnancy. These needs and their metabolic rationale have been discussed in previous chapters. However, a basic mineral related to water balance in pregnancy, also erroneously restricted in prior obstetrical practices, is sodium. When the total extracellular fluid is increased as it is in pregnancy, the total amount of its major cation sodium must also be increased to maintain a normal ionic concentration. In toxemic patients the increased sodium retention is in direct relation to the increased edema. Decreased edema and with

it decreased retention of sodium follows the establishment of normal circulating blood volume through correction of the hypoalbuminemia and hence better operation of the failing capillary fluid shift mechanism. Pike and Gursky[40] have demonstrated that sodium restriction serves only to compound the problem by stressing the renin-angiotensin-aldosterone system, leading to hypertrophy and hyperplasia of the adrenals and exhaustion of the secretory cells therein. In addition, the use of diuretics along with even a mildly restricted salt intake can have serious impact on the renin secretion by the kidney and on the structure and function of the adrenals.

Vitamins. Again, the full spectrum of vitamins is also required during pregnancy, as has been discussed. Basic to the full use of needed protein and other nutrients during pregnancy are those vitamins especially related to protein and energy metabolism. Vitamins A, C, and D have particular structural functions, and the B-complex vitamins are closely related to protein and energy metabolism through their roles as coenzyme factors. For example, vitamin B_6 has numerous functions related to amino acid metabolism, and deficiency states have been observed in pregnant women and in infants. During pregnancy there is an increased fetal and placental demand for vitamin B_6. Recent studies of placentas from toxemia patients showed that these placentas contained only about one third the normal content of vitamin B_6, and they also demonstrated greatly reduced activity of pyridoxal kinase, the enzyme necessary to convert the vitamin to its active form, pyridoxal phosphate.

Prevention and treatment

Certainly the best approach to clinical management of toxemia in pregnancy is its *prevention,* and primary among those factors related to its prevention is good prenatal care based on sound nutrition. It is evident from accumulating research that vigorous nutritional support is basic to a healthy pregnancy and the avoidance of complications. Maintenance of good nutritional status can be achieved through sound nutritional knowledge applied in a culturally acceptable manner to meet individual needs of all pregnant women.

MEDICAL COMPLICATIONS DURING PREGNANCY

During their pregnancies women with existing medical conditions require special care. Two of these major clinical conditions encountered in maternity care are diabetes mellitus and heart disease. Another area of need, less often encountered, is that of pulmonary disease. In all instances careful individual attention is mandatory, and nutritional components of care are vital.

Diabetes mellitus

Care of the diabetic patient during her pregnancy requires a full knowledge not only of the normal physiological adaptations of pregnancy but also of the altered metabolism of the diabetic state and the interrelationships of both states. Essentially, the metabolic processes involved with energy and growth systems provide the physiological environment that both supports the pregnancy and controls the diabetes. Here, then, we can better understand and meet these objectives of care by looking first at the energy metabolism adaptations in pregnancy in terms of the maternal-fetal-placental fuel and

hormone relationships, comparing them with changes taking place in the diabetic state and then basing plans for patient care on these principles.

Energy metabolism in pregnancy

In pregnancy energy needs are increased and thus the fuel requirements to meet these needs are also increased. In the human energy system, glucose and fatty acids provide the main fuel sources, with some additional supply from deaminated amino acids. However, glucose is the primary fuel. This is especially true in the developing fetus, which seems to depend heavily on glucose to meet growing energy demands, energy needed not only for tissue protein synthesis but also for conversion to fat and glycogen.[2] Fetal stores of glycogen, for example, are relatively greater per gram of tissue than those of an adult. To meet this energy demand the rate of fetal uptake of glucose is at least twice that of the adult. At term the fetal glucose uptake has been estimated to be 20 mg/min, a glucose utilization rate of approximately 6 mg/kg of body weight per minute.[39] This rate of glucose use by the fetus is much greater than that of the adult, in whom the glucose turnover rate is 2 to 3 mg/kg of body weight per minute.[10]

Fetal-maternal fuel–insulin relationships. The relatively large glucose requirement of the fetus to meet its energy needs is facilitated by the rapid transfer of glucose from the mother to the fetus in two ways: (1) Since fetal blood glucose levels are usually 10 to 20 mg/100 ml lower than those of the maternal circulation, simple diffusion would account for movement of glucose across the placental membranes; (2) since glucose is the only significant fuel used by the fetus and vital to its survival, additional rapid absorption is ensured by carrier-mediated diffusion or active transport. However, maternal insulin does not cross the placental membrane.[3] Thus the fetus is dependent on its own supply of insulin for development. Fetal insulin is already present at twelve weeks' gestation, stimulated by increased glucose available from maternal circulation as well as by increased amino acids present.[37] Amino acids are actively transported by the placenta from maternal to fetal circulation. The amino acids not only serve vital tissue synthesis needs in the fetus but also provide energy support. Thus fetal demands for glucose and key glucose precursor amino acids, notably alanine, pose a constant pull on maternal metabolic supply.

Maternal fasting blood glucose levels. As a result of rapid fetal uptake of glucose and glucose precursor amino acids, there is a fall in the maternal fasting levels of blood glucose. At fifteen weeks' gestation, for example, maternal glucose levels after an overnight fast are 15 to 20 mg/100 ml lower than levels of the nonpregnant woman. If fasting extends beyond 12 hours, the maternal blood glucose may drop as low as 40 to 45 mg/100 ml. In turn, this drop in maternal blood glucose brings a decrease in the fasting insulin level, which leads to a "starvation ketosis." Thus the net exaggerated response of the mother to even brief fasting periods is evidenced by hypoglycemia, hypoaminoacidemia, hypoinsulinemia, and finally hyperketonemia.[23] Maternal ketone fasting levels of beta-hydroxybutyric acid and acetoacetic acid can be two to four times higher than those of the nonpregnant woman. Moreover, these ketones can be taken up by the fetus in situations of limited glucose availability as an alternative fuel source. However, such recourse brings risk of damage to fetal neurophysiological development. Significant reduction in IQ in offspring has been associated with maternal ketonuria, whether from ketones, per se, or from accompanying metabolic alterations.[16] In the lack of available glucose, the fetus turns to ketones because these metabolites do cross the placental membrane, whereas fatty acids do not.[33]

Insulin antagonism effect of placental hormones. Changes in maternal levels of glucose and other metabolites and substrates in the fasting state are not only due to fuel drainage by the fetus but also to increased secretion of placental hormones, which reach maximum levels during the latter stages of pregnancy. These hormones affecting glucose and insulin metabolism include human chorionic somatomammotropin (HCS), estrogen, progesterone, and maternal cortisol.

Human chorionic somatomammotropin (HCS). The placental hormone HCS is also called human placental lactogen (HPL) or chorionic growth hormone-prolactin (CGP), since it is a polypeptide that is similar in structure and function to growth hormone but at term reaches maternal circulating levels a thousand times that of growth hormone. It has several functions similar to those of growth hormone: (1) stimulates protein metabolism—anabolism; (2) alters carbohydrate metabolism by diminishing the action of maternal insulin —insulin antagonism; and (3) causes a significant increase in mobilization of free fatty acids from peripheral fat depots—lipolysis. Secretion of HCS occurs mainly in the third trimester of pregnancy, when growth demands of the fetus are accelerated. This condition has the net effect of increasing the maternal glucose and amino acid supply available to the fetus to support that accelerated growth process. Only minute amounts of HCS enter the fetal circulation. Rather, it acts as a maternal anabolic, glucogenic, lipolytic agent in late pregnancy to ensure fetal growth and survival.[29] Moreover, its additional lactogenic effect on mammary glands is also designed to ensure nutrition for the newborn infant.

Estrogen and progesterone. In the developing pregnancy placental secretion of estrogen and progesterone, which easily enter maternal circulation, also affects maternal glucose metabolism, especially in late pregnancy. Estrogen acts as an insulin antagonist rather than as an inhibitor of insulin secretion, thus contributing to diabetogenic tendencies.[34] To a lesser degree progesterone also affects glucose metabolism. It acts as an insulin antagonist by diminishing the effectiveness of insulin in peripheral tissues, even though it does augment initial secretion.[35]

Cortisol. Plasma concentrations of free cortisol and cortisol-binding protein transcortin are elevated in pregnancy. Cortisol, or hydrocortisone, is a hormone secreted by the middle zone of the adrenal cortex in response to stimulation by adrenocorticotrophic hormone (ACTH) from the anterior pituitary. It acts to elevate blood glucose levels by stimulating gluconeogenesis from amino acids and antagonizing insulin action in muscle and fat tissue. It also may have glucogenic effects by enhancing glucagon secretion.[58] In contrast, however, to the increased activity of cortisol during pregnancy, growth hormone, which is an important insulin antagonist in the nonpregnant state, is inhibited, probably in response to the presence of the placental hormones HCS and progesterone.

Maternal insulin secretion. As pregnancy progresses, despite the altered hormonal setting described, carbohydrate homeostasis and normal glucose tolerance is maintained throughout. This is accomplished by an increased maternal secretion of insulin. Hyperinsulinemia has been observed in response to intake of glucose and of amino acids.[53] However, although there is an increase in postprandial insulin levels, the fasting level of insulin is reduced because of the fasting hypoglycemia tendency that persists throughout pregnancy.[25]

Diabetic state in pregnancy

In comparison with the normal energy metabolism adapted for pregnancy, the diabetic state during pregnancy is varied, depending on the individual nature of the diabetes. Thus the classification and definition of diabetes in pregnancy as originally presented by White still provides a helpful guide. This classification is given in Table 5-6.

Definitions of diabetic states. Various terms are in general use that refer to stages of diabetes and these terms need to be understood.

Prediabetes. Prediabetes is the state in which glucose tolerance is normal in an individual destined by genetic makeup to become diabetic at a later time, given additional stress factors. Of course, in the main, this is a retrospective diagnosis. Per-

Table 5-6. Classification of maternal diabetes*

Class	Onset	Duration	Symptomatology
A			Slightly abnormal glucose tolerance test during pregnancy; usually no insulin required
B	Age 20 years or after	Less than 10 years	No vascular disease
C	Between ages 10 to 19 years	From 10 to 19 years	No vascular lesions or minimal manifestations, i.e., retinal arteriosclerosis, calcification of leg vessels alone
D	Before age 10 years	20 years or more	Vascular lesions: retinitis or calcified leg vessels; transitory albuminuria, transitory hypertension
E†	Before age 10 years	20 years or more	Calcification of pelvic arteries seen on x-ray film
F	Before age 10 years	20 years or more	All patients with diabetic nephropathy

*Modified from White, P.: Pregnancy and diabetes, medical aspects, Med. Clin. North Am. **49:**1015, 1965.
†This classification is generally not used in current practice.

sons are suspect, however, and should have closer monitoring in pregnancy if (1) a strong family history of diabetes is known or (2) there is a previous history of large babies (9 pounds or more) or of stillbirths.

Gestational diabetes. Gestational diabetes is the state in which abnormal glucose tolerance presents during pregnancy but reverts to normal post partum. Although only 20% to 30% of women with this condition subsequently develop diabetes, identification and close watching are important because of the higher risk of fetal damage.

Latent diabetes. Latent diabetes is the state in which the glucose tolerance is normal except in times of stress, such as surgery or infection. Gestational diabetes under the physiological stress of pregnancy could be viewed as a form of latent diabetes.

Chemical diabetes. Chemical diabetes is the state in which no diabetic symptoms are present, but an elevated fasting blood glucose or an abnormal glucose tolerance persists. Identification of women with chemical diabetes during pregnancy is also important in reducing perinatal risks.

Overt diabetes. Overt diabetes is the state in which frank symptoms of diabetes are present, evidenced by polydipsia, polyuria, polyphagia, or weight loss. During pregnancy women with overt diabetes require insulin therapy.

Diagnosis of diabetes in pregnancy. Screening for diabetes is done in most prenatal clinics by determining blood glucose levels for every patient who shows glycosuria or who gives a history of (1) familial tendency for diabetes, (2) previous unexplained stillbirths, (3) large babies weighing 9 pounds or more, (4) habitual abortion, (5) birth of infants with multiple congenital anomalies, and (6) excessive obesity. Usually a 2-hour, post–100 gram oral glucose test is used, since the fasting blood glucose level is frequently normal in early or latent diabetes. If the results of the 2-hour blood glucose test are in any way doubtful, a standard glucose tolerance test is done, and if nor-

mal, may be repeated every eight to ten weeks for monitoring. Since the renal threshold for glucose normally diminishes in pregnancy, glycosuria is not uncommon in the presence of normal blood glucose levels. One study reports an incidence of renal glycosuria in approximately 1.7% of the cases reviewed.[13] Moreover, follow-up glucose tolerance tests after asymptomatic glycosuria in another group of pregnant women revealed a normal response in 75% of the cases.[7] Thus gestational glycosuria or renal glycosuria during pregnancy is physiological, and alone it is not to be confused with diabetes but, rather, to be viewed as an important general monitoring tool.

Course of diabetes in pregnancy. Usually the course of diabetes in pregnancy follows a varying pattern from the first stages of the pregnancy, through the second half, and into the postpartum period.

Early stages and first half of pregnancy. The early stages of pregnancy are characterized by an increasing transfer of maternal glucose to the fetus to meet energy demands. This "siphoning" of glucose by the fetus, plus a lowered food intake because of nausea and vomiting of early pregnancy, may reduce insulin requirements. Thus this reduced insulin requirement is not the result of changed tissue sensitivity or altered diabetic status but, rather, of less available circulating blood glucose.

Second half of pregnancy. In the second half of pregnancy, the increased diabetogenic effects of the placental hormones outweigh the continuous drainage of glucose by the fetus, and insulin requirements are increased. This insulin requirement has been found to be increased by 65% to 70%.[52] At the same time that insulin effectiveness is diminished, the tendency to ketoacidosis is increased in the face of blood glucose levels that are not markedly increased. Some confusion may occur because the ketonuria may reflect a starvation ketosis rather than diabetic ketosis, indicating the need for glucose rather than insulin. Thus close monitoring of all parameters is important.

Post partum. After childbirth maternal levels of the gestational hormones HCS, estrogen, and progesterone fall rapidly, continued suppression of the growth hormone release is also seen. These hormonal changes cause a reduction in maternal insulin requirements, usually to levels below the prepregnant dose.

Planning care of the pregnant diabetic patient

Principles. Care of the pregnant patient with diabetes should be based on a full knowledge of both pregnancy and diabetes, and it involves three fundamental principles: (1) frequent evaluation during pregnancy, (2) team approach to care, and (3) personalized, individual therapy.

Frequent evaluation during pregnancy. Clinicians agree from experience that there is no substitute for frequent contacts with the patient and close observation of the changing course of metabolism and its effects during the pregnancy. In most prenatal clinics all diabetic patients, including Class A cases, are seen every two weeks until the twenty-sixth week and every week, or more frequently as needed, thereafter.

Team approach to care. Because of the variable aspects of diabetes and its course during pregnancy, as well as the altered course of pregnancy in the presence of diabetes, an interdisciplinary team of specialists, including internist, obstetrician, nurse, nutritionist, and pediatrician at birth, can better meet the changing needs of the patient. Since nutritional therapy is fundamental to sound and safe care in both diabetes and in pregnancy, the skilled clinical nutritionist becomes a highly significant member of the care team. With this approach the patient plays a central role; progress is continually assessed and recommendations for modifications in self-care are proposed as justified

on the basis of adverse clinical symptomatology.

Personalized individual therapy. Because diabetes, pregnancy, and people in general vary in their natures, it is imperative that close, supportive individual therapy be followed. A primary medical concern is adequate control of the diabetes, with optimum nutritional support and insulin coverage to prevent fetal damage. Obstetrical concern centers on timing of the birth to minimize risk to mother and infant but allow for sufficient pulmonary maturity to avoid hyaline membrane disease.

Basic components of care. The basic components of diet and insulin must be carefully and constantly controlled to ensure an optimum outcome of the pregnancy.

Diet. The fundamental cornerstone of management of diabetes at any time is dietary planning and control. This factor becomes even more important during pregnancy. At all times throughout the pregnancy, the needs of the fetus must be paramount. Since the concepts of management in both diabetes[4] and in pregnancy[18] have been reevaluated and changed recently, it is mandatory that all practitioners participating in the care of a woman with diabetes during her pregnancy know and follow these current principles and concepts.

In the care of diabetes, principles of diet management are based on the concept of balance:

1. *Total energy balance.* Energy input as measured by calories is balanced with energy needs to achieve and maintain ideal weight. In pregnancy total energy requirements are governed by the demands of maternal-fetal growth and overall heightened metabolic needs. Any indicated weight reduction should never be undertaken during the pregnancy but should await the postpartum period. This does not preclude lactation, since a sound diet plan can provide for both gradual weight reduction, if needed, and breast-

feeding. Average weight gains during pregnancy in the studies of Hytten and Thomson,[32] which were associated with optimum course of the pregnancy, were 27.5 pounds and hence were recommended by them as a physiological norm. On the average, as recommended by the National Research Council report and described in this manual, the pregnant woman with diabetes will require 2000 to 2400 calories, or approximately 30 to 35 cal/kg of actual body weight, since the support of the pregnancy takes precedence.

2. *Nutrient balance.* In diabetes the ratio of nutrients is important to meet metabolic needs. Contrary to some former practices, carbohydrate intake should *not* be disproportionately reduced. However, it is best that this carbohydrate be provided in complex forms that are digested and absorbed slowly like, such as starches, vegetables, and fruits. Concentrated sweets that are quickly digested and absorbed result in greater increments of blood glucose. There is some evidence that an isocaloric increase in the carbohydrate proportion of the diet may actually improve glucose tolerance.[8] In pregnancy therefore adequate carbohydrate is important to meet needs for diabetes control as well as to meet fetal demands for glucose. This need translates to approximately 45% of the total calories or a minimum of 200 grams of carbohydrate.

Protein needs are increased in pregnancy, as has been described in previous chapters. Optimum protein is also important in diabetes control. Hence the diet of the pregnant woman with diabetes should contain approximately 2 grams of protein per kilogram of body weight per day, or about 100 to 120 gm/day.

Fat needs in the diet of the diabetic woman during pregnancy are not primary, and so the amount should be kept at moderate levels. Thus the remainder of the calories, or approximately 30% to 35% of the total calories (about 60 to 80 grams) may come from fat.

3. *Distributive balance.* In diabetes the regular distribution of the total diet throughout the day to balance with insulin activity is necessary to avoid insulin reactions and provide for a sustained release of glucose. A pattern of three meals with midafternoon and evening snacks will usually suffice. Each meal and snack should contain both protein and carbohydrate to smooth out the resulting glucose release. Some women may also need a midmorning snack, especially if a portion of regular insulin is mixed with the morning longer acting insulin. Meals and snacks must not be missed and should be regular in pattern each day.

In planning such a diet for a woman with diabetes during her pregnancy, the usual food exchange system may be used for making food selections. The current

Table 5-7. Meal pattern in food exchanges

	Total	Breakfast	Lunch	Snack	Dinner	Snack
Milk (skim)	4	1	1	1		1
Meat (1-2 eggs)	8	1	2	1	3	1
Bread	8	2	2	1	2	1
Vegetables						
Starch group	2		1		1	
List A	As desired					
Fruit	8	2	1	2	1	2
Fat	8	2	2	1	2	1
		(0 if using whole milk)				
		(4 if using low fat milk)				

revised edition of the food lists in this exchange system incorporate principles of reduced saturated fat but retain the basic general food groupings used in the system for some years.[22]

A diet prescription and food exchange pattern applying the principles of diet management for diabetes in pregnancy for a woman weighing 150 pounds may be as follows:

Calories	2200
Protein	120 grams
Carbohydrate	250 grams
Fat	80 grams

The meal pattern in food exchanges may be as shown in Table 5-7.

Insulin. With the exception of Class A gestational diabetes, insulin is required throughout pregnancy. Usually in Class A patients the glucose tolerance returns to normal postpartum, but it should be tested again six weeks after birth. About 28% of these women develop abnormal glucose tolerance tests in the nonpregnant state within five years and are true diabetic patients.[38] During pregnancy most diabetic patients can be controlled with a single dose of intermediate-acting insulin (NPH or lente). Occasionally a second dose may be required in the evening to prevent hyperglycemia during the night and early morning. As indicated, insulin requirements usually fall during the first half of pregnancy because of continuous fetal use of glucose, and the mother may need no more than two thirds of her prepregnant amount. In the second half of pregnancy, the progressive rise of the placental hormones HCS and progesterone and of maternal cortisol create the need for more insulin, with dosage requirements increasing approximately 70% to 100% above prepregnancy needs. This mean increase in insulin requirement has been shown to be approximately 1 unit per week.[47]

Although opinions vary, a reasonable goal of insulin therapy for the diabetic woman during pregnancy is to maintain blood glucose levels below 150 mg/100 ml in the fasting state and 2 to 3 hours after meals. This can generally be achieved without risking hypoglycemia. In any event, ketoacidosis must be avoided or, if present, promptly treated because the fetal death rate in such instances may increase to 50% or more. However, in pregnancy, starvation ketosis must be distinguished from diabetic ketoacidosis.

Starvation ketosis may occur more readily in pregnancy because of the accelerated fetal uptake of glucose and accentuated by early nausea and vomiting or by self- or physician-inflicted calorie restriction. In such cases, after overnight or extended fasts, blood ketone levels may rise to two or three times the normal nonpregnant level, but hyperglycemia is *not* present. This lack of hyperglycemia, characteristic of diabetic ketoacidosis, is the distinguishing feature. Thus treatment consists of glucose solutions and foods rather than supplemental insulin.

Diabetic ketoacidosis, to the contrary, occurs in the face of elevated blood glucose levels. Thus treatment consists of administering rapid-acting regular insulin, usually in an initial dose of 50 to 100 units intravenously, along with hypotonic fluids (4.5% of saline) and potassium supplements.[24] Bicarbonate therapy is only given to patients with an arterial pH below 7.25 or a bicarbonate level below 5 mEq/L or to those in a comatose condition. Continued monitoring of blood glucose levels, blood ketones, and arterial pH provide a basis for determining additional insulin needs.

Schedule for plan of prenatal care. At the first visit, as part of the complete history, physical examination, and laboratory workup, a nutritional history and assessment should be included, using guidelines outlined in Chapter 4. On the basis of this nutritional, physical, medical-obstetrical, and personal-social assessment, an individual problem-oriented plan of care, including an individually adapted diet prescription and food plan, should be developed by the care team. At each subsequent visit (every two weeks until the twenty-sixth week and every week thereafter), the patient is evaluated by the medical-obstetrical-nutritional team of specialists. Four urine samples, taken before each meal and at bedtime the previous day, are examined for glucose, acetone, and albumin. The patient's own record of fractional urine tests for glucose and acetone is also reviewed carefully, as well as intermittent food records. Weight, blood pressure, and signs of edema are checked. Hemoglobin is tested monthly. The ocular fundus is examined frequently.

Birth and postpartum care. The birth is timed carefully to protect the fetus. The incidence of stillbirths to diabetic mothers increases after thirty-six weeks' gestation, yet immaturity creates risks of respiratory distress syndrome (RDS) secondary to hyaline membrane disease. Thus most pregnancies of diabetic mothers are terminated during the month before term, with delivery planned at thirty-six to thirty-eight weeks' gestation or twenty-eight days before term, if all factors are favorable. A variety of parameters, such as tests of estriol levels, HCS, and lecithin/sphingomyelin (L/S) ratios in amniotic fluid, are used for individual assessment and timing of birth. Delivery is usually by induction and vaginal mode or by cesarean section if indicated. On the day of delivery the patient is given only one third to one half of her usual dose of insulin and an intravenous infusion of 5% dextrose at a maximum rate of 200 to 300 ml/hr to minimize maternal hyperglycemia and resulting neonatal hypoglycemia. After birth supplemental doses of regular fast-acting insulin are used according to fractional urine tests for glucose. In some clinics the patient's regimen is changed to regular insulin two days before birth, with the dose adjusted to the degree of glycosuria found in fractional urine tests.

After the birth, because of the rapid clearing of the placental hormones HCS

and progesterone and their insulin antagonism effect, as well as the continued suppression of maternal growth hormone, less insulin is required. Thus initially only about two thirds of the prepregnancy dose is given. Resumption of the woman's full diet is encouraged as soon as possible to initiate restoration of nutrition reserves and support lactation, should the mother choose to breast-feed her baby. Breast-feeding presents no problem in maternal diabetes. During the postpartum period and continuing, the dose of insulin varies but is adjusted rapidly according to blood and urine glucose determinations.

Heart disease

In the United States the incidence of diagnosed heart disease in pregnancy varies from 1.2% to 3.7%.[54] With good care the majority of these women carry their pregnancies to successful conclusions with no deterioration of their heart conditions. By and large, this improvement in care is the result of advances in medical and surgical treatment of heart disease in general, as well as more knowledge and better understanding of the normal cardiovascular adaptations to pregnancy. These physiological adaptations of cardiovascular dynamics designed to support and sustain the pregnancy have been reviewed in Chapter 3 and are basic to planning care.

Normal cardiovascular system during pregnancy

In pregnancy the maternal cardiovascular system makes basic physiological adjustments to support the changed metabolism of the maternal-fetal-placental synergistic *whole* organism. Essentially, these adjustments are involved in four areas of cardiovascular operation: blood volume, heart action, systemic regulatory agents, and blood pressure.

Total blood volume. To support the increased metabolic work of pregnancy, the total body water increases. Of this total increase, the plasma compartment expands also in proportion so that the total circulating blood volume increases 50% or more as in multiple pregnancies, for example, with twins.

Heart action. Beginning early in the pregnancy there is an increase in heart rate and in cardiac output, the elevated output sustained by an increased stroke volume. As the pregnancy progresses these actions gradually rise, reaching a peak six to eight weeks before term and declining significantly before labor begins.

Systemic regulatory agents. Both plasma renin and blood aldosterone levels increase. These regulatory agents are related to water and sodium metabolism, as has been described (Chapter 3), and to arterial pressures through the action of the vasopressor angiotensin. In addition to reactions to changes in vascular pressures as a cause of renin secretion, renin stimulation and plasma increase have been attributed to prior estrogenic stimulation of renin substrate (angiotensinogen) production by the liver.[49]

Blood pressure. The systolic blood pressure shows little change, but diastolic pressure falls somewhat, reaching its lowest value about the thirtieth week of pregnancy. In relation to the increases in cardiac output, this represents in effect a decreased systemic vascular resistance during pregnancy to facilitate circulation.

Heart disease in pregnancy

Confusion may arise in identifying heart disease in pregnancy because there is difficulty in differentiating between mild organic heart disease and the physiologically overacting heart of a normal pregnancy. Moreover, only about one half of the women found to have heart disease during pregnancy are aware of any preexisting heart problem, and only a tiny portion—about 5%—of all the disorders seen during pregnancy begin as a result of the pregnancy. Thus careful screening of all patients through meticulous histories and examinations is important in detecting underlying need and preventing problems. Such defining of need and classifying of disease according to cause, changed anatomy, and physiological state are basic to planning care during pregnancy.

Signs and symptoms of heart disease during pregnancy. Four basic criteria have served well as indications of heart disease in pregnancy to guide clinical care: (1) the presence of a diastolic murmur, (2) significant cardiac enlargement as shown by x-ray examination, (3) the presence of a systolic murmur of at least grade III intensity, and (4) the presence of a severe arrhythmia.

Classification of heart disease. In identifying need and planning individual care, it is important to relate nature and degree of the heart disease present to the patient's functional and therapeutic capacities. Such a standardizing of criteria for planning care has been developed by the Criteria Committee of the New York Heart Association and is in general use as a clinical guide (Table 5-8). The functional classifications are graded from Classes I to IV and refer to the type of activity that results in symptoms. The therapeutic classifications from Classes A to E refer to those activities that the patient may safely include in her daily life. This guide provides an important basis for all members of the health team in planning care, but especially to the nutritionist and the nurse in helping the mother adjust her activities at home or work.

Planning care of pregnant heart disease patient

Principles. Care of the pregnant patient with heart disease should be based on the same general principles of wise care planned for the woman with diabetes: (1) frequent evaluation, (2) team care, and (3) individualized therapy. Here, in caring for the woman with heart disease, the basic objectives are (1) cardiac rest and (2) nutritional support of the pregnancy. To this end, therefore, careful initial assessment is important. Since many women enter pregnancy unaware of any heart distur-

Table 5-8. Functional and therapeutic classification of heart disease*

Functional classification	Therapeutic classification
Relation of heart disease to heart function and activities that bring on symptoms	Relation of heart disease to permissible activities of daily living
Class I — No resulting limitations on physical activity; ordinary activity causes no undue fatigue, dyspnea, palpitation, or anginal pain	Class A — Physical activity need not be restricted (This is seldom the case, however, when applied to pregnancy because of the added physiological burdens involved.)
Class II — Slight limitation on physical activity; comfortable at rest, but ordinary activity causes fatigue, dyspnea, palpitation, or anginal pain	Class B — Ordinary physical activity need not be restricted, but patient should be advised against severe or competitive efforts
Class III — Considerable limitation of physical activity; comfortable at rest, but less than ordinary effort causes symptoms	Class C — Ordinary physical activity should be moderately restricted and more strenuous effort discontinued
Class IV — Unable to carry on any physical activity without discomfort; symptoms of cardiac insufficiency or of anginal syndrome present even at rest, and any physical activity increases discomfort	Class D — Ordinary physical activity should be greatly restricted
	Class E — Complete rest, confined to bed or chair

*Modified from Criteria Committee, New York Heart Association.

bance, the history should probe for any related prior experiences. For example, has the woman ever had rheumatic fever, chorea, or congenital heart disease? Has she had high blood pressure? Was her activity ever restricted because of "weak heart" or a heart murmur? Does she get short of breath after mild effort or note palpitations?

Basic components of care. To provide needed physical, physiological, emotional, and nutritional support for the woman with heart disease during her pregnancy, the basic components of diet and rest will require consideration as a focus for planning care for each patient.

Diet. Using the general outline given in Chapter 4 for nutritional needs during pregnancy, an individual food plan can be developed with the woman. In addition to these basic needs of pregnancy, two factors should be evaluated to help avoid heart problems.

1. *Energy balance in terms of weight control.* As with any woman during pregnancy, adequate weight gain to support the pregnancy should be encouraged. However, the woman with heart disease must be guided to plan her diet carefully so as to secure all the protective nutrients required and at the same time avoid the burden of *excessive* weight. The quality of the diet is the primary consideration, with excess quantities of food being unnecessary.

2. *Sodium intake.* Sodium is a necessary mineral element for the health of the pregnant woman, as has been indicated in previous discussions (p. 102). However, because the woman with heart disease is vulnerable to cardiac stress or failure, guidance can be given to her concerning ways to avoid excess sodium and keep her intake within moderate limits. Usually, the mildly restricted level of 2000 mg of sodium will suffice to meet needs. This general level

can be achieved by following two basic rules: (a) *light* use of salt in cooking, but none added at the table; and (b) no obviously salty foods, such as those processed in salt or salty condiments. During the initial nutrition assessment interview therefore, it is important to inquire concerning the patient's habits in regard to salt use in cooking or at the table or use of salty foods. Many alternative modes of seasoning can be explored together.

Despite these two moderate considerations in energy and sodium balance, a positive nutritional approach as described in Chapter 4 must be maintained. Also, counsel may be given concerning practical aspects of food marketing and preparation to conserve personal energy.

Rest. Adequate rest is imperative to reduce cardiac demands. This means both physical and mental rest. Thus it is helpful to enlist the support of family members in meeting these needs. The mother must get adequate sleep at night, rest at intervals during the day such as after meals, and sit while working whenever possible.

Postpartum period. Perhaps the greatest problem the mother with heart disease may face in the pregnancy–birth cycle is going home with her new baby. Some outside help is essential. The nutritionist and the nurse may provide much assistance in helping her plan home activities that will not place a strain on her heart. The pamphlet, "The Heart of the Home," published by the American Heart Association, is a good resource for finding easier and more pleasant ways of accomplishing household tasks and pacing the work so as to avoid fatigue. It includes a pictorial supplement of a kitchen designed to illustrate practical ways of saving time and energy. Also, patients may be referred to the local heart association homemaker program.

Pulmonary disease

Care of the woman with pulmonary disease during her pregnancy also presents problems in medical management. An understanding of the normal maternal physiological adjustments in respiratory function that are designed to support the pregnancy provides a basis for planning care. In the previous discussion presented in Chapter 3, a physiological basis for nutritional needs during pregnancy has been provided, including adjustments of the respiratory system. Thus reference is made to that discussion with a brief summary here as background for planning care. A number of pulmonary problems may be present during a woman's reproductive years and complicate a pregnancy. As they relate to the pregnancy in terms of pulmonary function, these problems require special care. The clinical condition of pulmonary tuberculosis may be used as a model.

Normal respiratory system during pregnancy

In pregnancy the maternal respiratory system makes basic physiological adjustments to meet the changed metabolism that develops to provide nourishment and nurturing of new life. Essentially, adjustments occur in two basic areas: (1) the mechanics of breathing and (2) lung functions of ventilation and gas exchange. All of these changes are designed for the basic purpose of facilitating an ample supply of oxygen to meet enhanced metabolic needs.

Mechanics of respiration. The most important muscle of inspiration is the diaphragm. Other inspiratory muscles include the external intercostal muscles and accessory muscles such as small muscles of the head and neck. In early pregnancy there is an upward displacement of the diaphragm of approximately 4 cm,[50] long before any displacement pressure of the uterus could occur. This raising of the diaphragm muscle in effect allows for a greater gas exchange and less volume of gas remaining in the lung after a normal expiration (functional residual capacity). Thus diaphragmatic breathing seems to play a more primary role than costal breathing during pregnancy. The expiratory muscles are the internal intercostal and abdominal wall muscles. With the stretch involved in pregnancy by the increased abdominal volume of the enlarging uterus, the action of these abdominal muscles is facilitated. Working together with a characteristic flaring of the lower rib cage during pregnancy, these muscles of respiration can contract more forcefully, especially during expiration, thus expelling more carbon dioxide and enabling more intake of oxygen on inspiration.

Lung functions. Changes in lung functions during pregnancy also facilitate oxygen supply. Without any appreciable change in respiratory rate, significant increases in ventilation, volume, and gas exchange occur.

Ventilation. During pregnancy the ventilation rate increases about 43%, from about 7 L/min to about 10 L/min.[19]

Volumes. Although the total lung capacity does not change significantly during pregnancy, there are several important changes in the respective volumes of the various lung compartments. Increases and decreases occur indicating greater volume exchange as follows:

Increases
1. *Tidal volume*—amount of gas inspired or expired with each breath (normal breathing)
2. *Vital capacity*—amount of gas that can be expired after a maximal inspiration
3. *Inspiratory capacity*—amount of gas inspired in a maximal inspiration

Decreases
1. *Residual volume*—amount of gas remaining in the lung at end of expiration
2. *Functional residual capacity*—amount of gas remaining in the lung after a normal expiration
3. *Expiratory reserve volume*—maximal amount of air expired from the resting end-expiratory position

Gas exchange. The primary function of the lung is the exchange of carbon dioxide and oxygen between the capillary blood and the gas in the distal air spaces across the alveolar-capillary membranes, thus maintaining normal oxygen–carbon dioxide tensions in the arterial blood. This vital alveolar ventilation, gas exchange, is regulated by the arterial blood carbon dioxide tension, oxygen tension ("tension" referring to the respective gas pressures), and the blood pH. Of these factors, the carbon dioxide tension is the most important. During pregnancy the increase in blood levels of progesterone from the placenta increases ventilation (gas exchange) probably by acting on the respiratory center to lower its threshold to carbon dioxide.[57] Thus there is increased oxygen consumption, more efficient mixing of gases, and an "overbreathing," or hyperventilation, that washes out carbon dioxide from the alveoli.

Dyspnea of pregnancy. Along with all of these lung function changes normal to pregnancy, there occurs a characteristic consciousness of the need to breathe—dypsnea. This "strain to breathe" seems more apparent at rest than with exertion. It is an interesting natural phenomenon of pregnancy and may represent, as Campbell and Newsom Davis[11] suggest, an awareness by the maternal organism that the dyspnea of overbreathing is due to "an appreciation that chest wall movements are inappropriate in terms of past experiences." It is as if the adaptations, being made, must be used—the scene is set so the drama must be played!

Pulmonary disease in pregnancy: tuberculosis

Nature of disease process. Historically, tuberculosis has flourished to epidemic proportions in the midst of overcrowding, poverty, poor hygiene, stress of varying kinds, and malnutrition. However, with an increasing standard of living reinforced by the advent of effective antituberculosis chemotherapy (1945), the incidence rate has dropped remarkably. A quarter of a century ago, about 80% of the United States urban population were tuberculin positive compared with only 15% to 20% now.

Human tuberculosis results from infection by the *Mycobacterium tuberculosis*— the tubercle bacillus. It is primarily an airborne disease that may develop when the tubercle bacilli are deposited in the distal air spaces of the lung (alveoli). The organisms are transmitted from an infected person by coughing or sneezing, with the subsequent inhalation by others present of minute droplet nuclei containing the bacilli. Initial lesions in the lung produce a lobular tuberculous pneumonia. At this active stage the disease may spread to other body tissues. General classifications of tuberculosis according to activity of the disease process have been used to guide treatment. A new United States classification for tuberculosis has recently been adopted (1974) by the American Lung Association. It identifies four classes as follows:

Class A: No tuberculosis exposure, not infected (no history of exposure, negative tuberculin skin test)
Class B: Tuberculosis exposure, no evidence of infection (history of exposure, negative tuberculin skin test)
Class C: Tuberculosis infection without disease (positive tuberculin skin test, negative bacteriological test if done, no x-ray findings compatible with tuberculosis, no symptoms due to tuberculosis)
Class D: Tuberculosis, infected with disease, to be characterized by location of the disease, bacteriological status, and chemotherapy

Planning care of the pregnant tuberculosis patient

Principles. Care of the pregnant patient with tuberculosis should incorporate the same fundamental triad of principles as used for the patient with heart disease: (1) frequent evaluation, (2) team care, and (3) individualized therapy. The basic objectives are the control of infection and support of the pregnancy. Adequate chemotherapy during pregnancy has largely eliminated risk factors. Moreover, patients with inactive disease who are receiving adequate chemotherapy should not be discouraged from breast-feeding their infants.

Basic components of care. Tuberculosis occurs in pregnant women in the United States in approximately 3% of the patients studied, according to several reports.[45] Thus it continues to be a significant problem encountered during pregnancy. Careful assessment at the outset is fundamental to planning adequate therapy. The majority of women found to have tuberculosis during pregnancy are discovered by routine x-ray examination and are asymptomatic. Whatever the stage of the disease, three components of care are essential: chemotherapy, diet, and rest.

Chemotherapy. Because of the infectious nature of the disease and its potential for development without adequate treatment, the cornerstone of care, whether the disease is active or inactive, is continuous close working relationship among the specialists providing care and the patient. In this kind of a supportive environment of mutual confidence, positive reinforcement can be given to the need for long-term, daily, uninterrupted antituberculosis chemotherapy where it is indicated. Many misconceptions and much anxiety exists concerning a fear of the effects of the disease, especially on the newborn infant. Empathetic, knowledgeable, and supportive discussions with the patient and her family can allay many of these anxieties. A number of drugs are available now for treatment of tuberculosis and are generally used in combinations to counteract growth of drug-resistant bacilli present. These drugs include isoniazid (INH), rifampin (RM), ethambutol (ETH), streptomycin (SM), para-aminosalicylic acid (PAS), and others.

Diet. Optimum nutritional support is necessary to counteract the disease process and promote healing, as well as to sustain the growth and energy needs of the pregnancy. A diet such as the one outlined in Chapter 4 for pregnancy will also meet healing needs of the disease. The diet should contain increased amounts of protein, vitamins and minerals, and calories.

Individual planning with the patient and her family can provide a variety of foods to stimulate appetite or meet variances in food toleration related to drug therapy.

Rest. Adequate rest balanced with activity that is not overtaxing to the patient is a helpful adjunct to therapy. Relaxation and breathing exercises may also be integrated into the care program to facilitate pulmonary function and allay anxieties. Such basic exercises can be taught to the patient so that she may practice them at home.

Smoking and pulmonary function

A final note may be added concerning the relation of smoking, pulmonary health, and pregnancy. Respiration is affected adversely by smoking, as is the health of lung tissue. Moreover, the oxygen-carrying capacity of the blood in both the mother and the fetus is decreased in women who smoke during pregnancy.[17] These factors may contribute to the increased incidence of low birthweight, prematurity, stillbirth, and late fetal and infant mortality reported in offspring of women who smoke. Certainly during pregnancy, but otherwise as well, smoking should be discouraged because of adverse effects on the lungs.

REFERENCES

1. Acosta-Sison, H.: Clinicopathologic study of eclampsia based upon 38 autopsied cases, Am. J. Obstet. Gynecol. **22:**35, 1936.
2. Adam, P. A. J.: Control of glucose metabolism in the human fetus and newborn infant, Adv. Metab. Disord. **5:**183, 1971.
3. Adam, P. A. J., Teramo, K., Raiha, N., Gitlin, D., and Schwartz, R.: Human fetal insulin metabolism early in gestation, Diabetes **18:**409, 1969.
4. Bierman, E. L., Albrink, M. J., Arky, R. A., et al: Special report: principles of nutrition and dietary recommendations for patients with diabetes mellitus, Diabetes **20:**633, 1971.
5. Brewer, T. H.: Limitations of diuretic therapy in the management of severe toxemia: the significance of hypoalbuminemia, Am. J. Obstet. Gynecol. **83:**1352, 1962.
6. Brewer, T. H.: Metabolic toxemia of late pregnancy: a disease of malnutrition, Springfield, Ill., 1966, Charles C Thomas, Publisher.
7. Brundenell, M., and Beard, R.: Diabetes in pregnancy, Clin. Endocrinol. Metab. **1:**673, 1972.
8. Brunzell, J. D., Lerner, R. L., Hazzard, W. R., Porte, D., Jr., and Bierman, E. L.: Improved glucose tolerance with high carbohydrate feeding in mild diabetes, N. Engl. J. Med. **284:**521, 1971.
9. Burrow, G. N., and Ferris, T. F.: Medical complications during pregnancy, Philadelphia, 1975, W. B. Saunders Co.
10. Cahill, G. F., Jr., and Owen, O. E.: Some observations on carbohydrate metabolism in man. In Dickens, F., Randle, P. J., and Whelan, W. J., editors: Carbohydrate metabolism and its disorders, vol. 1, New York, 1968, Academic Press, Inc.
11. Campbell, E. J. M., and Newsom Davis, J.: Respiratory sensations. In Campbell, E. J. M., Agostoni, E., and Newsom Davis, J., editors: The respiratory muscles—mechanics and neural control, ed. 2, Philadelphia, 1970, W. B. Saunders Co.
12. Chanarin, I.: Diagnosis of folate deficiency in pregnancy, Acta Obstet. Gynecol. Scand. **46:**39, 1967.
13. Chen, W. W., Sese, L., Tantakasen, P., and Tricomi, V.: Pregnancy associated with renal glucosuria, Obstet. Gynecol. **47:**37, 1976.
14. Chopra, J., Noe, E., Matthew, J., Dhein, C., Rose, J., Cooperman, J. M., and Luhby, A. L.: Anemia in pregnancy, Am. J. Public Health **57:**857, 1967.
15. Christakis, G., editor: Nutrition assessment in health programs, Am. J. Public Health **63**(supp.): 1, Nov., 1973.
16. Churchill, J. A., Berendes, H. W., and Nemore, J.: Neurophysiological deficits in children of diabetic mothers, Am. J. Obstet. Gynecol. **105:**257, 1969.
17. Cole, P. V., Hawkins, L. H., Roberts, D.: Smoking during pregnancy and its effects on the fetus, J. Obstet. Gynaecol. Br. Commonw. **79:**782, 1972.
18. Committee on Maternal Nutrition, Food and Nutrition Board, National Research Council, National Academy of Sciences: Maternal nutrition and the course of pregnancy, Washington, D.C., 1970, Government Printing Office.
19. Cugell, D. W., Frank, N. R., Gaensler, E. A., and Badger, T. L.: Pulmonary function in pregnancy. I. Serial observations in normal women, Am. Rev. Tuberc. **67:**568, 1953.
20. DeLeeuw, N. K. M., Lowenstein, L., and Hsieh, Y. S.: Iron deficiency and hydremia of normal pregnancy, Medicine **45:**291, 1966.
21. Eastman, N. J., and Hellman, L. M.: Williams' obstetrics, ed. 13, New York, 1966, Appleton-Century-Crofts.
22. Exchange lists for meal planning, Chicago, 1976, American Diabetes Association–American Dietetic Association.
23. Felig, P.: Maternal and fetal fuel homeostasis in human pregnancy, Am. J. Clin. Nutr. **26:**998, 1973.

24. Felig, P.: Current concepts: diabetic ketoacidosis, N. Engl. J. Med. **290:**1360, 1974.

25. Felig, P., and Lynch, V.: Starvation in human pregnancy: hypoglycemia, hypoinsulinemia, and hyperketonemia, Science **170:**990, 1970.

26. Ferguson, J. H.: Maternal death in the rural South, J.A.M.A. **146:**1388, 1951.

27. Friedman, E. A.: Effects of blood pressure on perinatal mortality, In Vollman, R., editor: International workshop on the clinical criteria of toxemia, Springfield, Ill., 1975, Charles C Thomas, Publisher.

28. Gant, N. F., Daley, G. L., Chand, S., Whalley, P. J., and MacDonald, P. C.: A study of angiotensin II pressor response throughout primigravid pregnancy, J. Clin. Invest. **52:**2682, 1973.

29. Grumbach, M. M., Kaplan, S. L., Sciarra, J. J., and Burr, I. M.: Chorionic growth hormone prolactin (CGP): secretion, disposition, biologic activity in man, and postulated function as the "growth hormone" of the second half of pregnancy, Ann. N.Y. Acad. Sci. **148:**501, 1968.

30. Harper, H.: Review of physiological chemistry, ed. 12, Los Altos, Calif., 1969, Lange Medical Publications.

31. Holly, R. G.: Dynamics of iron metabolism in pregnancy, Am. J. Obstet. Gynecol. **93:**370, 1965.

32. Hytten, F. E., and Thomson, M. A.: Maternal physiological adjustments. In Committee on Maternal Nutrition, National Research Council, National Academy of Sciences: Maternal nutrition and the course of pregnancy, Washington, D.C., 1970, Government Printing Office.

33. James, E., Meschia, G., and Battaglia, F. C.: A-V differences in FFA and glycerol in the ovine umbilical circulation, Proc. Soc. Exp. Biol. Med. **138:**823, 1971.

34. Javier, Z., Gersberg, H., and Hulse, M.: Ovulatory suppressants, estrogens, and carbohydrate metabolism, Metabolism **17:**443, 1968.

35. Kalkhoff, R. K., Jacobson, M., and Lemper, D.: Progesterone, pregnancy, and the augmented plasma insulin response, J. Clin. Endocrinol. **31:**24, 1970.

36. Kitay, D. Z.: Folic acid deficiency in pregnancy, Am. J. Obstet. Gynecol. **104:**1067, 1969.

37. Obershein, S. S., Adam, P. A. J., King, K. C., Teramo, K., Raivio, K. D., Raiha, N., and Schwartz, R.: Human fetal insulin response to sustained maternal hyperglycemia, N. Engl. J. Med. **283:**566, 1970.

38. O'Sullivan, J. B., Gellis, S. S., Dandrow, R. V., and Tenney, B. O.: The potential diabetic and her treatment in pregnancy, Obstet. Gynecol. **27:**683, 1966.

39. Page, E. W.: Human fetal nutrition and growth, Am. J. Obstet. Gynecol. **104:**378, 1969.

40. Pike, R. L., and Gursky, D. S.: Further evidence of deleterious effects produced by sodium restriction during pregnancy, Am. J. Clin. Nutr. **23:**883, 1970.

41. Pritchard, J. A.: Changes in the blood volume during pregnancy and delivery, Anesthesiology **26:**393, 1965.

42. Ross, R. A.: Factors of probable significance in causation of toxemias of pregnancy, South. Med. Surg. **102:**613, 1940.

43. Rothman, D.: Folic acid in pregnancy, Am. J. Obstet. Gynecol. **108:**149, 1970.

44. Scott, D. E., and Pritchard, J. A.: Iron deficiency in healthy young college women, J.A.M.A. **199:**897, 1967.

45. Selikoff, I. J., and Dorfmann, H. L.: Management of tuberculosis, In Guttmacher, A. F., and Rovinsky, J. J., editors: Medical, surgical, and gynecologic complications of pregnancy, ed. 2, Baltimore, 1965, The Williams & Wilkins Co.

46. Sheehan, H. L., and Lynch, J. B.: Pathology of toxemia of pregnancy, Baltimore, 1973, The Williams & Wilkins Co.

47. Spellacy, W. N., and Cohn, J. E.: Human placental lactogen levels and daily insulin requirements in patients with diabetes mellitus complicating pregnancy, Obstet. Gynecol. **42:**330, 1973.

48. Strauss, M. B.: Observations on the etiology of toxemias of pregnancy: The relation of nutritional deficiency, hypoproteinemia, and elevated venous pressure to water retention during pregnancy, Am. J. Med. Sci. **190:**811, 1935.

49. Tapia, H. R., Johnson, C. E., and Strong, C. G.: Effect of oral contraceptive therapy on the renin-angiotensin system in normotensive and hypotensive women, Obstet. Gynecol. **41:**643, 1943.

50. Thomson, K. J., and Cohn, M. E.: Studies on the circulation in pregnancy. II. Vital capacity observations in normal pregnant women, Surg. Gynecol. Obstet. **66:**591, 1938.

51. Tompkins, W. T., et al.: The underweight patient as an increased obstetrical hazard, Am. J. Obstet. Gynecol. **69:**114, 1955.

52. Tyson, J. E., and Felig, P.: Medical aspects of diabetes in pregnancy and the diabetogenic effects of oral contraceptives, Med. Clin. North Am. **55:**947, 1971.

53. Tyson, J. E., and Merimee, T. J.: Some physiologic effects of protein ingestion in pregnancy, Am. J. Obstet. Gynecol. **107:**797, 1970.

54. Ueland, K.: Cardiac surgery and pregnancy, Am. J. Obstet. Gynecol. **92:**148, 1963.

55. United States Department of Health, Education, and Welfare, National Center for Health Statistics: Blood Pressure of Adults, by Age and Sex, United States 1960-1962, PHS Pub. No. 1000, Ser. 11, No. 4, Washington, D.C., 1964, Government Printing Office.

56. Wallerstein, R. O.: Iron metabolism and iron deficiency during pregnancy, Clin. Haematol. **2:**453, 1973.

57. Wilbrand, V., Parath, C. H., Matthaes, P., and Jaster, R.: Der Einfluss der Ovarialsteroide auf die Funktion des Ztemzentrums (Effect of ovarian steroids in the function of the respiratory centre), Arch. Gynakol. **191:**507, 1959. Cited in Hytten, F. E., and Leitch, I.: The physiology of human pregnancy, ed. 2, Oxford, 1971, Blackwell Scientific Publications, Ltd.

58. Wise, J. K., Hendler, R., and Felig, P.: Influence of glucocorticoids on glucagon secretion and plasma amino acid concentrations in man, J. Clin. Invest. **52:**2774, 1973.

59. Zuzpan; F. P., Long, W. N., Russell, J. K., Stone, M. L., and Tarlow, A. R.: Anemia in pregnancy, J. Reprod. Med. **6:**13, 1971.

6

Nutritional needs of the pregnant adolescent

Bonnie S. Worthington

Human reproduction in the adolescent is a topic of increasing concern to obstetricians, pediatricians, and other health care professionals. In 1975 about 1 out of 5 babies were born to mothers under 19 years of age or younger, and of these mothers, more than one tenth were under 16 years of age. Pregnancy in the teenage girl is especially distressing because frequently she presents with a variety of serious health and social problems. These basic problems may be further complicated by psychological, educational, nutritional, and vocational difficulties, all of which need attention if the stress of pregnancy is to be minimized.

For many reasons, therefore the pregnant adolescent is viewed as a high-risk patient. She is "vulnerable" to the social, emotional, and biological stresses of pregnancy and is consequently highly susceptible to suboptimal pregnancy outcome. Identification of needy pregnant adolescents and management of their problems and concerns should be a primary goal of community health organizations. Interdisciplinary programs designed to meet the adolescent's need and those of her infant have operated with some success during the past decade; such programs have

served to improve prenatal conditions and prepare young mothers to cope with the problems of parenthood under adverse circumstances. Guidance in diet planning is an important component of successful programs for pregnant teenagers, and sincere efforts by skilled clinicians can help to improve the overall nutritional support available to both mother and child.

SCOPE OF THE PROBLEM
Demographic considerations

A variety of factors are believed to be responsible for the increasing trend in adolescent pregnancies, despite a declining birth rate in the general population. Significant among these factors are the following:

1. There was a sudden rise in the teenage population as an aftermath of the post–World War II "baby boom".[2] From 1950 to 1969 the number of youths 15 to 19 years of age in the United States increased from 10.6 to 18.6 million. In 1960 these youths represented 7.4% of the United States population, whereas in 1969 the figure was 9.1%, which is a 23% increase in the proportion. Since 1969 little additional change has been noted in these percentages.

119

2. Among females there was a declining age of maturation. Tanner[48] observed that the decrease in age of maturation in the United States has leveled off in the past fifteen years after dropping from about 14.25 years in 1900 to about 12.5 years in 1955. The average age of menarche is now 12.5 to 13 years of age. Tanner and others claim that the major factor responsible for the decline in age of menarche is an improvement in nutrition and health, which leads to an increase in rate of physical growth.

3. An increasing adolescent age-specific fertility is evident. The augmentation is related both to earlier age at marriage than before[10,36] and younger age at first pregnancy.[52]

4. An increase in sexual freedom has occurred. It is generally believed that the changing attitudes of today's youth coupled with the so-called "sexual revolution" have contributed in some degree to rising numbers of adolescent pregnancies in all cultural, racial, and socioeconomic groups.[32]

Adolescent maternal mortality

Maternal mortality rates have declined remarkably during the past fifty years in the United States.[2] Pregnancy and birth were more than twice as safe for women in 1970 than for their mothers in 1950 or their grandmothers in 1930 (Table 6-1). Maternal mortality rates for women under 20 years of age have declined more rapidly than for any other age group.[43]

It is important to recognize, however, that although the rates are low, the number of teenage maternal deaths is appreciable (Table 6-2). Since many small and large studies of maternal populations reveal few maternal deaths among young subjects,[2,25,39] it is surmised that mortality among pregnant adolescents occurs largely in situations other than well-supervised health care facilities or in connection with inappropriately performed abortions.[33,35,49]

In efforts to assess the reasons for adolescent maternal mortality, agreement is widespread that socioeconomic factors play a significant if not dominate role. Most of the deceased girls were single and non-white, and often the deaths were from preventable causes. In general, delayed diagnosis and delayed treatment were common faults in those cases in which the preventable factors were in the hands of professionals.

It is well recognized that adolescent pregnancies are fraught with potential risk. A large number of surveys have been conducted in an attempt to detect and describe

Table 6-1. Maternal mortality rates per 10,000 live births, United States and California, 1930 to 1970*

Year	United States	California
1970	3.0†	2.7†
1964	3.3	2.8
1960	3.7	2.9
1950	8.3	5.5
1940	36.4	28.4
1930	67.3	52.5
1920		70.5

*From Vital statistics of the United States, National Center for Health Statistics, Public Health Service, Washington, D.C., annual volumes, Government Printing Office; and California public health statistical report, 1964 vital statistics, Sacramento, Calif., 1964, State of California Department of Public Health.
†Estimated.

Table 6-2. Maternal mortality by age in the United States, 1973

Age group (yr)	Number of deaths
10-14	6
15-19	72
20-24	102
25-29	116
30-34	97
35-39	56
40-44	25
45-49	2
Total	477

From Vital Statistics of the United States, 1973, Vol II, Mortality, Part B, Public Health Service, National Center for Health Statistics, 1973.

this risk and to determine what factors are most responsible. The results have not been conclusive; observations and statistics presented in many reports are contrary to the results of other studies. According to Ballard and Gold,[2] this discrepancy among studies can be accounted for largely by variables other than maternal age; inherent selective factors in the study groups and a wide variety of other parameters, such as race, age differences, socioeconomic patterns, cultural factors, and nutritional status, could not be controlled. In reviewing the data, it is surprising that so few deaths have been documented when the morbidity information shows that the pregnant adolescent is subject to considerable risk of pregnancy complications.[25]

Maternal morbidity

A number of problems have been described as common and significant for pregnant adolescents. The most frequently mentioned complications include acute toxemia, uterine dysfunction, contracted pelvis, premature labor, prolonged labor, fetopelvic disproportion, vaginal infection, vaginal laceration, and heart disease.[2,46] The most consistent high-risk characteristic, noted by virtually every observer of adolescent pregnancies, is toxemia. Both preeclampsia and eclampsia occur with greater frequency among teenagers than in older women.[*] It is worth noting that with the addition of other variables reflecting poor nutrition, particularly nonwhite race and poverty, the incidence of toxemia in the subgroup formed is even higher.[18,25] The highest rates of toxemia reportedly occur in the youngest adolescents. Battaglia and co-workers[3] noted that among patients younger than 15 years of age, the rate of toxemia was 29.2%; this figure is significantly higher than the 21.1% seen in the 15- to 19-year-olds and the overall clinic rate of 11.2%. Similar findings have also been reported by Marchetti and Menaker[31]

and Clark.[11] In Marchetti's population the toxemia rate was 42% in the 13-year-olds and dropped to 16.1% in the 16-year-olds; in addition, eclampsia was seven times more frequent in the youngest group compared with the older patients.[31] Clark[11] found that girls under 16 years of age had toxemia five times as frequently as older patients.

Although toxemia during pregnancy may not seriously compromise the health of the infant, permanent damage may be done to the afflicted mother. The early (and often repeated) insult of toxemia on the cardiovascular-renal system of a young woman may contribute substantially to the increased severity of toxemia with subsequent pregnancies and the appearance of chronic disease later in life. Since pregnant teenagers are now known to be statistically destined to have more than the average number of pregnancies, the potential for repeated toxemia is great and the probability of development of long-term cardiovascular damage is sizable. It is obvious therefore that if the debilitating effects of frequent pregnancies are added to the nutritional burden already carried by the growing adolescent, the conditions are established for a rapid and irreversible slide from simple toxemia to renal damage and hypertensive disease.

The offspring

The outcome of a pregnancy cannot be measured in terms of maternal health alone. It is mandatory also to consider carefully the fate of the infant, and it is here that the greatest risks associated with adolescent pregnancy become glaringly apparent. Examination of the infant and perinatal mortality and morbidity in adolescent pregnancies strikingly point up the continuing excessive loss of human life in the form of pregnancy wastage. The majority of this wastage has preventable components, found mainly preconceptionally and/or prenatally.[16,41,49,53]

Perinatal deaths have declined drasti-

---

*See references 1-3, 10, 11, 18, 23, 25, 30, 35, 36.

cally in recent years; most physicians agree, however, that more improvement is possible if widespread availability of high-quality manpower and facilities can be achieved. Beyond this it is commonly believed that further improvement in both maternal and infant survival and health can come from early diagnosis and treatment of adverse socioeconomic conditions in the individual, the family, and the community. With this intent, identification and treatment of generalized overnutrition or undernutrition may be helpful in improving both preconceptional and prenatal conditions of young women from diverse socioeconomic circumstances.

Prematurity has long been recognized as the leading cause of perinatal mortality among the poor and is second on the list (exceeded only by Rh incompatibility) in private patient services where income level is more satisfactory. Prematurity is mentioned as frequently as toxemia by authors describing the characteristics of adolescent births.[10,18,22,25] Like toxemia the rates are highest in the youngest patients,[11] and existence of both problems in the same pregnancy is not uncommon. According to population surveys, a mother under 15 years of age is at twice the average risk of having a premature infant as the older woman.[11,18]

Although the etiology of prematurity remains unresolved, numerous characteristics other than age and race can be ascribed to groups of women with highest rates. Included in the list of characteristics are multiple births, parity of zero or over three, spacing of pregnancies less than two years apart, lower social class, poor economic status, inadequate prenatal care, and a host of medical conditions such as toxemia, cardiovascular-renal conditions, metabolic diseases, and others.[2] It has been proposed that the thread which ties these seemingly unrelated factors together is the nutritional status of the mother.[1,12] Nutritional status is a forgotten detail, often overlooked by investigators who study and describe selected groups of pregnant adolescents. In

the opinion of some health professionals, better prenatal care is the variable responsible for improved pregnancy outcome in special programs for adolescents; other concerned individuals recognize the clear association of poor diet with obstetrical complications. The devastating effect of overt malnutrition on fetal welfare is most clearly seen in underdeveloped areas of the world. Bishop[6] and others have shown, however, that undernutrition in any setting is accompanied by relatively high prematurity rates, and presumably the two circumstances are closely related.

One further area of concern related to the offspring is the problem of congenital abnormalities or "quality" of the newborn. Although the adolescent is at slightly greater risk of having a baby with a birth defect than is a woman of 20 to 30 years of age, the total and overall rate of abnormalities in children born to women over 30 years of age far exceed those of younger women. It is apparent, however, as seen in Table 6-3, that when anencephaly, spina bifida, and meningomyelocele are examined separately, the offspring of the teen-age mother is at equal or even higher risk of being born with one of these conditions when compared with babies born to older mothers.[8] In addition, malformations of other organ systems are commonly associated with neural tube defects. These

Table 6-3. Incidence of babies dying with selected neural tube defects by age of mother (rates per 1000 live births)*

Abnormality	Age of mother (yr)		
	<20	25-30	40+
Anencephalus	3.5	2.0	3.3
Spina bifida	1.7	0.9	1.5
Occipital meningocele	0.35	0.2	0.35
Hydrocephalus	0.28	0.32	0.70

*From Butler, N. R., Alberman, E. D., and Schatt, W. H.: The congenital malformations. In Butler, N. R. and Alberman, E. D., editors: Perinatal problems. Edinburgh and London, 1969, E. & S. Livingstone Ltd.

nclude cardiovascular defects, skeletal deformities, renal malformations, gastrointestinal abnormalities, and mental retardation, including Down's syndrome. When these conditions occur alone, however, they usually are associated with older maternal age.

Overall assessment of the problems of anencephaly and spina bifida necessitates consideration of the issue or parity. Both of these abnormalities occur more frequently in first births, less often in second births, and then at a progressively higher rate with higher parity.[8] The pregnant adolescent therefore is disadvantaged twice, once by being subjected to the higher rates just mentioned and, secondly, in later life by the increased rates associated with higher parity eventually expected among women starting childbearing at younger ages.[2]

In considering the offspring of adolescent mothers, a major concern relates to the postnatal environment of the infant, especially if the infant was unplanned, unwanted, and is without the support of a parent who is knowledgeable in child care and home management. This set of adverse circumstances often prevails, and often a long list of other related problems can also be developed. In dealing with the teenage mother therefore, attention must be given not only to her medical, obstetrical, and nutritional problems but also to the wide range of social, financial, legal, educational, vocational, and other difficulties that exist. It is a well-known fact that success in management of the nutritional defects apparent in a pregnant adolescent *cannot* be achieved unless the health care professional or team is able to define and attend to the total needs of the patient through the establishment of priorities and definition of a systematic approach to optimizing the patient's circumstance.

NUTRITIONAL CONCERNS
General

Adolescence is a time of great physical growth and development; to support its normal progress, substantial nutritional input is required. During adolescence therefore, increased amounts of food are needed and specific nutritional requirements relate directly to the time and degree of pubertal growth spurt. As one would expect, nutritional demands are greatest when growth is most rapid; when growth rate slows down, nutritional needs gradually taper off. Because the pubertal acceleration in growth generally occurs in girls (10½ to 13 years of age) before it occurs in boys (12½ to 15 years of age), separate dietary recommendations are proposed for boys and girls after 9 years of age.

Character and timing of physical growth and sexual maturation differ greatly among individuals, but in general, the adolescent girl does not complete linear growth until four years' postmenarche.[12] Teenagers who become pregnant during the four years after menarche are considered to be biological risks because they are anatomically and physiologically immature. Since these girls are generally still growing, their nutritional requirements exceed those of adult women. When the period of growth is complete (usually about 17 years of age), the adolescent is considered physiologically mature and similar to other "adult" women in her nutritional demands for normal pregnancy.

Since little information is available on nutritional needs of pregnant adolescents, *estimates* of needs are typically formulated by adding the pregnancy Recommended Dietary Allowances (RDA) for adult women to the RDA specifications for nonpregnant teenagers 15 to 18 years of age (Table 6-4). This method of approximation may overestimate total pregnancy requirements for some individuals. For example, the metabolic alterations promoted by pregnancy may promote the *retention* of essential nutrients by decreasing nutrient catabolism or by increasing the efficiency of nutrient absorption. Beaton[4] has shown in animals that growth hormone acts to decrease protein catabolism; human studies by Finch[15]

Table 6-4. Estimates of dietary needs for pregnant teenagers*

Nutrient	Recommended intake for nonpregnant teenagers, 15-18 years†	Recommended increment for adult pregnancy	Recommended intake for pregnant teenagers
Energy (kcal/kg‡)	40	5	45
Protein (gm/kg)	0.9	0.4	1.3
Calcium (gm)	1.2	0.4	1.6
Phosphorus (gm)	1.2	0.4	1.6
Iron (mg)	18	0	18¶
Magnesium (mg)	300	150	450
Iodine (μg)	115	25	140
Zinc (mg)	15	5	20
Vitamin A (IU)	4,000	1,000	5,000
Vitamin D (IU)	400	0	400
Vitamin E (IU)	11	3	14
Ascorbic acid (mg)	45	15	60
Niacin (mEq)	14	2	16
Riboflavin (mg)	1.4	0.3	1.7
Thiamin (mg)	1.1	0.3	1.4
Folacin (mg)	0.4	0.4	0.8
Vitamin B_6 (mg)	2.0	0.5	2.5
Vitamin B_{12} (μg)	3	1	4

*Modified from King, J. C., and Jacobson, H. N.: Nutrition and pregnancy in adolescence. In Zackler, J., and Brandstadt, W., editors: The teenage pregnant girl, Springfield, Ill., 1975, Charles C Thomas, Publisher.
†The value recommended for teenagers 15 to 18 years of age.
‡Intake for pregnant teenagers is 10.9 mj (millijoules), for nonpregnant teenager, 10.0 mj, and for pregnant adults, 9.2 mj.
¶Supplemental iron is recommended for pregnant teenagers.

have shown that the efficiency of iron absorption increases progressively during pregnancy. In addition, the raised circulating levels of estrogen that develop in pregnant teenagers may promote closure of epiphyseal plates and termination of growth; if this should occur, nutritional requirements allotted for growth would be unnecessary. Finally, if reduction in maternal physical activity level is substantial, energy needs may not differ greatly from those of nonpregnant adolescents. Recognizing all of the potential that may exist in the aforementioned additive approximation of nutritional needs therefore, the resultant values are probably the best possible figures to use if the pregnant girl is still growing. If, however, she is obviously mature, her nutritional requirements probably resemble more closely those defined for pregnant adults.

Energy

Since individual adolescents differ markedly in their growth patterns, body builds, and exercise routines, it is extremely difficult to predict energy requirements with great accuracy. The most sensible approach to the situation is to obtain information on body weight and height for each individual in question. Height data are probably most helpful in predicting total energy needs, but weight information is also useful in reflecting both growth rate and body build. Prediction of energy requirements can be further improved by evaluating the changes in height and weight that the given adolescent has demonstrated over the entire childhood period. Such a practice allows the professional to estimate the present growth rate of the child and to plan for necessary energy needs with growth rate in mind. Girls ten to reach puberty sooner than boys and thus have an increase in energy requirements at an earlier age. In addition, since the growth spurt for girls is relatively short, they typically demonstrate a rather rapid decrease in energy requirements *after* puberty.

The increased energy requirements during rapid growth are generally met without concentrated effort on the part of the adolescent. Appetite usually increases at this time, and increased food intake is a normal response to this circumstance. It is known, however, that young girls proceeding through adolescence under today's pressures for maintenance of slim physique frequently limit their food consumption to levels significantly less than those required to meet demands for normal growth. In one study the average energy intake of girls 9 to 11 years of age was found to be 2000 cal/day, whereas girls 12 to 17 years of age took in 2100 cal/day.[50] Since the recommended caloric need of a young girl 9 to 14 years of age is 2400 calories, approximate deficits of 400 and 300 cal/day, respectively, were apparent in the groups studied.

The long-term effects of calorie restriction by adolescent girls in developed societies are still unknown, since strict control of weight gain in this population has existed for only a decade or thereabouts. The permanent effects on the individual girl will relate directly to the particular time during her growth period when serious calorie restriction is imposed. Calorie deprivation during the period of rapid growth in height may compromise normal growth of the skeletal system. Under such circumstances long bones would be especially affected, and dimensions of the pelvic girdle may also be altered adversely.[5] Calorie restriction *after* the height spurt has been completed will not have such a devastating impact on normal growth processes in adolescent girls. Under such conditions, however, nutritional status may deteriorate, and tolerance to stress, disease, and other insults may decline. Pregnancy under such adverse circumstances is accompanied by considerable risk to both mother and fetus.

Pregnancy in the adolescent girl increases her calorie requirement to a level significantly above that of the nonpregnant teenager. Hytten and Leitch[24] suggest that the metabolizable energy needs average about 330 cal/day during the last three fourths of pregnancy. If this increment is added to their recommendation for nonpregnant teenagers, the estimated needs for the pregnant teenager become 2730 calories, or 47 cal/kg for a 58 kg girl. The RDA of the National Research Council is 45 kcal/kg for the pregnant teenager.[37]

Of additional interest, however, is the issue of energy expenditure. In a study by Blackburn and Calloway,[7] energy expenditure was assessed in pregnant adolescents. They found that during pregnancy, basal metabolic rate (BMR) was 1.11 kcal/min compared with 0.98 kcal/min at six to ten weeks' postpartum. Unexpectedly, however, when corrections were made for body weight, the differences in BMR between the two periods disappeared. These data suggest that the increase in body *mass* during pregnancy accounts for most of the increase in BMR. Blackburn and Calloway confirmed this idea by measuring energy expenditure of pregnant adolescents during activities unrelated to body weight (quiet sitting, combing hair, cooking at stove, etc.) and compared these figures with energy expended in activities affected by body weight (treadmill running, sweeping, bedmaking, etc.). Results suggested that energy expenditure during the latter group of activities was significantly greater during pregnancy than in the nonpregnant state, whereas energy expenditure in the former activities varied little from one circumstance to the other. Energy needs during pregnancy therefore appear to relate directly to the cost of weight movement that accompanies increase in body mass. Since the typical woman increases body mass about 20% during pregnancy, activities that demand a lot of movement must require as much as 20% more energy to accomplish.

One further point of interest, however, is

the modification in activity pattern typically demonstrated by pregnant adolescents. Blackburn and Calloway[7] recorded activity patterns of 12 pregnant teenagers and found that activity was distributed for most girls in the following categories:

Sleeping or lying in bed with magazine	40%
Quiet seated activities	40%
Eating	4%
Doing hair and other similar activities	5%
Light activities	9%
Total	98%

It can be seen that most girls spent the vast majority of their time in sedentary activities. Although the most active girl in the group utilized 50 kcal/kg/day, 7 of the 12 girls observed expended approximately 38 kcal/kg/day. It is apparent therefore that energy expenditure may be highly variable from individual to individual, and assessment of this factor along with all others will be necessary in approximating daily calorie requirements for pregnant adolescents. The best assurance of adequate intake is a satisfactory weight gain over time.[28]

Protein

Growth is accompanied by considerable nitrogen retention, and normal growth progress can be achieved only if adequate protein is provided in the diet. Protein deposition (and nitrogen retention) is greatest during the period of most active growth in the adolescent girl; as growth slows down, protein deposition diminishes.[19]

Protein intake by typical adolescent girls has been studied by several researchers.[12] It has been found that protein generally accounts for more than 10% of calories consumed, and frequently the level of intake is even higher. National Research Council reports suggest that average protein intake of adolescent girls exceeds the 44- to 54-gram level which they recommend; daily protein intakes of 75 to 80 grams frequently are consumed by girls in the 11- to 13-year-old age group. Evalua-

tion of dietary records clearly indicates tha adolescent girls prefer protein foods with a low caloric content. In many circumstances representative diets are reasonably high in protein and low in calories such that some dietary protein is used for energy and less remains for building body tissues. Unde conditions of rigorous calorie restriction the amount of protein available for production of lean body tissue may be inadequate and retardation in physical growth may occur. For this reason adolescent girls should be encouraged to plan diets tha contain enough energy to allow for use o an adequate amount of protein for tissue synthesis.

During pregnancy the adolescent girl' protein needs increase in line with the protein requirements of the growing fetus and accessory maternal tissue. Animal studie have clearly shown that birth weight declines when the mother's protein intake falls below a critical level.[34] The precise protein needs of the pregnant woman ar still unknown. Recommendations hav been based largely on the amount of protein deposited in maternal and fetal tissu during pregnancy. According to Hytter and Leitch,[24] dry protein stores averag approximately 925 grams for the entir pregnancy; daily deposition is estimated t be 5.4 grams during the later half of preg nancy. How these figures relate to dail dietary protein needs of the pregnan woman is unclear, but a series of nitroge balance studies has been completed wit the hope that specific requirements can b more clearly defined. According to Callo way,[9] the protein storage rate is about 6. gm/day, a figure approximately 1.5 gram more each day than has been accounte for by previous estimates of dry protei stores in maternal and fetal tissue. Thes recent findings of Calloway indicate tha protein (or nitrogen) retention is appre ciably larger than previously believed an probably is less variable from the first tr mester to the third trimester than former] recognized.

Recent work by King and associates[28] involved estimation of protein requirements of pregnant adolescents. In this study nitrogen retention was measured in a group of pregnant girls who resided in a metabolic research unit during the third trimester of their pregnancy. It was determined that when 15- to 19-year-olds were fed the 1968 National Research Council protein recommendation of 65 gm/day, they retained 1.4 gm/day of nitrogen (8.17 gm/day of protein). In addition, as nitrogen was increased from 9.3 to 20.0 gm/day (58 to 125 gm/day of protein) without variation of the energy input (43 kcal/kg), nitrogen retention increased linearly according to the following equation: nitrogen retention (gm/day) = 0.3 (nitrogen intake) − 1.73. King concluded from her findings that the 1968 National Research Council protein recommendation does not permit maximum protein storage during the third trimester in young primiparas. For this reason a protein intake of 75 gm/day is recommended along with an energy input of approximately 2700 calories.

Iron

Iron needs of the growing adolescent are sizable and relate to a requirement for iron by the enlarging muscle mass and blood volume.[19] Additionally, since the maintenance of adequate iron stores is considered desirable, extra iron is needed for this purpose. Because the adolescent girl loses body iron each month during menstruation, this loss must also be made up for by provision of iron from exogenous sources. Balance studies by Schlaphoff and Johnson[38] indicate that 11 to 13 mg/day of iron are needed to cover growth and menstrual losses. In 1973 the National Research Council recommended that adolescent girls and women consume 18 mg/day of iron[37]; it is generally believed that intake of iron at this level will allow for buildup of sufficient iron stores such that iron supplementation during pregnancy should be unnecessary.

Since dietary sources of iron are rather limited, fulfillment of the iron specifications may be difficult, if not impossible. Schorr and co-workers[40] reported that the iron intake of typical adolescent girls in New York State was 8.8 mg/day; Hampton and colleagues[17] determined the iron intake of teenage girls in California to be 9.5 mg/day; Van de Mark and Wright[51] reported that pregnant teenagers in a high-risk clinic population in Alabama consumed 6 to 8 mg/day of iron. Although the incidence of obvious iron deficiency anemias in these groups is not excessively high, the problem of low iron stores is believed to be widespread. Such a circumstance places a young girl at distinct risk for development of anemia when iron needs increase markedly during times of stress, like pregnancy.

According to estimates by Shank[42] and others, approximately 4.7 mg/day of iron must be stored over the last 140 days of pregnancy to meet the needs of the mother and fetus. Because menstruation ceases during pregnancy, the specific iron increment for pregnancy cannot be added to the nonpregnant requirement. Since the menstruating adolescent's average iron loss is 0.4 mg/day,[51] the increase in daily iron need for the last half of pregnancy is reduced to 4.3 mg.

Since the efficiency of iron absorption is believed to increase progressively during pregnancy,[24] the additional 4.3 mg of iron needed each day by the pregnant adolescent would likely be absorbed from diets containing 18 mg or more of iron. If the daily diet contains *less* than 18 mg of iron, supplementation with 30 to 60 mg of elemental iron (ferrous sulfate, ferrous fumarate, ferrous gluconate) would easily satisfy the iron needs of the healthy adolescent.

Calcium

Balance studies with adolescents have recently shown that calcium absorption and retention are increased prior to menarche and the growth spurt. According to Ohlson and Stearns,[34a] when calcium intakes range from 1.0 to 1.6 gm/day and vitamin D intakes are about 400 IU/day, retention of approximately 400 mg/day of calcium is allowed. This level of daily calcium retention during the several years of rapid growth appears to be necessary if adequate mineralization of the skeleton is to take place. It is interesting to note, however, that *evidence* of calcium deficiency in the United States is hard to come by, even though calcium intakes of 0.4 to 0.8 gm/day have been reported in teenage girls in several parts of the country.[12] Although the skeletal systems and height status of these girls appear normal, much remains to be learned about the long-term effects of low calcium consumption on skeletal disorders later in life.

The need for extra calcium during pregnancy relates largely to the development of the fetal skeletal system. According to Hytten and Leitch,[24] approximately 28 grams of calcium are stored in the fetus at birth. In addition, small quantities of calcium are deposited in maternal supporting tissues and fluids. Overall, calcium deposition during pregnancy is about 30 grams. Since the healthy adolescent contains approximately 1120 grams of calcium in her "body stores," the additional calcium required during pregnancy could likely be derived from this source if the dietary provisions were inadequate. Under such circumstances, however, demineralization of maternal bone is an inevitable consequence, and the possibility that this might prove detrimental to the young girl is worth recognizing.

In those young women whose calcium intakes have been low throughout childhood and adolescence, tissue stores of calcium are low and likely insufficient to meet the needs of a developing fetus during pregnancy. If such a woman continues to consume a diet with inadequate calcium content, fetal skeletal development and maternal skeletal integrity will be seriously compromised. Marginal calcium intake during pregnancy may also prevent adequate preparation of the maternal body for lactation. It is believed therefore that to provide sufficient calcium for normal fetal development *without* depleting maternal tissues, an additional intake of 400 mg/day of calcium is recommended for the pregnant adolescent.[37] Overall, to meet the calcium needs for her own growth and for that of the fetus, the pregnant adolescent needs to consume from 1.2 to 1.6 gm/day of calcium. The most appropriate level of intake for the *individual* girl will depend on her rate of growth at the time of the pregnancy.

Other nutrients

The restricted diets consumed by many adolescents frequently contain inadequate amounts of vitamins and trace minerals. Attention to this problem during pregnancy is important if the maternal and fetal tissues are to receive sufficient amounts of each nutrient for maintenance of metabolic processes and support of normal growth. Vitamins that are frequently found in short supply in the diets of adolescents include vitamins A, D, and C and folic acid. In girls who consume vegetarian diets, vitamin B_{12} intake may be seriously restricted. Evaluation of dietary patterns of pregnant adolescents should serve to expose potential dietary deficits. A skilled professional should be prepared to make appropriate recommendations for dietary improvement *when and if they can be adapted to the life-style of the individual without provoking undue stress on her or her family.* Nutritional supplements can be used when dietary adaptation appears impossible. A variety of vitamin and/or mineral supplements are available for purchase, and care should be taken to select the product that best meets the needs of the particular individual under consideration.

DIETARY PATTERNS IN THE ADOLESCENT

By the time a young girl has grown into adolescence, her dietary patterns are well established. By and large, her general preferences and dislikes relate to family circumstances she has been exposed to throughout childhood. In addition, however, adolescent food patterns always are influenced by living habits and daily routines, which vary according to individual interests during the busy high school years. Schedules will differ on weekdays and weekends, and activity patterns will vary from one time of the year to another. Attention to food may be excessive if the environment is food oriented. Meals and eating, on the other hand, may be put off if the busy schedule cannot accommodate them. Emotional problems commonly associated with adolescence may influence eating behavior in a variety of ways. Hinton and associates[20] have shown that girls who score best in emotional stability, conformity, adjustment to reality, and family relationships miss fewer meals, are familiar with a wider variety of foods, and have generally better diets than other girls. They also found that girls who mature late or early often have emotional problems accompanying this developmental characteristic and frequently have poorer eating habits than those girls maturing at normal rates.

Irregular eating habits are now known to be characteristic of most adolescents.[14,44,45] According to several surveys, as many as one fifth of all adolescent girls skip breakfast, and another 50% have poor breakfasts. Edwards and co-workers[14] reported that as students advanced from the seventh to the twelfth grade, the percentage who missed meals increased from 10% to 25%; in addition, twice as many missed breakfast in twelfth grade as in seventh grade. Many factors are involved in promoting alterations in meal patterns of the type described. For the adolescent girl significant factors certainly include busy schedules and motivation for weight control.

It should be recognized that along with a pattern of skipping meals frequently comes the pattern of increased snacking. Snacking should be considered a normal practice among teenagers, and diet plans should be made with this in mind. According to Hampton and colleagues[17] as much as one fourth of the total daily caloric consumption of adolescent girls typically comes from snacks, and those who snack frequently (in moderation) are also likely to eat meals of good quality and to have overall good diets. In planning the diet for a pregnant adolescent, it should consequently be remembered that moderate snacking is not to be outlawed. On the contrary, a diet plan will be accepted by the pregnant girl only if it fits her life-style closely; such a plan of necessity includes snacks, and the type of snack will be dictated by the environment in which it is obtained and/or consumed.

Although nutritionists and other health professionals may place much time and effort in nutrition counseling of pregnant adolescents, changes in dietary patterns may not be observed in some girls. This is to be expected, and according to several researchers,[17,39] food patterns of adolescent girls are not related to their knowledge of nutrition or to the number of nutrition information resources to which they have access. Since adolescents ultimately determine their own behavioral patterns and since these behaviors develop from a number of motivational forces, one can only hope that the information they acquire is accurate and the adult examples to which they are exposed are sensible and of obvious merit.

Unfortunately, there is no secret formula for motivating adolescent girls to adopt healthful dietary habits. Many approaches have proved successful in home and clinical circumstances, and every health professional and parent finds certain tactics superior to others. Of great importance in any consultation setting is the establishment of rapport with the teenager. Unless a relaxed and nonthreatening atmosphere is created for discussion, little successful interchange can take place. It may develop that the concerns of the adolescent involve issues other than diet; the skilled health professional should stand prepared to provide guidance in important areas like social skills, complexion management, hygiene, and figure control. Not infrequently, the pregnant adolescent is in great need of "an understanding friend to talk to." The health professional who is not prepared to provide a listening ear may well find that the specific "nutrition or diet goals" she is pushing are totally ignored by the girls who see her as an authoritarian rather than as a friend.

SPECIAL PROGRAMS FOR PREGNANT ADOLESCENTS

Since the pregnant teenager is considered "high risk" educationally, medically, socially, and nutritionally, a variety of comprehensive community programs have been developed with the intention of optimizing progress and happiness of mother and infant. A wide range of program models has been initiated, and each community has been responsible for defining its own pattern of operation and scope of services.[21,26,29,47,54] Support for these programs has been handled in a variety of ways, and the quality and scope of service and training provided in any setting are often determined by level of funding and requirements of funding agencies. Despite the variability in program design and individualized funding patterns, almost all programs have at least three common service components[21]: (1) early and consistent prenatal care, (2) continuing education on a classroom basis, and (3) counseling on an individual or group basis. Sometimes all three services are provided by one community agency; more frequently, however, the services are offered through cooperative efforts of several organizations.

According to Howard,[21] most programs for pregnant adolescents have both long- and short-term goals and objectives. Long-range goals frequently aim at promoting competent motherhood, good health of the mother and infant, high school graduation, stable family life, maturity and independence, and avoidance of further out-of-wedlock (or unwanted) pregnancies. While

seeking to accomplish long-range goals, attention to immediate problems and needs may be necessary. Efforts are made to provide for continuation of regular education during pregnancy and reentry into regular school as soon as possible. Health care is provided during and after the pregnancy, and the expectant mother is taught how to care for the infant after birth. Counseling is offered as appropriate and necessary to help the young girl cope with the problems that led to or have been caused by her pregnancy. Of interest along this line is a recent study by Duenhoelter and associates[13] in which pregnant adolescent patients differed significantly from older patients in their involvement in a greater number of *recurring* pregnancies within eighteen months of the initial one. Attention to this potential problem by the skilled counselor should be of primary concern in programs for pregnant teenagers, since available data strongly suggest that the biological and sociological consequences of short interconception period in the young woman are often highly unfavorable for both mother and offspring.

The plan of attack therefore, in programs for pregnant adolescents, is to deal with pressing problems first and then move to more general goals. General goals relate basically to management of medical, social, and educational circumstances that will determine the long-range health and welfare of mother and child. Among the many issues requiring attention is the role of diet (or nutrition) in promoting growth and health in mother and baby. The pregnant adolescent should leave the program with an appreciation for the important part she plays in providing satisfactory nutritional support to the young family for which she is responsible.

Although well-planned programs for pregnant adolescents are relatively new in most communities, their importance in improving maternal and child health is well recognized. In most situations where good programs have been established, efforts are ongoing to upgrade and improve program design and to campaign vigorously for continued financial support from private and public sources. The number of girls served annually by such programs has risen gradually over the past decade.[54] It is still apparent, however, that considerable variability exists from one community to another, and in many areas the establishment of minimal services has not yet been accomplished. Available data strongly suggest that improvement of discrepant conditions around the United States is desperately needed. The challenge of the future for most communities is to describe community strengths and deficits and to establish comprehensive interdisciplinary services in accordance with needs of the population served.

REFERENCES

1. Aznar, R., and Bennett, A. E.: Pregnancy in the adolescent girl, Am. J. Obstet. Gynecol. **81:**934, 1961.
2. Ballard, W. M., and Gold, E. M.: Medical and health aspects of reproduction in the adolescent, Clin. Obstet. Gynecol. **14:**338, 1971.
3. Battaglia, F. C., Frazier, T. M., and Hellegers, A. E.: Obstetric and pediatric complications of juvenile pregnancy, Pediatrics **32:**902, 1963.
4. Beaton, G. H.: Nutritional and physiological adaptations in pregnancy, Fed. Proc. **20**(suppl. 7): 196, 1961.
5. Bernard, R. M.: The shape and size of the female pelvis, Edinburgh Med. J. **59:**1, 1952.
6. Bishop, E. H.: Prematurity, etiology and management, Postgrad. Med. **35:**185, 1964.
7. Blackburn, M. L., and Calloway, O. H.: Energy expenditure and pregnant adolescents. In Protein requirements of pregnant teenagers, final report to National Institutes of Health, Division of Research Grants, Grant No. H.D. 05246, 1973.
8. Butler, N. R., Alberman, E. D., and Schatt, W. H.: The congenital malformations. In Butler, N. R., and Alberman, E. D., editors: Perinatal problems, Edinburgh and London, 1969, E. & S. Livingstone, Ltd.
9. Calloway, O. H.: Nitrogen balance during pregnancy. In Winick, M., ed.: Nutrition and fetal development, New York, 1974, John Wiley & Sons, Inc.
10. Claman, A. D., and Bell, H. M.: Pregnancy in the very young teenager, Am. J. Obstet. Gynecol. **90:** 350, 1964.
11. Clark, J. F.: Toxemia is major complication in teen pregnancy, Obstet. Gynecol. News **5:**35, June 15, 1970.
12. Committee on Maternal Nutrition, Food and Nutrition Board, National Research Council, National Academy of Sciences: Maternal nutrition and the course of pregnancy, Washington, D.C., 1970, Government Printing Office.
13. Duenhoelter, J. H., Jimenez, J. M., and Baumann, G.: Pregnancy performance of patients under fifteen years of age, Obstet. Gynecol. **46:**49, 1975.
14. Edwards, C. H., Hogan, G., Spahr, S., and Guilford Co. Nutrition Committee: Nutrition survey of 6200 teenage youth, J. Am. Diet. Assoc. **45:** 543, 1964.
15. Finch, C. A.: Iron deficiency anemia, Am. J. Clin. Nutr. **22:**512, 1969.
16. Gold, E. M., and Ballard, W. M.: The role of family planning in prevention of pregnancy wastage, Clin. Obstet. Gynecol. **13:**145, 1970.
17. Hampton, M. C., Huenemann, R. L., Shapiro, L. R., and Mitchell, B. W.: Caloric and nutrient intakes of teenagers, J. Am. Diet. Assoc. **50:**385, 1967.
18. Hassan, H. M., and Falls, F. H.: The young primipara: a clinical study, Am. J. Obstet. Gynecol. **88:**256, 1964.
19. Heald, F. P.: Adolescent nutrition, Med. Clin. North Am. **59:**1329, 1975.
20. Hinton, M. A., Eppright, E. S., Chadderson, H., and Wolins, L.: Eating behavior and dietary intake of girls 12 to 14 years old, J. Am. Diet. Assoc. **43:**223, 1963.
21. Howard, M.: Comprehensive community programs for the pregnant teenager, Clin. Obstet. Gynecol. **14:**473, 1971.
22. Hulka, J. F., and Schaaf, J. T.: Obstetrics in adolescents: a controlled study of deliveries by mothers 15 years of age and under, Obstet. Gynecol. **23:**678, 1964.
23. Hsia, D. Y.: Human developmental genetics, Chicago, 1968, Year Book Medical Publishers, Inc.
24. Hytten, F. E., and Leitch, I.: The physiology of human pregnancy, ed. 2, Oxford, England, 1971, Blackwell Scientific Publications, Ltd.
25. Israel, S. L., and Woutersz, T. B.: Teenage obstetrics, Am. J. Obstet. Gynecol. **85:**659, 1963.
26. Kappelman, M., Kahn, M., Washington, V., Stine, O., and Cornblath, M.: A unique school health program in a school for pregnant teenagers, J. School Health **44:**303, 1974.
27. King, J., and Jacobson, H. N.: Nutrition and pregnancy in adolescence. In Zackler, J., and Brandstadt, W., eds.: The teenage pregnant girl, Springfield, Ill., 1975, Charles C Thomas, Publisher.
28. King, J. C., Calloway, O. H., and Margen, S.: Nitrogen retention, total ^{40}K and weight gain in teenage pregnant girls, J. Nutr. **103:**772, 1973.
29. Klaus, H., Meurer, J., and Sullivan, A.: Teen-

age-pregnancy: multidisciplinary treatment and teaching, J. Med. Educ. **48:**1027, 1973.

30. Lewis, B., Victor, M. B., and Nash, P. J.: Pregnancy in patients under 16 years, Brit. Med. J. **2:**733, 1967.
31. Marchetti, A. A., and Menaker, J. S.: Pregnancy and the adolescent, Am. J. Obstet. Gynecol. **59:**1013, 1950.
32. Minkler, D. H.: Fertility regulation for teenagers, Clin. Obstet. Gynecol. **14:**420, 1971.
33. Montgomery, T. A., Lewis, A., and Hammersly, M.: Maternal deaths in California, 1957-1962, Calif. Med. **100:**412, 1964.
34. Nelson, M. N., and Evans, H. M.: Relation of dietary protein levels to reproduction in the rat, J. Nutr. **51:**71, 1953.
34a. Ohlson, M. A., and Stearns, G.: Calcium intake of children and adults, Fed. Proc. **18:**1076, 1959.
35. Osofsky, H. J.: The pregnant teenager, a medical, educational and social analysis, Springfield, Ill., 1968, Charles C Thomas, Publisher.
36. Population profile: the teenage mother, Washington, D.C., June 3, 1962, Population Reference Bureau, Inc.
37. Recommended dietary allowances, Washington, D.C., 1974, National Academy of Sciences, National Research Council.
38. Schlaphoff, D., and Johnson, F. A.: Iron requirements of six adolescent girls, J. Nutr. **39:**67, 1949.
39. Schneider, J.: Identification of high risk pregnancy, Ob-Gyn Dig., p. 31, July, 1970.
40. Schorr, B. C., Sanjiir, D., and Erickson, E. C.: Teenage food habits, J. Am. Diet. Assoc. **61:**415, 1972.
41. Semmens, J. P.: Implications of teenage pregnancy, Obstet. Gynecol. **26:**77, 1965.
42. Shank, R. E.: A chink in our armor, Nutr. Today **5:**5, 1970.
43. Shapiro, S., Schlesinger, E. R., and Nesbitt, R. E.

L.: Infant, perinatal, maternal and childhood mortality in the United States, American Public Health Association Vital and Health Statistics Monographs, 1968.
44. Spindler, E.: Eating habits in teenagers, Food Nutr. News **39:**1, 1968.
45. Spindler, E. B., and Acker, G.: Teenagers tell us about their nutrition, J. Am. Diet. Assoc. **43:**228, 1963.
46. Stepto, R. C., Keith, L., and Keith, D.: Obstetrical and medical problems of teenage pregnancy. In Zackler, J., and Brandstadt, W., eds.: The pregnant teenager, Springfield, Ill., 1975, Charles C Thomas, Publisher.
47. Stine, O. C., and Kelley, E. B.: Evaluation of a school for young mothers, Pediatrics **46:**581, 1970.
48. Tanner, J. M.: Earlier maturation in man, Sci. Am. **218:**26, 1968.
49. Tompkins, W. T.: National efforts to reduce perinatal mortality and morbidity, Clin. Obstet. Gynecol. **13:**44, 1970.
50. United States Department of Agriculture, Agricultural Research Service: Food intake and nutritive value of diets of men, women, and children in the United States, Spring, 1975: A preliminary report, ARS 62-18, Washington, D.C., 1975, Government Printing Office.
51. Van de Mark, M., and Wright, A. C.: Hemoglobin and folate levels in pregnant teenagers,
52. Wallace, H. M.: Teenage pregnancy, Am. J. Obstet. Gynecol. **92:**1125, 1965.
53. Wallace, H. M.: Factors associated with perinatal mortality and morbidity, Clin. Obstet. Gynecol. **13:**13, 1970.
54. Wallace, H. M., Gold, E. M., Goldstein, H., and Oglesby, A. C.: A study of services and needs of teenage pregnant girls in the large cities of the United States, Am. J. Public Health **63:**5, 1973.

7

Lactation, human milk, and nutritional considerations

Bonnie S. Worthington

Lactation is an ancient physiological process accomplished by females since the origin of the human race. Today, as in times past, the process of breast-feeding is successfully initiated by at least 99% of women who try. All that is required of the lactating mother is an intact mammary gland (or preferably two) and the presence and operation of appropriate physiological mechanisms which allow for adequate milk production and release. The establishment and maintenance of lactation in the human is determined by at least three factors:

1. The anatomical structure of the mammary tissue and the adequate development of alveoli, ducts, and nipples
2. The initiation and maintenance of milk secretion
3. The ejection or propulsion of milk from the alveoli to the nipple

A thorough understanding of each of these factors is essential for proper and effective lactation management and for prevention of lactation failure in today's inexperienced mother.

MAMMARY GLAND

The mammary gland of the human female consists of glandular epithelium and a duct system embedded in interstitial tissue and fat (Fig. 7-1). The size of the breast is variable, but in most instances it extends from the second through the sixth rib and from the sternum to the anterior axillary line. The mammary tissue lies directly over the pectoralis major muscle and is separated from this muscle by a layer of fat, which is continuous with the fatty stroma of the gland itself.[22,35]

The center of the fully developed breast in the adult woman is marked by the areola, a circular pigmented skin area from 1.5 to 2.5 cm in diameter. The surface of the areola appears rough because of the presence of large, somewhat modified sebaceous glands, which are located directly beneath the skin in the thin subcutaneous tissue layer. The fatty secretion of these glands is believed to lubricate the nipple. Bundles of smooth muscle fibers in the areolar tissue serve to stiffen the nipple for a better grasp by the suckling infant.[22,35]

The nipple is elevated above the breast and contains fifteen to twenty lactiferous ducts surrounded by fibromuscular tissue and covered by wrinkled skin. Partly within this compartment of the nipple and partly below its base, these ducts expand to form

133

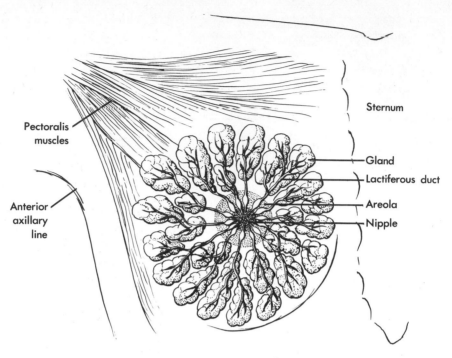

Fig. 7-1. General anatomical features of the human breast showing its location on the anterior region of the thorax between the sternum and the anterior axillary line.

the short lactiferous sinuses in which milk may be stored. The sinuses are the continuations of the mammary ducts, which extend radially from the nipple toward the chest wall with numerous secondary branches. The ducts end in epithelial masses, which form lobules or acinar structures of the breast (Fig. 7-2). The number of tubules and size of the acinar structures vary greatly in different women and at different ages. In general, the terminal tubules and glandular structures are most numerous during the childbearing period and reach their full physiological development only during pregnancy and lactation.[22,35]

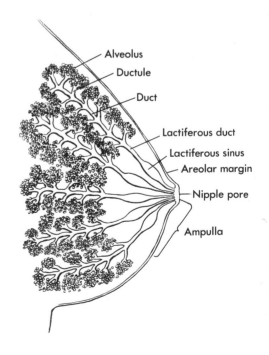

Fig. 7-2. Detailed structural features of the human mammary gland showing the terminal glandular (alveolar) tissue of each lobule leading into the duct system, which eventually enlarges into the lactiferous duct and lactiferous sinus. The lactiferous sinuses rest beneath the areola and converge at the nipple pore.

Wide variation in the structural composition of the human breasts has been observed in women after childbirth. Some breasts contain little secretory tissue; some large breasts contain less glandular tissue than much smaller organs. Engel[13] reported that in a series of 26 lactating breasts, only 16 showed what appeared to be adequate amounts of alveolar tissue. It is well known, however, that neither size nor structural composition of the breast significantly influences lactation success in the average woman. Almost all women who want to breast-feed find that they can.

BREAST DEVELOPMENT

In the human newborn the mammary glands are developed sufficiently to appear as distinct, round elevations, palpable as movable soft masses. Histologically, the future milk ducts and glandular lobules can be easily recognized. In many infants an everted nipple is apparent, and in about 10% a greatly enlarged gland can be palpated. These early glandular structures can produce a milklike secretion ("witches milk"), starting two or three days after birth. All of these neonatal phenomena related to the mammary glands probably result from the intensive developmental processes that occur in the last stages of intrauterine life; usually they subside in the first few weeks after birth. Some involution in the breast then takes place, and this is followed by the "quiescent" period of mammary growth and activity during infancy and childhood.[2,38]

With the onset of puberty and during adolescence, ovarian maturation and follicular stimulation are accomplished by an increased output of estrogenic hormone (Fig. 7-3, *A*). As a result of the response, the mammary ducts elongate and their lining epithelium reduplicates and proliferates at the ends of the mammary tubules. The growth of the ductal epithelium is accompanied by growth of periductal fibrous and fatty tissue, which is largely responsible for the increasing size and firmness of the adolescent female gland. During this period the areola and nipple also grow and become pigmented.

BREAST MATURATION

As the developing woman matures and ovulation patterns become established, the regular development of progesterone-producing corpus lutea in the ovaries promote the second stage of mammary development (Fig. 7-3, *B*). Lobules and acinar structures gradually appear, giving the mammary gland the characteristic lobular structure found during the childbearing period. This differentiation into a lobular gland is finished approximately twelve to eighteen months after the first menstruation, but further acinar development continues in proportion to the intensity of the hormonal stimuli during each menstrual cycle and especially during pregnancies. Fat deposition and formation of fibrous connective tissue contribute to the increasing size of the gland in the adolescent period.[22]

The mammary gland of a nonpregnant woman is inadequately prepared for secretory activity. Only during pregnancy do those changes occur which make milk production possible (Fig. 7-3, *C*). In the first trimester of pregnancy, the terminal tubules sprouting from the mammary ducts proliferate to create a maximum number of epithelial elements for future acinar formation. In the mid-trimester the reduplicated terminal tubules group together to form large lobules. Their lumina begin to dilate, and the acinar structures thus formed are lined by cuboidal epithelium. In the last trimester the existent acini progressively dilate in final preparation for the lactation process.[2]

The placenta has been found to play an important role in mammary growth in pregnancy. It is known that in some animals hypophysectomy, ovarectomy, or both can be performed after a certain stage of gestation without interrupting pregnancy and mammary development. The placenta has been found to secrete ovarian-like hor-

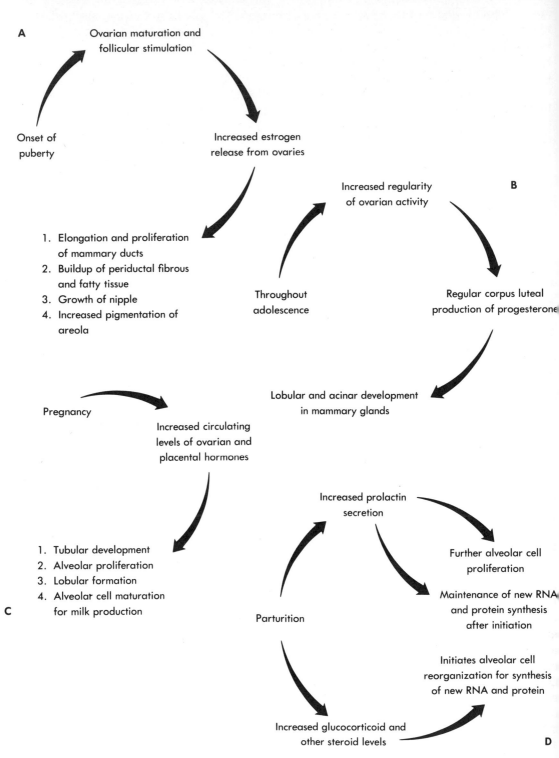

A

Ovarian maturation and follicular stimulation

Onset of puberty

Increased estrogen release from ovaries

Increased regularity of ovarian activity

B

1. Elongation and proliferation of mammary ducts
2. Buildup of periductal fibrous and fatty tissue
3. Growth of nipple
4. Increased pigmentation of areola

Throughout adolescence

Regular corpus luteal production of progesterone

Lobular and acinar development in mammary glands

Pregnancy

Increased circulating levels of ovarian and placental hormones

Increased prolactin secretion

1. Tubular development
2. Alveolar proliferation
3. Lobular formation
4. Alveolar cell maturation for milk production

C

Further alveolar cell proliferation

Maintenance of new RNA and protein synthesis after initiation

Parturition

Initiates alveolar cell reorganization for synthesis of new RNA and protein

Increased glucocorticoid and other steroid levels

D

Fig. 7-3

mones in large quantities. Human chorionic somatomammotropin (HCS) has been found to promote mammary growth and lactation in experimental animals and presumably is secreted in sufficient amounts to act with placental progesterone and estradiol to stimulate breast development in pregnancy. Mammotrophic activity has been detected in the placentas of rats, mice, and goats, and presumably it is also found in the placentas of humans.[2]

Although mammary growth and development occur rapidly throughout pregnancy, additional proliferation of parenchymal cells takes place shortly after parturition (Fig. 7-3, *D*). The proliferation of epithelial cells that begins just before parturition in response to increasing titers of prolactin results in daughter cells with a new complement of enzymes. The expression of new enzyme activities is the result of production of a new species of messenger RNA. A glucocorticoid is required for the synthesis of several enzymes involved in carbohydrate metabolism. An adrenocortical steroid is necessary also for redistribution of free ribosomes into the rough endoplasmic reticulum (RER). Once the RER is formed, prolactin is required for sustained RNA synthesis and subsequent casein synthesis.[2] Cowie and Tindall[9] suggest that both a mineralocorticoid and a glucocorticoid are necessary for optimal milk secretion.

PHYSIOLOGY OF LACTATION

Full lactation does not begin as soon as the baby is born. During the first two or three days after birth, a small amount of colostrum is secreted. In subsequent days a rapid increase in milk secretion occurs, and in usual cases lactation has become reasonably well established by the end of the first week. In primiparas, however, the establishment of lactation may be delayed until the third week or even later. Generally, therefore, the first two or three weeks are a period of rapid lactation initiation, and this is followed by the longer period of

maintenance of lactation. These two phases are not caused by precisely the same stimuli, but the basic physiological mechanisms that are operative are similar in both cases.

Initiation and maintenance of lactation is a complex neuroendocrine process. It involves the sensory nerves in the nipples and adjacent skin of the breast and chest wall, the spinal cord, the hypothalamus, and the pituitary gland with its various hormones, particularly prolactin, ACTH, glucocorticoids, growth hormone, and oxytocin.[2,22,35] The process of milk production occurs in two distinct stages, including the stage of secretion of milk into the alveolar lumen and the stage of propulsion, or ejection, whereby the milk passes along the duct system. Although the two events are closely related and often occur simultaneously in the nursing mother, they are best discussed separately for greatest clarity.

The secretion of milk involves both the synthesis of the milk components and the passage of the formed product into the alveolar lumen (Fig. 7-4). These events may be under independent control, since the accumulation of both lipid and protein, as observed by electron microscopy, reaches a high level during the latter part of pregnancy. Shortly before parturition the accumulated secretory products begin to be passed into the lumen, leaving the epithelial cells essentially devoid of biosynthetic products. Transport mechanisms for the milk components vary with the type of product secreted. Apocrine secretion of lipid droplets from the alveolar cells has been observed, but protein droplets appear to be released by a form of reverse pinocytosis. Fat is synthesized within the rough endoplasmic reticulum and is extruded as a droplet at the apical surface; it is synthesized primarily from free fatty acids and triglycerides derived from the bloodstream. Triglycerides as such as not absorbed directly into the mammary tissue cells, but these cells efficiently take up fatty acids and glycerol from the extracellular space. Additionally, short chain fatty acids may be

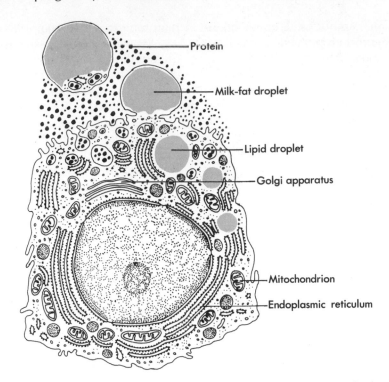

Protein

Milk-fat droplet

Lipid droplet

Golgi apparatus

Mitochondrion

Endoplasmic reticulum

Fig. 7-4. Diagrammatic representation of a mammary gland cell showing the basic cuboidal shape with typical microvillus border and basal nucleus. Cytoplasmic organization is characteristic of cells undergoing active protein synthesis and secretion. The synthetic apparatus consists of many free ribosomes and an extensive system of rough endoplasmic reticulum. A large Golgi body is located above the nucleus, and associated with it are some vacuoles containing fibrillar or particulate material that condenses into a central core or granule. Toward the apex the granules become progressively larger and contain more dense protein granules. The vacuoles fuse with the surface membrane and liberate their contents intact into the lumen. Fat droplets are found throughout the cell but are largest near the apex. They protrude into the lumen and appear to pinch off from the cell proper along with a small bit of cytoplasm. Other cytoplasmic structures include large mitochondria with closely packed cristae, lysosomes, and a small number of smooth membranous tubules and vesicles. (Modified from Lentz, T. L.: Cell fine structure: an atlas of drawings of whole cell-structure, Philadelphia, 1971, W. B. Saunders Co.)

manufactured from the glucose and acetate within the mammary cells, and enzymes associated with these reactions are greatly increased in their level of activity during lactation.[2,35]

Ultrastructural studies have clearly shown that the abundant rough endoplasmic reticulum is the site of protein synthesis in the secretory cell. Protein granules accumulate within the Golgi complexes in the form of macromolecular particles prior to transport through the cell and release into the lumen by reverse pinocytosis. The proteins in milk are derived from two sources: some are synthesized de novo in the mammary gland and others are derived as such from plasma. Inclusion of plasma-derived proteins in the milk secretion occurs primarily in the early secretory product colostrum. Thereafter, the three main proteins in milk (casein, α-lactalbumin, and β-lactalbumin) are synthesized within the gland from amino acid precursors. All of the essential and some of the nonessential amino acids are taken up directly from plasma, but some of the nonessential amino acids are synthesized by the alveolar cells of the gland.[2,22]

The predominant carbohydrate in milk is lactose, and its synthesis occurs within the Golgi apparatus of the alveolar cell in the presence of the enzyme lactose synthetase. Lactose synthetase is a unique enzyme with two protein components, the A and B proteins, production of which is under hormonal regulation, and both must be present before lactose synthesis can occur. Because of the constancy of concentration of lactose in milk, it has been suggested that the lactose concentration cannot vary under physiological conditions and therefore must play a decisive role in the control of the volume of milk secretion. Progesterone apparently inhibits milk secretion by inhibiting one component of lactose synthetase. Once synthesized within the Golgi complex, lactose is attached to a protein and released from the surface of the cell by vesicular transport and exocytosis as occurs with several other milk components.[22]

The stimulus for active milk secretion derives largely from the hormone prolactin (Fig. 7-5), which acts on mammary alveolar cells and promotes continual milk production and release. *Maintenance* of milk secretion, however, requires other galactopoietic factors from the anterior pituitary. If sucking is discontinued during the lactation period, pituitary release of these necessary hormones ceases and milk secretion usually stops in the following few days with accompanying atrophy and sloughing of alveolar cells.[2,35]

A variety of other hormones and exogenous stimuli are known to affect the process of milk secretion in humans. Estrogens, for example, affect milk secretion, probably by acting through the pituitary.

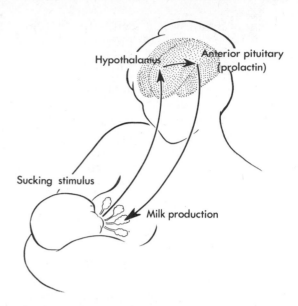

Fig. 7-5. Diagrammatic representation of the basic physiological features of milk production. The sucking stimulus provided by the baby sends a message to the hypothalamus. The hypothalamus stimulates the anterior pituitary to release prolactin, the hormone that promotes milk production by alveolar cells of the mammary glands.

The type of effect promoted by estrogens, however, has been shown to relate to the level of estrogens in the blood. When the blood estrogen level is low, as in the virgin, there is no prolactin in secretion. If the blood level is suitable, as occurs in parturition, the pituitary gland can discharge prolactin. When the estrogen level is raised beyond the point of adequacy, as occurs in pregnancy, the output of prolactin is inhibited. For this reason estrogens are used to arrest lactation where it is undesirable, as in the case of severe engorgement of the breast. The inhibitory effects of estrogens on milk production are less in the period of established lactation than in the early weeks of the initiation period.[22]

The effect of oral contraceptive use on lactation has received considerable attention in recent years. Filer[15] evaluated milk production in lactating women by assessment of infant weight gain in the first few months of life. Growth progress of infants fed by women using oral contraceptives was compared with growth progress of infants nursed by women not using the "pill." The average growth of breast-fed infants nursed by mothers not using oral contraceptives was 30 gm/day. In contrast, infants nursed by mothers using oral contraceptives gained only 20 gm/day. Similar results were reported by Miller and Hughes[33] and Koetsawang and co-workers.[30] There seems to be little question therefore that oral contraceptives at hormone levels utilized in these studies reduce milk production to a significant degree.[8]

Reported data, however, are not without disagreement. Barsivala and Virkar[4] reported that the use of low-dosage progestogen or long-acting progestogen does not result in reduced weight gain by infants. According to their observations, women taking a combination type of oral contraceptive and those taking low-dosage progestogens produced milk lower in protein, fat, and calcium content. Changes in composition of human milk were of statistical significance only for those samples obtained from women receiving the combination type of oral contraceptives. Comparable effects of oral contraceptives on human milk composition were reported by Abdel-Kader and associates[1] who found that a combined estrogen-progestogen tablet given to lactating women raised the fat content of breast milk and lowered its protein content. Observations of this type provoke considerable concern in proposing oral contraceptive use in developing countries; in these areas family planning is highly desirable, but infants are solely dependent on breast milk for initial survival and subsequent growth and development.

Active inhibition or suppression of lactation may be required for patients who may not or will not breast-feed. Estrogen preparations have been used for this purpose for some time, but side effects from this procedure have provoked continual concern.

An increased incidence of thromboembolism has been reported by several researchers,[10,27] and problems with abnormal uterine bleeding associated with gross endometrial hyperplasia have also been observed.[32] Recently the use of high doses of pyridoxine (600 mg/day) has been tested for its effect on suppression of lactation[18,32]; a high percentage of women exposed to this means of treatment have responded favorably within one week of administration, and additional work is under way to examine further the basis and acceptability of this antilactogenic procedure.

Once milk production and secretion have been accomplished, the baby may then obtain this milk by promoting its "ejection" from the alveoli and ducts. The "milk ejection," or "let-down reflex," is a neurohor-

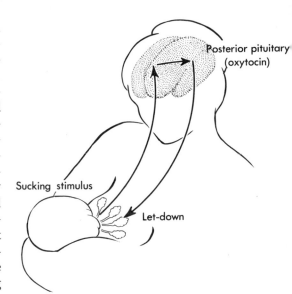

Fig. 7-6. Diagrammatic representation of the basic features of the "let-down reflex." The sucking stimulus arrives at the hypothalamus, which promotes the release of oxytocin from the posterior pituitary. Oxytocin stimulates contraction of the myoepithelial cells around the alveoli in the mammary glands. Contraction of these musclelike cells causes the milk to be propelled through the duct system and into the lactiferous sinuses, where it becomes available to the nursing infant.

monal mechanism regulated in part by central nervous system factors (Fig. 7-6). The primary stimulus is sucking on the nipple, which triggers the discharge of oxytocin from the posterior pituitary. Oxytocin is carried in the bloodstream to the myoepithelial cells around the alveoli, causing them to contract; contraction of these small musclelike cells pushes the milk out of the alveoli and along the duct system, where it is easily available to the nursing baby (Fig. 7-7).

The milk ejection reflex appears to be sensitive to small differences in circulating oxytocin level; minor emotional and psychological disturbances may influence the degree to which breast milk is "released" to the baby. The psychological importance of the milk ejection reflex in humans has been demonstrated by numerous case histories, which illustrate the fact that milk ejection can be inhibited by embarassment or stress and can be conditioned so that it is "set off" by the mere thought of the baby or the sound of his cry. This observation has been confirmed by experimental stimulation (or inhibition) of the milk ejec-

tion reflex so that it is now known to be easily accomplished. Signs of successful let down are easily recognized by the nursing mother. Common and significant occurrences include (1) milk dripping from the breasts before the baby starts nursing, (2) milk dripping from the breast opposite to the one being nursed, and (3) uterine cramps during nursing due to the action of oxytocin of the uterus.

The "draught reflex" also contributes to successful propulsion of milk through the ducts. Within several minutes after the baby starts to feed, most mothers experience a prickly sensation in the breast, which is called the draught. Milk is not always easily eliminated from the more distal parts of the duct system to the lactiferous sinuses where it is readily withdrawn by the baby. If the child is not allowed to nurse after the draught, he may have difficulty getting enough milk, since the draught reflex may not be obtained again for some time.

Sucking stimulation is widely accepted as the most effective means of maintaining adequate lactation. It is believed to be of even greater significance than the milk ejection reflex itself. There is considerable evidence in human subjects that the restriction of sucking significantly inhibits lactation. Artificial sucking stimulation in the form of manual expression or a breast pump has repeatedly been recommended as a means of increasing milk yield or maintaining yield in the absence of the baby.

By reducing feedings from six to five daily, Egli and colleagues[12] recognized a "not enough milk syndrome" in about one third of the observed primiparas and in several multiparas. Salber[39] subsequently studied 1057 newborns and determined that babies on a true self-demand feeding showed the most rapid weight gain and were nearest their birth weight at one week when compared with the 3- to 4-hour scheduled infants. Illingworth and Stone[25] also reported that self-demand newborns

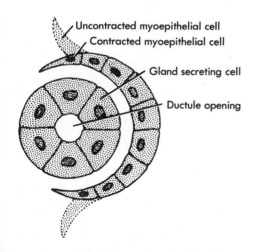

Uncontracted myoepithelial cell
Contracted myoepithelial cell
Gland secreting cell
Ductule opening

Fig. 7-7. Diagram of the mammary alveolus surrounded by a long, thin myoepithelial cell. Contraction of the myoepithelial cell promotes a "squeezing" pressure on the gland cells so that milk is forced to move along the attached duct system.

compared with newborns on a rigid schedule ate more frequently, gained significantly more weight by the ninth day, caused only half as much nipple soreness in the mothers, and were significantly more likely to be breast-fed beyond one month.

Local and cultural patterns of infant feeding are of great significance in determining the duration of breast-feeding for a given mother. Although successful lactation can continue as long as adequate sucking stimulation is maintained, a gradual fall in the amount of milk produced generally develops after twelve months. This drop in milk output largely relates to reduction of demand and cessation of recurrent stimulation of the nipple by the infant. In a survey of forty-six pre-literate cultures, Ford[17] found that in none of them did weaning occur before 6 months of age. In thirty-one of the cultures the earliest recorded age of weaning any infant from the breast was 2 or 3 years. It is clear from these and many other observations that the potential duration of lactation in most women is significantly greater than the period actually selected.

The phenomenon of lactation without pregnancy has been recognized as possible for many centuries. The Talmud describes a poor man whose wife died in childbirth leaving him without a means of feeding the infant. Miraculously he grew breasts and nursed the child through infancy. Other case studies have periodically appeared in the literature involving lactation by virgin girls and nonpuerperal women who have responded to vigorous suckling by infants with the resulting mammary growth and lactation. In these interesting cases it is likely that the ovarian or testicular hormones were present in sufficient amounts to initiate the developmental process.

Induced lactation in nonpuerperal women is still, in some areas, a well-recognized and accepted method of feeding infants whose mothers could not breast-feed or who have died in childbirth.[34,41] Breast-feeding of adopted children has been successfully carried out by mothers in the United States, Australia, and other parts of the world. Many cases of lactation persisting for long periods after pregnancy result from continued stimulation of the breasts. This phenomenon has been recognized since the Middle Ages, when grandmothers frequently maintained employment as wet nurses by putting suckling puppies to their breasts between jobs.

COMPOSITION OF HUMAN MILK
General

Large numbers of investigations during the past decade have been aimed at defining the biochemical and nutritional properties of different types of mammalian milk. It is clear from these efforts that each type of milk is unique and consists of a highly complex mixture of organic and inorganic compounds. Reports during the past ten years on the biochemical composition of human milk have included over 300 publications; large numbers of new components continue to be characterized such that more than a hundred constituents are now recognized.[28,29]

Basically, human milk consists of a solution of protein, sugar, and salts in which a variety of fatty compounds are suspended (Table 7-1). The composition varies from one human to another, from one period of lactation to the next, and even hourly during the day. The composition of a given milk sample is related not only to the amount secreted and the stage of lactation but also to the timing of its withdrawal and to the individual variations among lactating mothers. These latter variations may be affected by such variables as maternal age, parity, health, and social class. Although much data have been recorded on the differences in samples of human milk, the general picture is the same throughout the world. Except for vitamin and fat content, the composition of human milk appears to be largely independent of the state of nutrition of the mother. Even after prolonged lactation for two years or more, the quality

Table 7-1. Composition of mature human milk and cow's milk*†

Composition	Human milk	Cow's milk	Composition	Human milk	Cow's milk
Water (ml/100 ml)	87.1	87.2	Fatty acids (% un-	47	32.5
Energy (kcal/100 ml)	75	66	saturated)		
Total solids (gm/100 ml)	12.9	12.8	Major minerals per liter		
Protein (gm/100 ml)	1.1	3.5	Calcium (mg)	340	1170
Fat (gm/100 ml)	4.5	3.7	Phosphorus (mg)	140	920
Lactose (gm/100 ml)	6.8	4.9	Sodium (mEq)	7	22
Ash (gm/100 ml)	0.2	0.7	Potassium (mEq)	13	35
Proteins (% of total protein)			Chloride (mEq)	11	29
Casein	40	82	Magnesium (mg)	40	120
Whey proteins	60	18	Sulfur (mg)	140	300
Nonprotein nitrogen (mg/	32	32	Trace minerals per liter		
100 ml)			Chromium (μg)	—	8-13
(% of total nitrogen)	15	6	Manganese (μg)	7-15	20-40
Amino acids (mg/100 ml)			Copper (μg)	400	300
Essential			Zinc (mg)	3-5	3-5
Histidine	22	95	Iodine (μg)	30	47‡
Isoleucine	68	228	Selenium (μg)	13-50	5-50
Leucine	100	350	Iron (mg)	0.5	0.5
Lysine	73	277	Vitamins per liter		
Methionine	25	88	Vitamin A (IU)	1898	1025§
Phenylalanine	48	172	Thiamine (μg)	160	440
Threonine	50	164	Riboflavin (μg)	360	1750
Tryptophan	18	49	Niacin (μg)	1470	940
Valine	70	245	Pyridoxine (μg)	100	640
Nonessential			Pantothenate (mg)	1.84	3.46
Arginine	45	129	Folacin (μg)	52	55
Alanine	35	75	B₁₂ (μg)	0.3	4
Aspartic acid	116	166	Vitamin C (mg)	43	11¶
Cystine	22	32	Vitamin D (IU)	22	14‖
Glutamic acid	230	680	Vitamin E (mg)	1.8	0.4
Glycine	0	11	Vitamin K (μg)	15	60
Proline	80	250			
Serine	69	160			
Tyrosine	61	179			

*From Foman, S.: Infant nutrition, Philadelphia, 1974, W. B. Saunders Co., pp. 362-363.
†Data on proximate composition from Macy and Kelly (1961) for human milk, and from Watt and Merrill (1963) for cow's milk; percent of proteins from casein and whey and content of nonprotein nitrogen from Macy and Kelly (1961); concentrations of amino acids from Food and Nutrition Board (1963) except for alanine, aspartic acid, glutamic acid, glycine, proline, and serine, which are from Macy and Kelly (1961); concentrations of calcium, phosphorus, sodium, and potassium in cow's milk from Watt and Merrill (1963), whereas concentrations of other major minerals from Macy and Kelly (1961); iron and trace minerals from sources identified in Chapters 12 and 13 of Foman; concentrations of vitamins from Hartman and Dryden (1965) except those of folacin and vitamins E and K, which are from sources identified in Chapter 9 of Foman.
‡Range 10 to 200 μg/liter.
§Average value for winter milk; value for summer milk, 1690 IU/liter.
¶As marketed; value for fresh cow's milk 21 mg/liter.
‖Average value for winter milk; value for summer milk, 33 IU.

of milk produced by Indian and African women appears to be well maintained, although the quantity may be small. It is well known, in addition, that severely undernourished women during times of famine often manage to feed their babies reasonably well.[24]

Colostrum

In the first few days after birth of the baby, the mammary glands secrete a small amount of thick fluid called colostrum. It is yellowish and transparent and contains more protein, less sugar, and much less fat than milk produced thereafter. The energy value of human colostrum is lower (60 cal/100 ml) than that of mature milk (71 cal/100 ml), and the ash content of colostrum is relatively high.[22] Since the globulin content is also high, colostrum is frequently described as an extremely rich solution of globulin in a fluid that otherwise resembles milk (Table 7-2). Compositional analyses of human colostrum show striking variability during any one day and from day to day; it is likely that this circumstance partially reflects the unstable secretory patterns which exist in the mammary apparatus as it begins active production, secretion, and ejection of milk.

Colostrum changes to milk between the third and the sixth day, at which time the protein content is still rather high. By the tenth day the major changes have been completed, and by the end of the first month the protein content reaches a consistent level, which does not fall significantly again until near the end of lactation. As the content of protein falls, the content of lactose progressively rises. This is also the case for fat, which increases to typical levels as lactation becomes more firmly established.

Mature milk

Protein. It is well known that different animals show different rates of growth, and this appears to be related to the composition of their milk. The slowest rate of

Table 7-2. Composition of human colostrum (per 100 ml)*

Components	Quantities
Calories	60
Lactose (gm)	5.7
Total fat (gm)	2.5
Total cholesterol (mg)	13-36
Total protein (gm)	3.2
Casein (gm)	1.5
Whey protein (gm)	1.7
Calcium (mg)	27
Chlorine (mg)	88
Magnesium (mg)	3
Phosphorus (mg)	15
Potassium (mg)	74
Sodium (mg)	47
Sulfur (mg)	20
Copper (mg)	0.05
Iodine (μg)	12.2
Iron (mg)	0.1
Manganese (mg)	Trace
Zinc (mg)	0.57
Vitamin A (μg)	54-161
Carotenoids (μg)	85-137
Vitamin E (mg)	1.0-1.5
Vitamin C (mg)	1.4-7.2
Biotin (μg)	0.1
Nicotinic acid (μg)	75
Pantothenic acid (μg)	183
Vitamin B_6 (μg)	
Riboflavin (μg)	12-25
Thiamine (μg)	2-35

*Data from Macy, I. G., et al.: The composition of milk, Publication No. 254, Washington, D.C., 1953, National Research Council, National Academy of Sciences.

growth is found in humans, and human milk contains the lowest protein content. The major proteins found in breast milk are casein (curd protein) and lactalbumin (whey protein). It also contains a number of other simple proteins built only from amino acids and present in tiny amounts; the nutritional relevance of these small proteins has not been clearly determined. Overall, mature milk contains 1.5 grams of protein per 100 ml of whole milk compared with 3.5 grams in cow's milk. The differences largely relate to casein content, since human milk contains only one sixth that of cow's milk; the whey-protein content, both relative and absolute, is higher in breast milk.[22,29]

For many years it was generally assumed that the protein found in human milk was nutritionally superior to that of cow's milk. Lactalbumin (in whey) was thought to have a higher biological value than casein (in curd), largely because it contained more methionine and cystine. Amino acid analyses of the two milks, however, has revealed that they are similar, and both adults and babies have been kept in nitrogen balance when fed equivalent amounts of both casein and lactalbumin. Fomon[16] has shown, however, that 1-day-old breast-fed infants demonstrate a mean serum albumin concentration which is higher than that of evaporated milk–fed babies. Fomon maintains that human milk protein may, indeed, be superior and that serum albumin concentration may be a more sensitive index of protein quality than nitrogen balance studies or standard growth rate parameters.

Observations of many women in a variety of countries have shown that protein content of human milk is not reduced in mothers consuming a diet low in protein or poor in protein quality. A recent study in Pakistan supports this idea in that the protein quality and quantity of milk collected from women of a very low socioeconomic group in Karachi was similar to that of well-nourished women there and in other parts of the world.[31] Of interest, however, was the observation that the concentration of lysine and methionine in the free amino acid content of milk samples from malnourished women was reduced when compared with milk from healthy, well-nourished mothers. The investigators suggest that this finding could imply a reduction in nutritional *quality* of the protein in these milk samples. It seems important to recognize, however, that dietary amino acid deficits may be readily subsidized from maternal tissues as long as reserves are available from which to draw. Temporary fluctuations in free

amino acid levels may be apparent therefore, but alterations in quantity or quality of intact milk proteins are much less likely to occur until maternal protein stores are severely depleted.

Lipids. Nearly 90% of the lipid in human milk is present in the form of triglycerides, but small amounts of phospholipids, cholesterol, and free fatty acids are also found. The fatty acid composition of human milk differs greatly from that of cow's milk. The content of the essential fatty acid, linoleic acid, is considerably greater in human milk than in cow's milk; the content of oleic acid is also greater in human milk, whereas the content of shorter chain saturated fatty acids (C_4 to C_8) is greater in cow's milk. Of equal interest is the observation that human milk contains more cholesterol than cow's milk. A beneficial effect of this higher cholesterol content has been suggested by recent studies in experimental animals, which have shown that a dose of cholesterol seems to be required in the early weeks of life; otherwise, it appears there may be a risk of not acquiring the ability to maintain cholesterol homeostasis in later life, possibly because of inadequate development of necessary enzyme systems.[28]

The total lipid content of the milk varies considerably from one woman to another, and even more from one phase of nursing to another in the same woman. Several researchers have established that there is a diurnal variation in the fat content apart from the higher percentage found in the after-milk. After an ordinary period of milk release, about 20% of the milk remains in the gland, and this milk contains 50% of the fat. Hytten and Thomson[24] suggest that this phenomenon is due to the adsorption of the fat globules to the surface of the alveolar cells. It has recently been suggested that this changing fat composition of human milk during a feed may be one of the mechanisms of aiding appetite control of infants. The higher fat composition of the hind-milk in comparison with the fore-milk may serve to signal satiety in the infant and gradually motivate him to withdraw from the breast and cease feeding.

The composition of the fat in human milk varies significantly with the diet of the mother.[26,37] The fatty acid pattern of human milk can be changed significantly by modifying energy intake and fatty acid composition of dietary fat. Lactating women fed a diet rich in polyunsaturated fats, such as corn and cottonseed oil, will produce milk with an increased content of polyunsaturated fats. Such dietary changes do not affect the volume of milk produced or its total fat content. When calorie intake is severely restricted, fatty acid composition of human milk resembles that of depot fat. This circumstance is to be expected and represents fat mobilization in response to the reduction in energy intake. A substantial increase in the proportion of dietary calories from carbohydrate will result in an increase in milk content of lauric and myristic acids. The significance of this latter observation is unknown, but Sinclair and Crawford[40] reported increased mortality and reduced body size and brain cell number among rats nourished by dams whose milk contained a high content of short and medium chain fatty acids.

Of interest is a recent finding that human milk contains several fat-digesting enzymes or lipases. One is a serum-stimulated lipase (lipoprotein lipase) that may appear in the milk as a result of leakage from the mammary tissue. This lipase probably has no physiological function in the milk. The other lipase is inactive in milk, since it is secreted from the gland but becomes active when bile salts are exposed to it. This lipase, the bile salt–stimulated lipase, is believed to be present only in the milk of primates and is thought to serve some useful purpose for this species. Since the bile salt–stimulated lipase has been clearly shown to be stable and active in the intestine of infants, it may contribute significantly to the hydrolysis of milk triglycerides and partly account for the greater ease in fat digestion that is commonly demonstrated by breast-fed babies.[23,36]

Carbohydrate. Lactose is the main carbohydrate in human milk, and for a long time it was considered to be the only one present. Chromatographic processing of human milk samples, however, has revealed trace amounts of glucose, galactose, glucosamines, and other nitrogen-containing oligosaccharides. The role or significance of these minor carbohydrates has not been defined, but it is possible that one or more of them could contribute to the gut colonization by specific microorganisms with potentially beneficial effects to the infant. The nitrogen-containing oligosaccharides, for example, have a *Lactobacillus bifidus*–promoting activity. This organism has the property of breaking down lactose into lactic acid and acetic acid, and thus it is responsible for the acid reaction of the intestinal contents of breast-fed infants that may interfere with the growth of many enteropathogenic organisms.

The lactose found in human milk occurs in two forms, α-lactose and β-lactose. It is relatively insoluble and is slowly digested and absorbed in the small intestine. The presence of lactose in the gut of the infant stimulates the growth of microorganisms, which produce organic acids and synthesize many of the B vitamins. It is believed that the acid milieu that is created helps to check the growth of undesirable bacteria in the infant's gut and to improve the absorption of calcium, phosphorus, magnesium, and other metals. Since human milk contains much more lactose than cow's milk (7% and 4.8%, respectively), these gut-associated benefits of lactose are more significant in the breast-fed than in the bottle-fed infant.

The products of lactose digestion in the small intestine are glucose and galactose, and these monosaccharides are absorbed with ease into the portal circulation. The glucose component contributes to a variety of metabolic pathways; galactose can be converted to glucose in the liver or used as such for the synthesis of galactosides or cerebrosides of brain and medullary sheaths of nerve tissues. Galactose in some respects might be considered indispensable, and the contribution of galactose that is made by breast milk is probably of distinct significance.[2,22]

Minerals. The major minerals found in mature human milk are potassium, calcium, phosphorus, chlorine, and sodium. Iron, copper, and manganese are found in only trace amounts, and since these elements are required for normal red blood cell synthesis, infants fed too long on milk alone become anemic. Minute amounts of zinc, magnesium, aluminum, iodine, and fluorine are also found in breast milk. Infants who are not provided with fluoridated water in addition to breast milk may benefit from a daily oral fluoride supplement of regulated dosage predetermined by the physician and pharmacist.[28,29]

The total mineral content of human milk is fairly constant, but the specific amounts of individual minerals may vary considerably with the diet of the mother and the stage of lactation, although by no means is the variability as dramatic as that of the vitamins. Of all the minerals, iron and calcium appear to show the least variability from sample to sample, even though maternal diet may fluctuate markedly from day to day.[28,29]

One of the most striking differences between human and cow's milk lies in the mineral composition. As with protein, it is believed that this difference may be related to the rate of growth of the species for which the milk was intended. According to typical estimations, there is six times more phosphorus, four times more calcium, three times more total ash, and three times more protein in cow's milk than in human milk. The high mineral and protein composition of cow's milk distinctly affects the solute or osmolar load provided to the kidney. One might speculate that the kidney of the newborn infant is prepared to handle the solute load derived from breast milk but is "stressed" unduly by the requirements placed on it when cow's milk formulas are selected as an alternative.[28,29]

Vitamins. Breast milk is an important source of vitamins for the infant. All the vitamins required for good nutrition and health are supplied in breast milk, provided the diet of the mother is adequate. Movement of vitamins from the maternal serum into the milk product of the mammary gland is accomplished for most of the vitamins, but to varying degrees. In general, water-soluble vitamins move with ease from blood to milk, but fat-soluble vitamins encounter a little more resistance in transfer. This is especially the case for vitamins D, E, and K, which traverse the pathway with only limited success.

Until recently the vitamin D concentration in human milk was believed to be very low, yet breast-fed infants infrequently develop rickets. All of the early assays of vitamin D in human milk were made on the lipid fraction of the milk and the aqueous phase was discarded. It is now clear that most of the vitamin D in human milk is present as a water-soluble conjugate of vitamin D with sulfate. Such was the case in the milk of 22 women 3 to 8 days post partum and 14 women 4 to 6 weeks post partum. The vitamin D sulfate concentration in milk collected between the third and fifth days was 1.78 μg/100 ml, significantly higher than the 1.00 μg/100 ml for milk collected between the sixth and eighth days. After the eighth day there was no significant change.[30a]

Milk is a good source of vitamin A and its precursors. Its concentration in human milk is strongly influenced by the quality and quantity of the dietary elements consumed by the mother. The vitamin A content of breast milk is reportedly much lower in some developing countries than in the West; maternal serum vitamin A levels in these same regions are also typically low. Vitamin A (or carotene) intake of some Western mothers is higher in the spring and summer months because of greater supplies of green leafy and yellow vegetables; modern methods of preservation, however, have extended the length of seasons for many vegetables and fruits so that dietary differences from season to season may be minimal for many women with access to supermarkets, home freezers, and other such luxuries of modern society.

The vitamins whose content in the maternal diet is most greatly reflected in breast milk composition are ascorbic acid, riboflavin, and thiamine. Maternal dietary supplementation with each of these vitamins has been already shown to increase their content in breast milk. In well-nourished mothers human milk provides about 4 mg/100 ml of vitamin C. Unless the mother's diet is adequate in its content of vitamin C, the milk content of ascorbic acid will be low and infants may develop megaloblastic anemia because of the combined folic acid and vitamin C deficiencies. Likewise, maternal diet will significantly affect the levels of riboflavin, thiamine, pantothenic acid, pyridoxine, biotin, folic acid, and vitamin B_{12} in breast milk.

Resistance factors. A thorough discussion of the composition of breast milk of necessity must include mention of the beneficial components of human milk that are not classified as nutrients. One of the earliest resistance factors to be described in human milk was the bifidus factor, which as mentioned previously, is a nitrogen-containing polysaccharide that favors the growth of *Lactobacillus bifidus*. *L. bifidus* confers a protective effect against invasive enteropathogenic organisms, such as *Escherichia coli*. The stools of the breast-fed baby differ from those of the bottle-fed baby, not only in their appearance, odor, and consistency but also in their microbial population, which is dominated by *L. bifidus*.[29]

Various antibodies are also present in human milk, in particular the secretory IgA variety, which is found in large amounts in colostrum and in smaller, but still significant, levels in mature breast milk.[19] Secretory immunoglobulins have been shown to be a major host resistance factor against organisms that infect the gastrointestinal tract, in particular *E. coli* and the enteroviruses. In addition, a protective effect against other organisms has been demonstrated, and human milk clearly can be said to exhibit a prophylactic effect against septicemia of the newborn.

Some of the other host resistance factors in breast milk are also worthy of mention. Lysozyme, an antimicrobial enzyme, occurs at 300 times the concentration found in cow's milk. Lactoferrin has been described relatively recently as a compound with a "monilia-static" effect against *Candida albicans;* it inhibits the growth of staphylococci and *E. coli* by binding iron, which the bacteria require to proliferate. Lactoperoxidase, which has been shown in vitro to act with other substances in combatting streptococci, is also found in human milk. Of additional interest is the recent discovery that the lymphocytes in human milk produce the antiviral substance interferon. Macrophages are also found in colostrum and mature milk; 21,000/cu mm reportedly are present in a typical colostrum specimen. Macrophages are motile and phagocytic and have been shown to produce the antibody IgA. The role of the macrophages is still under investigation, but they undoubtedly have a protective function, both within the mammary lacteals and subsequently within the baby.[6,7,19-21]

Such host resistance factors as those described clearly have greatest significance in countries where infections are common and hygienic background is poor. Nevertheless, benefits have been observed in breast-fed infants in the so-called developed countries. In these areas the protective effects of human milk seem substantiated for necrotizing enterocolitis, acrodermatitis enteropathica, intractable diarrhea, and pathogenic *E. coli* infection. The incidence of these problems is clearly greater in babies who are not breast-fed.[2,15]

Diet for the nursing mother

The Committee on Recommended Dietary Allowances of the Food and Nutrition Board considers the optimal diet for the lactating woman to be one which supplies

Table 7-3. Recommended daily dietary allowances for lactation*

	Age (yr)			
	11-14	**15-18**	**19-22**	**23-50**
Body size				
Weight (kg)	44	54	58	58
(lb)	97	119	128	128
Height (cm)	155	162	162	162
(in)	62	65	65	65
Nutrients				
Energy (kcal)	2900	2600	2600	2500
Protein (gm)	64	68	66	66
Vitamin A (RE†)	1200	1200	1200	1200
(IU†)	6000	6000	6000	6000
Vitamin D (IU)	400	400	400	400
Vitamin E activity (IU)	15	15	15	15
Ascorbic acid (mg)	80	80	80	80
Folacin (μg)	600	600	600	600
Niacin (mg‡)	20	18	18	17
Riboflavin (mg)	1.8	1.9	1.9	1.7
Thiamine (mg)	1.5	1.4	1.4	1.3
Vitamin B_6 (mg)	2.5	2.5	2.5	2.5
Vitamin B_{12} (μg)	4.0	4.0	4.0	4.0
Calcium (mg)	1200	1200	1200	1200
Phosphorus (mg)	1200	1200	1200	1200
Iodine (μg)	150	150	150	150
Iron (mg)	18	18	18	18
Magnesium (mg)	450	450	450	450
Zinc (mg)	25	25	25	25

*Modified from Food and Nutrition Board, National Research Council, National Academy of Sciences: Recommended Dietary Allowances, ed. 8, Washington, D.C., 1974, Government Printing Office.
†RE = Retinal equivalent; IU = international unit. The recommended unit of measure is RE. 1 RE = 10 IU.
‡Although allowances are expressed as niacin, it is recognized that on the average, 1 mg of niacin is derived from each 60 mg of dietary tryptophan.

somewhat more of each nutrient, except vitamin D, than that recommended for the nonpregnant female (Table 7-3). The most significant increases are recommended for intake of protein and energy.

About 900 calories of energy are required for the production of 1 liter of milk by the adult female. During pregnancy, most women store approximately 2 to 4 kg of body fat, which can be mobilized to supply a portion of the additional energy for lactation. It is believed that storage fat will provide 200 to 300 cal/day during a lactation period of three months; this amount of energy represents about one third of the en-

ergy cost to produce 850 ml/day of milk. The remainder of the energy needs should derive from an additional 500 calories in the daily diet during the first three months of lactation. During this time, lactation can be successfully supported, and readjustment of maternal fat stores can take place. If lactation continues beyond the initial three months or if maternal weight falls below the ideal weight for height, the daily extra energy allowance should be increased accordingly. If more than one infant is nursed during the first few months of life, maternal calorie stores will be more quickly utilized and daily supplemental energy needs will double when maternal stores are depleted.[42]

For many women the usual slow rate of weight loss after childbirth may not satisfy their desires for immediate return to pre-pregnancy body weight. It is likely therefore that dietary restriction may be instituted, even though it is discouraged by health care professionals. It is important to recognize, however, that moderate to severe restriction of caloric intake during lactation will compromise the woman's ability to synthesize milk. This is especially significant in the early weeks of lactation initiation before the process is firmly established. As a result of this effect of caloric restriction on milk production, lactating women should be advised to accept a gradual rate of weight loss in the first six months after childbirth; otherwise, lactation success may be limited and the infant may suffer from insufficient milk supply to meet his needs.

The efficiency of milk production has been estimated by several researchers by the observation of energy intake and utilization of breast-feeding and nonbreast-feeding mothers. English and Hitchcock[14] compared the energy intake of 16 nursing mothers to 10 non-nursing mothers and found that the energy intake of breast-feeders in the sixth and eighth postpartum week was 2460 calories. The energy intake of non-nursing mothers during the same postpartum period was 1880 calories—a difference of 580 calories. In a later study by Thomson and co-workers,[42] lactating women were found to ingest 2716 cal/day and non-nursing mothers 2125 cal/day—a difference due to nursing of 590 calories. By adding the assumed energy equivalents of body weight being lost, total energy available to the two groups was 2977 and 2364 cal/day, respectively. If one assumes that the energy requirements for basal metabolism and activity are equivalent for the two groups, the energy needed for daily milk production is considered to be 560 calories; the production efficiency of human milk is therefore about 90%.

Along with the recommended energy increment, a 20-gram increase in daily protein intake is advised for lactating women. The extra protein is believed to be necessary to cover the requirement for milk production with an allowance of 70% efficiency of protein utilization. The increased needs for energy and protein can be easily met by consumption of about 3 to 3½ extra cups/day of whole milk. This will provide the needed protein and energy but will not cover the increased recommendations for ascorbic acid, vitamin E, and folic acid. It is therefore recommended that other foods such as citrus fruits, vegetable oils, and meat (or a suitable substitute) be increased slightly in the daily diet.

Maintenance of lactation while consuming a vegetarian diet can be managed nicely, providing all the basic principles of sensible vegetarian eating are followed carefully. The nutritional needs of the lactating vegetarian woman are the same as those of the lactating woman with a more traditional diet. Appropriate extra sources of calories and protein must be clearly defined; if dairy products are acceptable in the chosen dietary regimen, extra milk consumption is applicable here, as previously mentioned. If daily products are not included in the accepted list of foods, extra energy and high quality protein must be obtained from appropriately combined vegetables, grains, nuts, and other such sources. Calcium needs can be met by consumption of large quantities of green leafy vegetables and other significant sources of vegetable calcium. Dietary supplements may be unacceptable, and thus intelligent diet planning on a daily basis is of utmost importance for maintenance of successful lactation and health of the vegetarian mother.

Although lactation increases a woman's requirement for nearly all nutrients, these increased needs can be provided by a well-balanced diet. For this reason nutritional supplements are generally unnecessary except when there is a deficient intake of one or more nutrients. It is true, for example, if the lactating woman is intolerant of milk, that calcium supplementation (as well as alternative calorie and protein sources) would help to prevent unnecessary calcium loss from bones. Supplementation with iron is also advisable during lactation, not because of the increased needs during lactation, but for the purpose of replenishing her iron stores after their depletion during pregnancy.[24]

Whereas there is no evidence that calcium composition of human milk can be influenced by dietary intake of calcium, it is well known that dietary calcium deficiency promotes mobilization of calcium from bones to maintain milk calcium levels. Atkinson and West[3] have shown that healthy lactating women mobilize about 2.2% of femoral bone mineral in 100 days on a low calcium diet. If one assumes that this loss applies to the whole skeleton or body pool of calcium, which approximates 1.2 kg, the daily mobilization of calcium can be estimated as being 250 mg. It has been proposed that the relatively high incidence of osteomalacia and osteoporosis in the United States is partially related to the waning intake of milk and dietary calcium by adult women, particularly those who have supported multiple pregnancies and lactation experiences. Whether or not this is the case is still unknown. It stands to

reason, however, that prolonged lactation accompanied by poor calcium intake will significantly compromise the calcium status of the skeletal system and increase its susceptibility to fractures and other forms of trauma.

The cost of providing adequate nutritional support to the lactating mother depends heavily on what foods she selects to meet her nutritional needs. Some older studies suggest that human milk costs more than bottle feeding because of the extra nutrients the mother must consume. It is clear, however, in examining the costs of appropriate extra foods for the lactating mother that human milk is cheaper than proprietary cow's milk formulas if economical food choices are made (Tables 7-4 to 7-6). The present difference between the cost of cow's milk formulas and human milk undoubtedly will continue to increase in coming years, since the price of "double cycle" animal products (including cow's milk) continues to escalate. Beyond the price consideration, however, it is hard to justify "wastage" of human milk and the resultant unnecessary draw on the precious supply of other animal protein available to the world's population. Human milk represents a vital national resource, which if utilized to its fullest extent, could mark-

Table 7-4. Nutrients, amounts, and estimated cost of foods needed to meet additional nutritional requirements of a lactating woman: standard (nonbudget) plan

Suggested foods	Amounts	Cost*	Calories	Protein	A	C	B_1	B_2	B_3	Calcium	Iron
Milk, fresh, 2%	2 cups	0.21	290	18	700		0.14	0.82	0.4	576	
Meat (round steak)	2 oz	0.16	150	13	35		0.04	0.11	2.8	6	1.7
Vegetable, dark green or yellow, cooked (broccoli)	½ cup ¾ cup	0.12	20	2.5	1990	70	0.07	0.15	0.6	68	0.6
Other vegetable or fruit (grapefruit)	½	0.15	45	1	10	44	0.05	0.02	0.2	19	0.5
Citrus fruit (orange juice)	½ cup	0.07	60	1	275	60	0.11	0.01	0.5	12	0.1
Enriched (or whole grain) bread	1 slice	0.06	65	3			0.09	0.03	0.8	24	0.8
Totals		$0.77	630	38.5	3010	174	0.5	1.14	5.3	705	3.7

*Costs of June, 1976, Seattle, Wash.

Table 7-5. Nutrients, amounts, and estimated cost of food needed to meet additional nutritional requirements of a lactating woman: budget plan

Suggested foods	Amounts	Cost*	Cal-ories	Pro-tein	A	C	B₁	B₂	B₃	Cal-cium	Iron
Nonfat dry milk (prepared for drinking)	2 cups	0.05	180	18	20		0.18	0.88	0.40	592	
Peanut butter	2 oz	0.08	190	8			0.04	0.04	4.8	18	0.6
Vegetable, dark green or yellow, cooked (carrots)	½ cup ¾ cup	0.07	25	0.5	7610	4.5	0.04	0.03	0.04	24	0.45
Citrus fruit (tomato juice)	½ cup	0.05	25	1	970	20	0.06	0.04	0.95	86	1.1
Enriched (or whole grain) bread	2 slices	0.12	130	6			0.18	0.06	1.6	48	1.6
Totals		$0.37	550	33.5	8600	24.5	0.5	1.05	7.79	768	3.75

*Costs of June, 1976, Seattle, Wash.

Table 7-6. Cost per day of the most commonly used prepared formulas, basic equipment, and fuel

Formula	Cost*		Average cost per day	
Formula, 13 oz can, double strength (formula, ready-to-feed, 1 qt)	$0.57	($0.89)	$0.57	($0.89)
12 unbreakable bottles with nipples at 49 cents each	5.88		0.04	0.04
12 nipples at 3 for 51 cents	2.04		0.01	0.01
Energy, electricity			0.02	0.02
Total cost			$0.64 to	0.96

*Costs of June, 1976, Seattle, Wash.

edly improve not only the health and nutritional status of today's children but also the "natural resource base" of many underdeveloped countries.[5,43]

CONCLUSION

From many standpoints evidence supports the suitability of breast milk for the human infant. Nevertheless, bottle feeding prevails in the United States and is gaining widespread acceptance elsewhere. "Aside from the dedicated efforts of La Leche League members and their well-known counseling centers, little "national" effort is under way to assess critically the significance of this trend or to educate the public about the factors of importance in selecting the most appropriate means of nourishing young infants. The role of the health professional in filling this gap is only beginning to be recognized. Effective functioning as a breast-feeding counselor demands a thorough understanding of the process of lactation and a sincere desire to help inexperienced mothers decide for themselves about best approaches to infant feeding in their own circumstances.

REFERENCES

1. Abdel-Kader, M. M., Abdel-Hay, A., el-Safouri, S. et al.: Clinical, biochemical, and experimental studies, Am. J. Obstet. Gynecol. **105**:978, 1969
2. Arrata, W. S. M., and Chatterton, R. T.: Human

lactation: appropriate and inappropriate, Obstet. Gynecol. Annu. **3:**443, 1974.

3. Atkinson, P. J., and West, R. R.: Loss of skeletal calcium in lactating women, J. Obstet. Gynaecol. Br. Commonw. **77:**555, 1970.
4. Barsivala, V. M., and Virkar, K. D.: The effect of oral contraceptives on concentrations of various compounds in human milk, Contraception **7:**307, 1973.
5. Berg, A.: The nutrition factor, Washington, D.C., 1973, Brookings Institution.
6. Bullen, J. J.: Iron-binding proteins in milk and resistance to *Escherichia coli* infection in infants, Postgrad. Med. J. **51:**67, 1975.
7. Chandan, R. C., Shahani, K. M., and Holly, R. G.: The lysozyme content of human milk, Nature **204:**76, 1964.
8. Chopra, J. G.: Effect of steroid contraceptives on lactation, Am. J. Clin. Nutr. **25:**1202, 1972.
9. Cowie, A. T., and Tindall, J. S.: The maintenance of lactation in the goat after hypophysectomy, J. Endocrinol. **23:**79, 1961.
10. Daniel, D. G., Campbell, H., and Turnbull, A. G.: Puerperal thromboembolism and suppression of lactation, Lancet **2:**287, 1967.
11. Easthan, E., Smith, D., Poole, D., and Neligan, G.: Further decline in breast-feeding, Br. Med. J. **1:**305, 1976.
12. Egli, G. E., Egli, N. S., and Newton, M.: Influence of number of breast feedings on milk production, Pediatrics **27:**314, 1961.
13. Engel, S.: Anatomy of the lactating breast, Br. J. Child Dis. **38:**14, 1941.
14. English, R. M., and Hitchcock, N. E.: Nutrient intakes during pregnancy, lactation, and after the cessation of lactation in a group of Australian women, Br. J. Nutr. **22:**615, 1968.
15. Filer, L. J.: Maternal nutrition in lactation, Clin. Perinatol. **2:**353, 1975.
16. Fomon, S.: Infant nutrition, ed. 2, Philadelphia, 1974, W. B. Saunders, Co.
17. Ford, C. S. A.: Comparative study of human reproduction, New Haven, 1945, Yale University Press.
18. Foukas, M. D.: An antilactogenic effect of pyridoxine, J. Obstet. Gynaecol. Br. Commonw. **80:**718, 1973.
19. Goldman, A. S., and Smith, C. W.: Host resistance factors in human milk, J. Pediatr. **82:**1082, 1973.
20. Gothefors, L., Olling, S., and Winberg, J.: Breast feeding and biological properties of faecal *E. coli* strains, Acta Paediatr. Scand. **64:**807, 1975.
21. Hanson, L. A., and Winberg, J.: Breast milk and defenses against infection in the newborn, Arch. Dis. Child. **47:**845, 1972.
22. Harfouche, J. K.: The importance of breast-feeding, J. Trop. Pediatr., p. 135, Sept. 1970.
23. Hernell, O.: Human milk lipases. III. Physiologi-

cal implications of the bile salt-stimulated lipase, Eur. J. Clin. Invest. **5:**267, 1975.
24. Hytten, F. E., and Thomson, A. M.: Nutrition of the lactating woman. In Kon, S. K., and Cowie, A. T., editors: Milk: the mammary gland and its secretions, Vol. II, New York, 1961, Academic Press, Inc.
25. Illingworth, R. S., and Stone, D. G. H.: Self-demand feeding in a maternity unit, Lancet **1:**683, 1952.
26. Insull, W., Jr., Hirsch, J., and James, T.: The fatty acids in human milk. II. Alterations produced by manipulation of caloric balance and exchange of dietary fats, J. Clin. Invest. **38:**443, 1959.
27. Jeffcoate, T. N. M., Miller, J., and Roos, R. F.: Puerperal thromboembolism in relation to the inhibition of lactation by oestrogen therapy, Br. Med. J. **4:**19, 1968.
28. Jelliffe, D. B.: Unique properties of human milk, J. Reprod. Med. **14:**133, 1975.
29. Jelliffe, D. B., and Jelliffee, E. F. P.: The uniqueness of human milk, Am. J. Clin. Nutr. **24:**968, 1971.
30. Koetsawang, S., Bhiraleus, P., and Chiemprajert, T.: Effects of oral contraceptives on lactation, Fertil. Steril. **23:**24, 1972.
30a. Lakdawala, D. R., and Widdowson, E. M.: Vitamin-D in human milk, Lancet **1:**167, 1977.
31. Lindblad, B. S., and Rahimtoola, R. J.: A pilot study of the quality of human milk in a lower socio-economic group in karachi, Pakistan, Acta Paediatr. Scand. **63:**125, 1974.
32. Marcus, R. G.: Suppression of lactation with high doses of pyridoxine, S. Afr. Med. J., p. 2155, Dec., 1975.
33. Miller, G. H., and Hughes, L. R.: Lactation and genital involution effects of a new low-dose oral contraceptive on breastfeeding mothers and their infants, Obstet. Gynecol. **35:**44, 1970.
34. Mobbs, G. A., and Babbage, N. F.: Breast feeding adopted children, Med. J. Aust. **2:**436, 1971.
35. Newton, M.: Human lactation. In Kon, S. K., and Cowie, A. T., editors: Milk: the mammary gland and its secretions, Vol. I, New York, 1961, Academic Press, Inc.
36. Olivecrona, T., Billstrom, A., Fredrikzon, B., Johnson, O., and Samuelson, G.: Gastric lipolysis of human milk lipids in infants with pyloric stenosis, Acta Paediatr. Scand. **65:**520, 1973.
37. Potter, J. M., and Nestel, P. J.: The effects of dietary fatty acids and cholesterol on the milk lipids of lactating women and the plasma cholesterol of breast-fed infants, Am. J. Clin. Nutr. **29:**54, 1976.
38. Raynaud, A.: Fetal development of the mammary gland and hormonal effects on its morphogenesis. In Falconer, I. R., editor: Lactation, London, 1971, Butterworth & Co. (Publishers), Ltd.
39. Salber, E. J.: Effect of different feeding schedules

on growth of Bantu babies in first week of life, J. Trop. Pediatr. **2:**97, 1956.

40. Sinclair, A. J., and Crawford, M. A.: The effect of low fat maternal diet on neonatal rats, Br. J. Nutr. **29:**127, 1973.

41. Smith, I. D., Shearman, R. P., and Korda, A. R.: Lactation following therapeutic abortion with prostaglandin F_{2a}, Nature **240:**411, 1972.

42. Thomson, A. M., Hytten, F. E., and Billewicz, W. Z.: The energy cost of human lactation, Br. J. Nutr. **24:**565, 1970.

43. Wade, N.: Breast-feeding: adverse effects of a Western technology, Science **184:**45, 1974.

General

Raphael, D.: The tender gift: breastfeeding, New York, 1973, Schocken Books.

8
Guidance for lactating mothers

Lynda E. Taylor and Bonnie S. Worthington

Until the last century the continuation of the human species depended on a mother's ability to provide nourishment for her newborn child until he was old enough to feed himself. She was confident of her ability to nourish the child, since there was no other way. Today the situation is different. In one generation we in the United States have gone from a predominantly breast-feeding to a predominantly bottle-feeding society. This chapter will examine the advantages of breast-feeding and the reasons for its decline. Attention will then be given to the role of the health professional in teaching lactation techniques to new mothers.

ADVANTAGES OF BREAST-FEEDING
Morbidity and mortality

Around the turn of the century there was little knowledge of microbiology or of immunology, and bottle-fed infants suffered from a much higher incidence of diarrhea and acute gastrointestinal infection and, indeed, experienced higher mortality rates than breast-fed infants. Throughout much of the United States and the industrialized West, techniques for microbial control of the artificial diet have lessened the differences in mortality and morbidity rates between bottle-fed and breast-fed infants.

In 1951 Robinson[22] conducted a well-controlled study of differences in morbidity and mortality among breast-fed, partly breast-fed, and bottle-fed infants between birth and 7 months of age. He found that the incidence of all types of infections and mortality rates from these infections were significantly higher among bottle-fed infants. The illnesses were less severe, and recovery tended to be more complete among breast-fed infants.

Several other researchers have also noted that breast-fed infants seem to be more resistant to gastrointestinal infections, particularly those caused by *Escherichia coli* organisms. In severe outbreaks of *E. coli*–induced diarrhea among artificially fed infants in nurseries, Svirsky-Gross[23] was able to halt cross-infections and noted significant improvement of symptoms by feeding breast milk to these infants. The mechanism by which breast milk promotes *E. coli* resistance in babies is poorly understood, but it is believed that breast milk contains a factor which encourages the growth of *Lactobacillus bifidus;* this organism produces metabolic end products, which cause the bowel contents to become more acidic, thus inhibiting the growth of *E. coli* organisms. In addition, however, it has been reported that breast milk contains

155

specific antibodies to diarrhea-producing forms of *E. coli.*[15]

Growth and development

Bottle-fed and breast-fed infants follow similar growth curves from birth until the third or fourth month of age.[12] From the fourth month on the bottle-fed infant gains weight at a faster rate. The growth of the breast-fed infant, although slower, generally continues at a sufficient rate for catch-up to occur later in the preschool period. Long-term studies tend to suggest that this slow steady growth pattern may be more desirable for overall health and well-being of the young child. This idea is supported by the observation that bottle-fed babies are more likely than breast-fed babies to become obese in infancy, childhood, and adolescence.[17] Obesity among breast-fed infants is rare, in particular if breast milk provides the major source of calories during the first year of life.

Of additional interest is a recent report of differences in maxillofacial development between bottle-fed and breast-fed infants.[6] According to Graber,[6] malocclusion and other orthodontic problems may be more common in bottle-fed infants for several reasons. Of greatest significance may be the increased incidence of finger sucking in this group and the specific character of the sucking pattern established by the bottle-fed baby to extract milk from the artificial nipple.

Allergy

Allergy to breast milk is extremely rare. Some researchers question whether it exists at all. Occasionally, allergic reactions in the infant may be triggered by a protein that has been ingested by the mother and enters the breast milk supply intact. This, too, is rare. Treatment is usually not complicated; the offending food is traced and eliminated from the maternal diet. In one study of 262 infants totally breast-fed for six months or more, only 4.2% of the infants developed allergies; none became

allergic without a family history of allergy. This contrasts with an incidence of 12% among infants who are breast-fed for less than four days.[16]

One possible mechanism for the low incidence of allergy among breast-fed infants is the proposed capability of colostrum to promote gut closure in mammalian infants.[8] Although this property of colostrum has not yet been adequately studied in human young, the colostrum of most animal species has been found to decrease the permeability of the gut to macromolecules. Intact proteins are macromolecules, and many are sufficiently antigenic to promote an allergic response if absorbed. Early and effective gut closure theoretically should decrease the possibility of allergy problems.

Psychological development

The period of breast-feeding has been referred to as the period of "exterior gestation" because it provides continuity with the intrauterine environment while providing security and nourishment. Recent work by Newton[19] suggests that prolactin, coupled with sensory input from the baby, produces "mothering" responses in most women. Many women who have raised both breast-fed and bottle-fed infants state that they feel a special closeness to the breast-fed child which has persisted into adult life.

Satisfactory mothering and psychological development can be accomplished during bottle-feeding if the infant is held and cuddled during feedings. Even on the busiest days, however, there is no tendency for the breast-feeding mother to "prop the bottle" for her baby.

Maternal benefits

One of the earliest documented maternal benefits of breast-feeding is the effect of oxytocin on involution of the uterus. Early breast-feeding, even on the delivery table, stimulates contractions of the uterus that help to control blood loss. An increased incidence of thromboembolism has been noted among women who do not lactate. This is particularly true of women who have operative deliveries. In many of these studies it is not clear, however, whether the embolism resulted from the decreased involution of the uterus and resultant venous stasis in the nonlactating woman, or whether stilbestrol administration to suppress lactation was a causative factor.

It is commonly recognized that a definite tendency exists toward decreased fertility as long as a woman is supplying total nourishment for her child.[12] The stimulation of the nipples and resultant secretion of prolactin is thought to suppress ovulation in many women. This phenomenon is believed to be of major significance in promoting short-term child spacing in the developing countries. When solid foods become a major source of nourishment, nipple stimulation and prolactin levels decrease in the lactating mother and ovulation and menstruation usually begin again.

One of the prime benefits expressed by most women who breast-feed is the ease with which feeding is managed, particularly at night. The actual time spent nursing the infant may be greater during the first two weeks for the breast-feeding mother, since the infant eats more frequently to build up the mother's milk supply. More total time is spent in "nursing" by the bottle-feeding mother, however, since she must make the formula, sterilize tools and bottles, and heat the feedings before serving them to the infant.

Economy can no longer be used as a *major* reason for breast-feeding in the United States. Evaporated milk formula costs about the same as the additional food required by the lactating woman. This is not true, however, for most other parts of the world. Even in the United States commercial formulas are more expensive than breast-feeding; ready-to-feed formulas, the only type that rivals breast-feeding in convenience, are not within economic capabilities of many families.

It has been reported that failure to lactate might be a contributing factor in the increased incidence of mammary carcinoma.[12] Although it is true that there is increased risk among women who do not marry and women of low parity,[11] available information suggests that limited breast-feeding of one to two years total duration offers little protection against the development of breast cancer in later life.

INCIDENCE OF BREAST-FEEDING

In spite of the recognized benefits of breast-feeding for the child as well as the mother, the number of babies in the United States who were *artificially* fed climbed to an estimated 82% in the two decades prior to 1970.[10] Comparable statistics were reported from England and France in the period after World War II.[19] A recent report from the American Hospital Association, however, indicates that this trend is beginning to reverse.[1] The number of mothers who breast-feed was reported as 23% in 1971. This increase is largely among upper middle class, college-educated women.

The trend toward artificial feeding has recently spread to the so-called "third world" nations, partly as a result of commercial propaganda.[4,7,14] Formula manufacturers have endowed bottle-feeding with an aura of "snob appeal" by suggesting that it is the preferred method of feeding in industrialized nations. Unfortunately, the upper class parents in these nations who can afford artificial feeding and who can provide a relatively sterile and hygienic environment for the child are not the only ones who are "propagandized." Families with fewer resources are also swayed by the propaganda and may attempt to provide artificial formulas to their infants even though funds and storage facilities are insufficient to justify such action. Overdilution and contamination of formulas are major problems that compromise growth and health of infants in these circumstances. Artificial methods of feeding infants have been termed one of the most deleterious exports from the West. The World Health Organization states that the trend toward bottle-feeding "should not be encouraged."

There have been several attempts to determine why the change to bottle-feeding has been so sudden and widespread. The change has been much too rapid to be attributed to hereditary factors or major physiological changes. Although the reasons are complex and are poorly understood, they have been classified in four major categories: (1) changes in economic and social development, (2) changes in the woman's role, (3) attitude of the medical profession, and (4) commercial propaganda.

Changes in economic and social development

Economic development (an improved standard of living, relative affluence, and a monetary-based economy) has been associated with a decreased incidence of breast-feeding. Historians have documented cycles in breast-feeding popularity from earliest recorded history.[5] Breast-feeding was unfashionable during periods of great wealth but always returned to vogue during what Toynbee has called "times of trouble."

Changes in woman's role

Particularly in the United States, and in countries under its social influence, the movement for women's rights and the push for reevaluation of women's traditional roles have caused many women to view their role as a mother to be less valuable than their role as a wife-mistress or career woman. For many of these women breast-feeding is not in keeping with their image of the "modern woman." Although many women state that they prefer bottle-feeding because they "don't want to be tied down" or that they "must return to work," Newton[19] believes that the primary reason is ignorance about breast-feeding coupled with fear of failure in this role which is so uniquely woman's.

Attitude of the medical profession

The medical profession should assume part of the responsibility for declining breast-feeding rates both in the United States and abroad. Prenatal clinics abound with information on how to bottle-feed an infant. In fact, medical school curricula and textbooks routinely cover bottle-feeding and formula preparation with little or no time devoted to the physiology and advantages of breast-feeding. The result is a generation of health professionals who are neither convinced of the superiority of breast-feeding nor knowledgeable enough on the subject to be supportive of mothers who would like to attempt breast-feeding. It has been shown that physicians and clinics that are supportive of breast-feeding have built up practices with a greatly increased incidence of successful lactation.

Another factor that has had a detrimental effect on lactation has been hospital routines to which mother and infant are subjected in the neonatal period. These include procedures that delay the first feeding and/or severely limit the number and duration of feedings, separate mothers and infants for prolonged periods, discourage night feedings, give supplemental glucose water or formula, and promote rigid feeding schedules that hinder the establishment of lactation. Even though these procedures have not been proved beneficial to the infant, altering them for the purpose of aiding the lactating mother is often an uphill battle. It has been shown that mothers who have their infants with them throughout the day produce more milk than mothers who see their infants only at feeding time. Hospitals that allow rooming-in or modified rooming-in will generally have a higher ratio of successful breast-feeding mothers.

Commercial propaganda

Pressure from the manufacturers of infant formulas is widely evident throughout the United States and is even apparent in remote areas of Africa and South America. Whereas there is no formula that is *better* than human milk, there are many brands of artificial milks that are equal to each other in value. Therefore manufacture and promotion of infant formulas has become a highly competitive and very profitable venture. Samples are often provided to the hospitals free of charge by the manufacturer. Often free samples are provided for bottle-feeding and breast-feeding mothers when they are discharged from the hospital. Pediatric literature, both professional and lay, abounds with pictures of babies being artificially fed. Photographs of women breast-feeding are sometimes taboo; in fact, breast-feeding, even discreetly, in public places is still considered indecent exposure and is punishable by imprisonment and fine in several states. In view of these facts some researchers have remarked that it is a wonder the incidence of breast-feeding has remained above 5% to 10%.

ROLE OF THE HEALTH PROFESSIONAL IN ESTABLISHING LACTATION

The nurse's role has become increasingly more important to successful lactation over the past few generations. When most women lived in an extended family setting, there were abundant "models" for the new mother to emulate. She did not doubt that she could breast-feed her infant; her grandmother, mother, and many of her friends had breast-fed children. The presence of these older women was also a source of supportive advice. Jelliffe and Jelliffe[14] have pointed out that the knowledge of how to suckle the young of the species is no longer instinctive in primates. Chimpanzees reared in captivity who have never observed a suckling pair of their species have considerable difficulty establishing lactation. Many women today live apart from their families; they may never have observed a mother breast-feeding her child. Therefore they may need considerable support and instruction from some *other* source if lactation is to be a successful undertaking. The logical place for this woman to turn is to the nurse. A few

women are determined to breast-feed; nothing anyone says could change their minds. But many more, perhaps most primiparas, know nothing about breast-feeding and would be willing to attempt lactation with the help of a knowledgeable and supportive nurse.

The remainder of this chapter provides the basic information, procedures, and techniques to be used in teaching lactation. Most instruction is provided on an individual basis, counseling one patient at a time. However, larger clinics may find it beneficial to use group discussion sessions for the prenatal and follow-up sessions. Good results have been obtained in group sessions when the nurse is skilled in managing discussion and is adequately prepared with factual material and teaching aids.

Rarely is the nurse who conducts the prenatal session the same one who provides instruction at the initial feeding session in the hospital. Extra care must be taken to provide continuity of advice and methods when many people are involved. Information that is contradictory is often little better than none at all. Through the use of in-service training sessions, standardized manuals of procedures, and printed instructions for the new breast-feeding mother, one can be assured that mothers obtain consistent advice. A pamphlet published by the International Childbirth Education Association entitled "Instructions for Nursing Your Baby"[9]* is useful for hospitals and clinics that have not developed their own materials.

PRENATAL VISITS

It is suggested that both parents be included in the instruction sessions if possible. Fathers tend to be more supportive if they know what to expect and understand the difficulties that might be encountered. The prenatal visit affords the nurse the opportunity to get to know the parents, to

*Copies available from ICEA Supplies Center, P.O. Box 70258, Seattle, Wash. 98107 (cost: about $5.00 per 100).

find out how much they know about breast-feeding, to determine what fears and apprehensions they may have, and to estimate how much help and support the mother is likely to need in the early weeks of breast-feeding. It is well to remember that there is no typical breast-feeding personality; women who appear to be "nervous" can learn to breast-feed successfully if they can cultivate a relaxed and confident attitude toward feeding. This is best accomplished by adequate instruction and professional support.

Physiology and diet

The nurse should discuss the advantages of breast-feeding; she should listen and respond to any concerns that the parents may have. The physiology of lactation should be covered in as much detail as the parents are able to handle. A good understanding of physiology is a great aid in promoting confidence in the ability to lactate. Simplified diagrams and explanations such as those provided on pp. 140 and 141 may be useful.

A brief discussion of the dietary requirements for lactation should be included in the prenatal visits. It is usually sufficient to stress that additional amounts of the same types of food that belong in any well-balanced diet, with special attention to fluid intake and a source of calcium and of vitamin C, will adequately provide the additional requirement for approximately 500 to 600 calories.

Nipple conditioning

During the prenatal session the nurse can also teach exercises for nipple conditioning that will help to prevent nipple soreness once lactation begins. In societies where the breast is uncovered or where clothing is loosely worn, nipple soreness is much less of a problem. The woman who plans to breast-feed should purchase a "nursing brassiere" which will suffice for the increased size required for the last few months of pregnancy as well as for lactation. If the woman's breasts are very heavy,

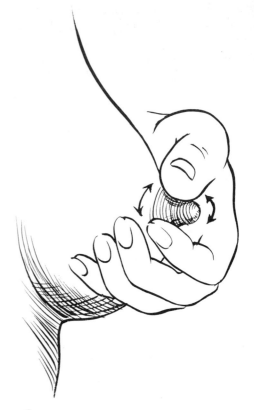

Fig. 8-1. Diagrammatic representation of a proposed method for preparation of nipples for breast-feeding.

or if she feels uncomfortable with the weight unsupported, the brassiere can be worn day and night. One of the easiest ways to get the nipples used to tactile stimulation is to leave the flaps on the brassiere open as much as possible during the day and at night. This allows the nipples to rub against clothing and gradually desensitizes them.

Some women have found a simple exercise to be of benefit (Fig. 8-1). The nipple is grasped gently but firmly between the thumb and index finger and is rolled back and forth between them while maintaining slight traction on the nipple. The grasp is then rotated one quarter turn so that all areas of the nipple are stimulated. The exercise is then repeated on the other side. It can be done two or three times a day during the last trimester and is particularly helpful for nipples that tend to invert. A few women have found that brisk rubbing of the nipple with a terry cloth towel after bathing is also useful in the process of desensitization. Attempts to express milk or colostrum manually before parturition accomplish little and may leave the breast open to infection.

No special ointments or preparations are generally required for nipple conditioning. Pure lanolin appears to be harmless, but products containing alcohol and petroleum-based products are too harsh for the nipple and areola. Since soap is drying and removes the natural lubricant of the areola, it is advisable to wash the nipple area with water only.

Effect of anesthetics

The last major consideration to be discussed during prenatal visits is the effect on early feedings of anesthetics and analgesics given during labor and birth. Recent research has indicated that even the nerve conduction anesthetics affect the reflexes in the newborn and may impair his ability to suck well. The baby may be lethargic and disinterested in feeding or may take the breast and suck only weakly until the effects of anesthesia have worn off. This information may be useful to the patient in selecting an anesthetic. If the baby is uncooperative because of sedation, he can still be breast-fed successfully; it will probably take a few days longer to establish a let-down reflex and to promote production of an adequate milk supply. The baby who is severely affected may not suck well until the third or fourth day of life. With the current trend toward early hospital discharges, it might be well to keep mother and baby in the hospital for an extra day or to provide good follow-up care at home to ensure that lactation gets off to a good start.

The mother should be encouraged to jot down questions that arise. Several excellent books on breast-feeding are referenced at the end of this chapter. Most are available in paperback and from public libraries. Some large clinics have established their own lending libraries. Some women will benefit from talking with mothers who are already successfully breast-feeding. If no suitable candidates can be found from office files, local chapters of La Leche League International will usually be able to assist the parents.

THE FIRST FEEDING

The most critical period in the establishment of lactation is the first few days. Fortunately, this is also the time when most new mothers are confined in a hospital and can receive almost continuous instruction and support from the hospital nurse who has been trained in the techniques of breast-feeding.

Timing

Although many hospital routines prohibit early feeding, the overwhelming bulk of recent research shows that the best time for the first feeding, providing that mother and baby are physically able, is within a half hour after birth. This can even be accomplished on the delivery table. A study by Archavsky[3] has shown that the sucking reflex is strongest twenty to thirty minutes after birth and that if the infant is not fed at this time, the vigorous sucking reflex diminishes and does not return until the end of the second day of life. The first few feedings will provide colostrum, which has been shown to be highly beneficial to the infant. Colostrum provides more protein, less sugar, less fat, and more of many minerals than does milk. The globulin content is high. The apparent resistance of many breast-fed infants to viral and bacterial infections has led researchers to speculate that some form of immunity may be conferred by colostrum in the early days of life. In addition to colostrum's nutritional bonus for the infant, drainage of this viscous material from the ducts in prelacteal feedings prevents problems of stasis and engorgement and stimulates milk production.

There is no scientific support for the practice of giving glucose water for the first feeding.

Breast-feeding will probably be a new experience for the mother as well as for the baby. The mother may be apprehensive and unsure of herself; she may need help and guidance in handling the infant. The nurse who is to instruct her at the first feeding should inquire as to her preference for privacy; try to make her feel as much at ease as possible. A matter-of-fact attitude on the part of the nursing staff will do much to break down inhibitions. The father should be encouraged to be present at feedings and during instruction if the hospital permits it and if the mother is comfortable with his presence. The father's support, knowledge, and understanding will be valuable later on; he may remember advice and techniques that she has forgotten.

Positions

There are two basic breast-feeding positions each of which is subject to a wide variety of individual adaptations. The chief requirements are the comfort of the mother throughout the feeding and the positioning of the baby so that the process of swallowing is not impaired. If the mother has had an episiotomy or operative delivery, she may be more comfortable breast-feeding lying down. She should position herself comfortably on her side, using pillows for additional support as required. The baby should be placed on his side with his mouth parallel to the nipple. A roll of receiving blankets makes a good support for baby's back (Fig. 8-2). The baby can then feed comfortably from the lower breast without undue nipple traction or unnecessary distortion of his alimentary tract. Both the baby and mother will probably need help in repositioning to feed from the other breast. A variation of this position is shown in Fig. 8-3 and can be used if the nipples become tender. Reversing the baby's position so that his feet are toward his mother's head will allow slightly different areas of the nipple to be stimulated and often affords some relief.

The second common position for breast-

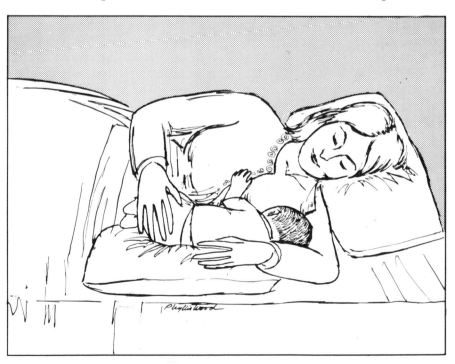

Fig. 8-2. Recommended recumbent positioning for breast-feeding.

feeding is for the mother to sit in a comfortable chair that provides good back support, arm rests, and if possible, foot and leg support. She then cradles the baby in her arm, placing his head over her elbow so that his mouth is adjacent to the nipple. A pillow may be required on her lap to support the baby's body and/or under her elbow to prevent her arm from becoming too tired while holding baby's head in the proper position for feeding. This procedure is illustrated in Fig. 8-4 and must be reversed for feeding on the opposite side. This position can be modified for use in the hospital bed (Fig. 8-5). If this is to be successful, the head of the bed should be raised fully and the foot adjusted to provide back and leg support. Pillows will be required to support the arm holding the baby's head. An additional blanket or pillow under the mother's knees may make the position more comfortable. The position should be checked after feeding has begun to make sure that nipple traction and distortion of the infant's alimentary tract are at a minimum.

Best results are obtained when both breasts are offered at each feeding. Once the infant has fed 5 to 10 minutes on one side, the position should be reversed and the other breast offered. Over the next couple of days the feedings can be lengthened to 10 to 15 minutes per side.

Taking advantage of reflexes

There are several reflexes operative in the process of breast-feeding, and most mothers will need to be taught to take advantage of these. The rooting, sucking, and swallowing reflexes are generally well developed in the full-term newborn at birth. Poor understanding of the rooting reflex in particular can create frustration for the mother and infant and may cause the nurse to advise bottle-feeding because the "infant fights the breast." The rooting reflex causes the infant to turn his face in the direction of the stimulation when his cheek is stroked. Thus pressure on the left side of his face by a well-meaning hand trying to turn his face to the right will actually produce the opposite result. The mother

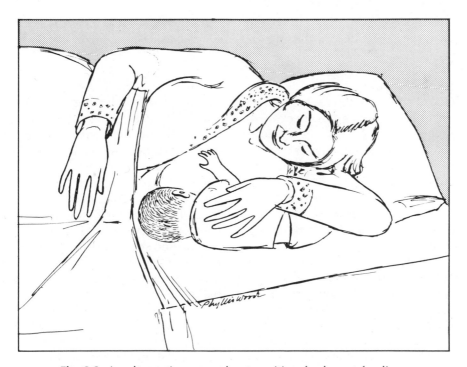

Fig. 8-3. An alternative recumbent position for breast-feeding.

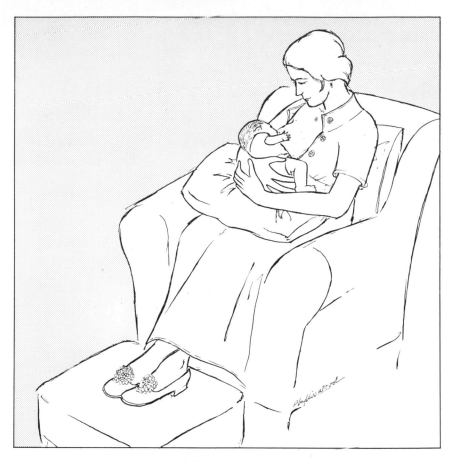

Fig. 8-4. Recommended positioning for breast-feeding while sitting in a comfortable chair.

can be taught to use this reflex to her advantage by gently stroking the cheek nearest the nipple with the nipple or her forefinger. The baby will automatically turn his head and open his mouth, eager for the waiting nipple. Sucking and swallowing reflexes occur naturally in most infants. If problems arise, most physical therapists can suggest simple exercises and procedures to promote proper function.

The prolactin and let-down reflexes generally need some conditioning before they occur spontaneously. Prolactin, the main hormone responsible for milk production, is stimulated by the infant's sucking. The let-down reflex is basically a psychosomatic reflex. Its somatic component functions much like the prolactin reflex. The infant's sucking causes the secretion of oxytocin, which, in turn, is responsible for contraction of the myoepithelial cells around the alveoli. This makes the milk available to the baby. This reflex is extremely sensitive to the mother's mood; anxiety, fear, and distraction impair its function. Newton and Newton[20] showed that in mothers who had established successful lactation, distraction before and during a feeding reduced the infant's available milk supply by almost one half. This may be even more critical in the woman for whom this reflex is not fully conditioned. For this reason confidence, support, and a proper psychological outlook are critical during this period. It may take

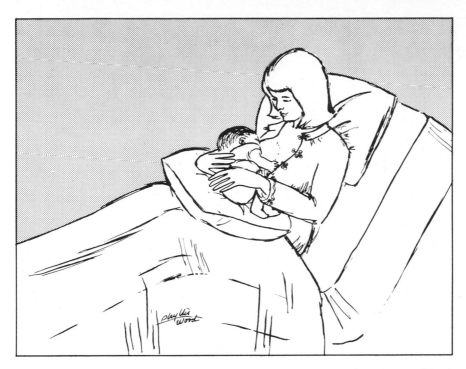

Fig. 8-5. Modified positioning for breast-feeding while sitting in a hospital bed.

several days or even weeks for the reflex to become fully functional. When it does, most women experience a tingling sensation in the breast, and milk may begin to drip from one or both breasts. Some women find that just thinking about feeding the baby or hearing him cry may cause a let-down reflex at an inappropriate time, particularly in the first couple of weeks. This can often be stopped by pressing hard against the nipples with the heels of the hands until the tingling stops. Soaking of clothing can be prevented by wearing cotton pads inside the nursing brassiere. Pads should be changed when they become damp. If allowed to dry, they may stick to the nipple and can cause nipple damage; also, the milk may be a source of bacterial growth. A soft cotton handkerchief provides a recyclable substitute for disposable pads. Pads with plastic backing should be avoided as these prevent air from circulating around the nipple and can cause nipple soreness and cracking.

Initiation and termination of feedings

Most new breast-feeding mothers will also benefit from a few hints on the initiation and termination of feedings. Poor techniques for nipple grasp and release are one of the main contributors to nipple discomfort. The areola should be grasped lightly between the forefinger and middle finger of the free hand and flattened slightly to correspond with the oval shape of the infant's mouth. This helps to ensure that a good portion of the areola, and not just the nipple, will be grasped by the infant (Fig. 8-6). The forefinger can be used to restrain breast tissue from blocking the baby's nostrils, particularly while the breast is full (Fig. 8-7). To release the suction before removing the nipple from the infant's mouth, the mother should insert the little finger of her free hand into the corner of the infant's mouth. This is one good reason to encourage the mother to wash her hands before each feeding. If the baby has a particularly tenacious grip and this technique

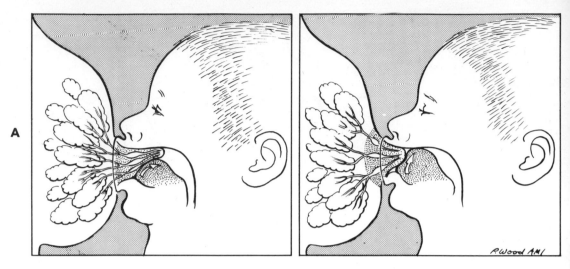

Fig. 8-6. Diagram showing adequate and inadequate methods of nipple grasp by the nursing infant. **A,** The nipple is drawn thoroughly into the mouth with the aid of the tongue. The baby's lips almost completely encompass the areola. **B,** The nipple is only partially grasped by the infant's mouth so that an adequate milking sequence cannot be established.

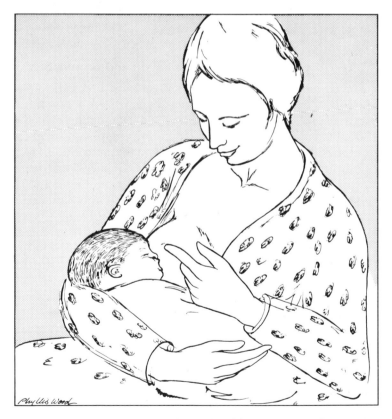

Fig. 8-7. Diagrammatic representation of a method for restraining breast tissue with the forefinger so that the baby's nostrils will not be blocked while nursing.

does not work, blocking his nostrils so that he must let go to take a breath will accomplish the same result. To attempt to pull the nipple from his mouth will cause pain and possible nipple damage.

Alternate massage

Iffrig[13] found that a technique of "alternate massage" was helpful to many of her patients in providing good milk drainage while the let-down reflex was being established. The mother needs to learn to distinguish the long, rhythmic suck and swallow when the infant is drawing nourishment from the short, choppy jaw movements when he is not. Once he has exhausted the readily available milk supply, the breast is gently massaged in a circular pattern by the fingertips of her free hand. This pushes more milk into the ducts and sinuses, which can then be readily removed by the infant. This massage should be done, one quadrant at a time, until the entire breast has been drained.

The uncooperative baby

There are many reasons why a baby may be an uncooperative feeder, even with the best efforts on his mother's part. A baby who is groggy with sedation will feed poorly, as will one who has been filled with water or formula in the hospital nursery in an attempt to placate him until it is "time for" a breast-feeding. A baby who is hysterical from hunger or for any other reason will also be difficult to feed. It may be well for the mother to try to settle him down before he is offered food. In any case if the mother is really trying and the baby is still uncooperative, the nurse should help the mother to realize that she is doing a good job and that the lack of success at this feeding is really not her fault. This mother will need additional help and support at the next feeding. Above all, the staff should try to minimize as many of the nursery-caused deterrents to lactation as possible before the next feeding.

Frequency and duration of feeding

Much research has focused on the frequency and duration of feedings during the first few days of life. A considerable amount of controversy exists even today, since many of the findings of this research directly conflict with hospital routine. Early recommendations to women in the United States advised four feedings during the first day of life, six on the second day, ten a day during the first month, eight a day for the second and third month, seven a day for the fourth and fifth months, and six a day until the eleventh month when gradual weaning took place.

Olmstead and Jackson,[21] who studied 100 newborn breast-fed infants on a self-demand schedule, found that the average number of feedings per day throughout the first week of life was as follows:

Day: 1 2 3 4 5 6 7
Feedings: 6.2 6.9 8.1 8.6 8.5 8.3 7.0

The wide variations observed between infants and variation in the pattern of any given infant from day to day could not be accommodated on a rigid feeding schedule.

Demand feedings have been shown to have a beneficial effect on the milk supply, since the breasts tend to be emptied more fully.[2] Demand feedings also reduce the incidence of engorgement, result in better weight gain by the infant, and reduce the frequency and severity of nipple discomfort. Routine administration of sleeping medication to breast-feeding mothers is not advisable, since night feedings are critical to the early establishment of the milk supply and the prevention of breast engorgement. It has been shown that even one bottle during the critical period of "imprinting" of feeding behavior can have an adverse effect on the sucking reflex.

There is also little scientific support for severely limiting the duration of feedings during the first few days. This merely delays, not prevents, the onset of nipple discomfort. Since it may take 2 or 3 minutes to establish a let-down reflex, removal of the infant from the breast before this has occurred will accomplish little. It has been shown that allowing the infant to suck on an empty breast causes more nipple discomfort than do feedings of moderate duration. The breast is usually empty after about 7 to 10 minutes of sucking. It is not necessary to prolong a feeding beyond this point if the nipples are tender.

Mothers should realize that infants are highly variable in their eating patterns but that it is not uncommon for the breast-fed infant to want to eat every 1½ to 2 hours. This is not surprising when one considers the infant's limited stomach capacity, the good digestibility of human milk, and the gradual process of establishing an adequate milk supply.

The new breast-feeding mother should be provided in printed form with reliable information on the maintenance of lactation (as covered in the following section). This will give her a reference for answers to some of the questions that have not yet come up. Also, it is often helpful if she has the name and telephone number of someone knowledgeable in breast-feeding techniques to whom she can turn in an emergency. Often the clinic or hospital nurse can fill this need. In some cities public health nurses routinely handle follow-up for new mothers. In any case the person assigned the follow-up duty should receive the same training as the clinic and hospital nurse so that continuity of advice is assured.

MAINTENANCE OF LACTATION

Even though the prenatal and early postnatal assistance with lactation may have been of high quality, it is likely that young mothers will have additional problems and questions during the occasional crisis periods of the first few weeks. During this time a variety of concerns often develop, and attention to them may well determine the duration of breast-feeding for the distraught mother.

Typical concerns of the new breast-feeding mother

Milk is produced to equal demand in almost all women. If the let-down reflex is functioning adequately, insufficient milk is rarely a problem. The reason for the mother's concern may derive from a well-meaning friend or relative who has said that breast-feeding is something that many women cannot do successfully. Nurses should try to impress on the new breast-feeding mother that in many societies *all* women breast-feed. Virtually all women in United States society who really want to breast-feed can do it too! If feeding sessions have been frequent and of adequate duration, the milk supply is probably ample.

Mothers may need to be reminded that babies do not always cry from hunger. Sometimes they may need to be "bubbled," or have diapers changed; often they require companionship, and sometimes a baby seems to need to cry—for no apparent reason. If the baby is growing well and has at least six wet diapers a day (assuming he is receiving no additional water or formula), the mother should be comforted by knowing that the milk supply is adequate and that this fussy baby might be even fussier if he were being bottle-fed.

Too many well-meaning "advisors" are quick to volunteer that "the milk obviously doesn't agree with him" or "he's got gas (or colic); it must be something *you* ate." This immediately endows the mother with a sense of guilt. The quality of mother's milk varies only slightly (some estimate less than 1%) among lactating women, and never has milk been "too rich" or "too thin" for an infant. Even malnourished mothers provide milk of high quality—often to the detriment of their own tissues. Allergy to human milk has never been satisfactorily documented; however, occasionally, allergy to foods in the maternal diet does occur. These foods are usually easy to identify and can be omitted from the maternal diet. Most foods that could be tolerated during pregnancy will be well tolerated by the mother and the infant during lactation. There is no basis for avoiding garlic, curry, sulfur-containing vegetables, or any other nourishing food because the woman is breast-feeding. If a food consistently seems to bother the mother or child, it can be omitted to see if relief, real or imagined, occurs. Likewise, there are no foods that must be eaten to ensure successful lactation. Substitutes for the common sources of all required nutrients are readily available in most diets.

Supplements

During the first couple of weeks it is wise to avoid supplemental feedings of formula, if possible, because it adversely affects the establishment of the milk supply. An occasional bottle will usually not significantly affect the supply after this period, especially if the milk from the missed feeding is expressed manually into a sterile container and frozen for the next bottle-feeding. Rare is the mother who does not want, indeed, need to be away from her infant for a brief period that will undoubtedly include a feeding. For this reason it is a good idea to introduce the baby to the occasional bottle at least by the end of the second month. Many infants do not accept a bottle from their mothers but will take it readily from the father or a sitter. The infant who is accustomed to breast-feeding will often swallow more air with a bottle-feeding and may need to be "bubbled" more frequently, particularly if he seems to take the milk very quickly.

Water is rarely required by the infant who is breast-fed on demand unless the outdoor temperature exceeds 90° F. Administration of additional fluid by teaspoon or dropper interferes least with the desirable sucking pattern in the very young infant.

Manual expression of milk

Manual expression of milk is a useful technique for the breast-feeding mother to learn. Although many women find it a labo-

rious procedure, there is often no substitute. The procedure is as follows: Placing the thumb on top and the forefinger under the nipple, gently push the finger and thumb back toward the chest to grasp behind the milk sinuses. Squeeze gently in a "milking" motion to remove the milk that has collected in the sinuses. Repeat the procedure, rotating the position of the grasp on the nipple occasionally so that all the sinuses are drained. Some women will find that milk flows freely once a let-down reflex occurs. Others will only be able to express a few drops at a time manually. Mothers who need to express milk for a period of days or weeks, such as in the case of a hospitalized infant where the regulations prohibit continued breast-feeding, might find it considerably more comfortable to use an electric breast pump. Many cities have rental sources; the local La Leche League chapter can usually provide information on suppliers. Manual breast pumps frequently do not work well and can cause considerable discomfort and even nipple damage because of the tremendous negative pressure required to extract milk.

Growth spurts

Infants' demands for food often do not increase at a constant rate. There may be periods of rapid growth accompanied by greatly increased appetite. These periods typically occur at around 6 and 12 weeks of age. More frequent feeding for a few days will increase the supply of milk to meet the increased demand.

Introduction of solids

Sooner or later, though, the baby will begin to indicate that he is ready for something else to eat. He will eagerly accept the breast but will look around in obvious expectation of "more" when he has finished. This usually happens around 4 to 6 months of age, and this is the time for the introduction of solids. Introducing solids much earlier than this will provide no nutritional advantage and may do harm. Early solids are a definite factor in childhood obesity and are the cause of many childhood allergies. Milk will continue to be the major source of protein and fluid for the infant for several months yet. Therefore breast-feeding should be offered before or at a separate time from solid food. Offering solids first will decrease the appetite and diminish the vigorous sucking reflex, eventually decreasing the milk supply. Once the infant is accepting a wide variety of solids, usually around 8 or 9 months of age, milk may be offered from a cup at one or more meals. The introduction of solid foods and eventual weaning to a cup are met with mixed emotions by most women who have experienced a pleasant breast-feeding relationship. Many mothers will maintain one feeding or more a day even after the bulk of the infant's needs are being met by table foods.

Weaning

Weaning actually begins the first time the infant receives supplemental or solid nourishment. Many researchers and pediatricians believe that the need for sucking and the sucking reflex persist well into the second year of life and that infants weaned from the breast before that time should be given a bottle. Many women, however, wean the child from the breast when he can take liquid well from a cup—usually about 1 year of age.

Weaning can be accomplished in a week or less, but most women have found that to drop one feeding at a time, with an interval of at least four or five days before omitting the next feeding results in the least amount of trauma for both mother and child. When the feedings have decreased to one a day, the duration of the feeding is reduced so that the infant is allowed to suck only enough to remove the sensation of fullness. Eventually one feeding in two or three days may be sufficient. Milk production will decrease to the point where the mother will "forget" a feeding and realize that weaning is complete.

Gradual weaning is so much more pleasant for most women than "drying up" after childbirth that one obstetrician produced a fourfold increase in breast-feeding in his practice by suggesting initial breast-feeding with gradual weaning to supplemental formula over a couple of weeks as an alternative to medication to suppress lactation. This does not seem unwise in view of the reported complications of many of these medications and the extreme discomfort noted by many women.

SPECIAL PROBLEMS AND CASES
Unusual conditions in the mother

Although each case must be evaluated on its own merit, there are very few conditions that automatically preclude breast-feeding. Mothers who have had operative deliveries usually find that they can breast-feed successfully after the effects of anesthesia have worn off for both mother and child. Heart disease, diabetes, hepatitis, nephrosis, and most other chronic medical conditions are not themselves a contraindication to breast-feeding. Generally, if the condition can be managed well enough to allow successful termination of pregnancy, breast-feeding may be the feeding method of choice because it is less tiring for the mother. Infectious diseases that would require isolation of the mother from other adults as well as from children often are a contraindication to breast-feeding. Active pulmonary tuberculosis is an example of such a condition. When the mother becomes pregnant again, it is usually considered necessary to wean the older infant, although this can be done gradually. The main reason for such weaning is the acute stress placed on maternal tissues by the demands of both pregnancy and lactation.

Much research has focused on excretion of drugs in breast milk. The current findings indicate that some drugs appear in the milk in sufficient quantity to be harmful to the infant and should be avoided.

1. Anticoagulants

2. Antibiotics with the capacity to sensitize, like penicillin, ampicillin
3. Antimicrobials such as sulfonamides and tetracyclines (These drugs are found in milk at less than therapeutic concentrations but at levels that may produce hyperbilirubinemia or calcium binding.)
4. Thiouracil
5. Radioactive substances such as ^{131}I, technetium, ^{24}Na
6. Aspirin
7. Antineoplastic agents

If such drugs are essential for maternal well-being, breast-feeding would be contraindicated. Maternal allergy is rarely, if ever, a reason not to breast-feed. On the contrary, considering the infant's chances for inherited allergy, breast-feeding would be the preferred method of feeding.

One of the most recent problems of concern has related to the identification of polychlorinated and/or polybrominated biphenyls (PCBs and PBBs) in milk of nursing mothers in some regions of the United States. These compounds have been shown to be carcinogenic and teratogenic in experimental animals and thus their potential effect on nursing babies provokes much anxiety. PCBs and PBBs are used in industry for plastics, adhesives, printer's ink, insecticides, and other products. Accidental spillage of waste from these industries was reported to cause contamination of the food supply in parts of Michigan and elsewhere.[16a] Samples of human milk from mothers in these regions were shown to contain a significant amount of these compounds. Thorough evaluation of the situation, however, has revealed that the contamination was limited in its scope and duration, even in the regions and duration of major involvement. These isolated reports do not constitute sound basis for discontinuance of breastfeeding in our society.[18a]

One factor that would definitely contraindicate breast-feeding is a negative attitude on the part of the mother. If the mother, after being given adequate information on breast-feeding, prefers to bottle-feed her baby, she should not be encouraged to do otherwise. Rarely is lactation successful when maternal desire to breast-feed is absent. If, on the other hand, a mother begins breast-feeding and finds that she lacks the support of her family or her physician and cannot continue, her decision to wean the infant to a bottle must be supported. It should be stressed again, however, that good professional support can often make a difference between success and failure.

Unusual conditions in the infant

Infants who are premature or who have heart anomalies or other debilitating conditions can usually be breast-fed successfully, providing obstetrical and nursery staff are willing to expend a little more effort to see that lactation gets off to a good start. Usually the mother will need to use an electric breast pump to express feedings until the infant is strong enough to suck. The milk is then stored for feeding to the infant. It has been suggested that the nursery is a good place for the breast pump to be set up for use while the mother is still hospitalized, since the sight and sounds of the infant are stimulating and reassuring to the mother. When she is released from the hospital, she will need access to an electric breast pump or instruction in the techniques of manual expression of milk. Care should be given to procedures for sterile storage and transportation of milk. If the hospital does not permit the infant to receive his mother's milk, the local milk bank will usually be glad to receive the supply until such time as the infant can be breast-fed.

Rh and other blood incompatibilities seldom preclude lactation. According to Meyer,[18] infants with erythroblastosis fetalis are not made worse by breast-feeding. Milk-induced physiological hyperbilirubinemia of the newborn is reported to be caused by high levels of pregnane-3α, 20β-

diol in the maternal system, which is passed to the infant in the milk supply. Previous use of oral contraceptives, diuretics, and the use of oxytocin during birth are all implicated in the failure of pregnane-3α, 20β-diol levels to drop after parturition. Some researchers have indicated that the incidence of this form of physiological jaundice may be as high as 80% in areas such as Scandinavia, South America, and The Netherlands, where most infants are breast-fed. The condition typically is mild and appears within the first few days of life. Untreated, it disappears by the tenth to fourteenth day. Treatment usually consists of withholding breast milk feedings for 24 to 48 hours. The condition generally clears up and does not return when breast-feeding is again instituted. Considering the mild form of the condition, its lack of complications, and self-limiting nature, many researchers believe that there is little scientific justification for withholding breast-feeding.

Infants with a cleft palate have been successfully breast-fed. The mother must have a strong desire to breast-feed and have good professional support if she is to overcome the numerous obstacles. The infant is usually fitted with an artificial palate, which allows for proper sucking technique. Manual expression and administration of milk by teaspoon and/or dropper have been reported to work well until satisfactory sucking can be initiated.

Twins

Many women have successfully breast-fed twins both with and without supplements. The milk supply ordinarily parallels demand well, and no unusual measures are needed. Adequacy of maternal dietary intake should be assured, however, because of the increased demands in feeding two infants. Twins can be fed simultaneously, reducing feeding time by one half. It may be helpful for the mother to talk with other mothers who have breast-fed twins. Clinical records or La Leche League are possible sources for women who could offer help and support.

Nipple soreness

Nipple soreness is a condition that is better prevented than treated. If it must be treated, it should be treated promptly rather than allowing the condition to progress to cracked and fissured nipples that are open to infection. In addition to the techniques already suggested for nipple conditioning and prevention of soreness, the following may prove helpful:

1. Be sure that the baby is fed on demand. If he gets too hungry, he may suck harder, causing further soreness.
2. Be sure that feedings are promptly terminated; allowing a baby to suck on an empty breast causes increased damage. Ten to twelve minutes on each side should be sufficient.
3. Be sure that nipples are dry before brassiere flaps are replaced and that air is allowed to circulate as freely as possible.
4. Avoid soaps, ointments, and especially petroleum-based products on the nipple area; they cause further irritation.
5. Mothers with sore nipples should begin each feeding on the breast that is least tender. Allow the baby to suck until the let-down reflex has occurred; then switch to the tender side and allow the baby to empty that breast. Promptly return to the less tender side to finish the feeding. Breast shields may be helpful during the first few minutes of vigorous sucking but should then be removed, since they prevent complete emptying of the breast.

Engorgement

Many physicians and nurses familiar with breast-feeding see engorgement as basically a hospital-acquired condition caused by infrequent feeding. The remedy is immediate and frequent feedings, day and night. Heat and moisture may relieve some of the discomfort between feedings.

Clogged milk ducts

Clogged milk ducts, sometimes called "caked breasts," are caused by incomplete emptying of one or more ducts. This sometimes occurs when the infant's feeding position does not allow him to draw equally on all of the milk sinuses, causing stasis. Usually a hard, painful lump may be felt in one area of the breast. The remedy, again, is more frequent feeding, especially on the affected side. If the mother can lie down and allow the infant to suck on that breast for half an hour or so, the improvement is often dramatic. Warmth and moisture may help to alleviate the discomfort when this is not possible. A warm, damp cloth can be placed in a small plastic bag and be applied to the affected area on the breast. If the mother must move about, the cloth may be held in place by the brassiere. If treatment is prompt, recovery should be nearly complete within twenty-four hours. If not, an infection should be suspected.

Mastitis

The symptoms of breast infection are similar to those of engorgement. The breast is tender, is distended with milk, and may feel hot to touch; fever may be present. Treatment consists of prompt medical attention, antibiotic therapy, bed rest, and continued breast-feeding. Discontinued feeding causes increased stasis and further pain. Frequently the source of the infection is an untreated infection in the infant. In any case, weaning should not be attempted until the infection has cleared up.

Colds and influenza

The presence of a cold or other mild viral infection such as influenza is seldom a reason to discontinue lactation. The infant has usually been exposed to the infection by the time the mother realizes that she is affected. There is good evidence that the infant has some immunity through maternal antibodies. If he comes down with the infection, it is often in a very mild form. When the infant has a cold, nasal congestion will make it difficult for him to breathe while sucking. Use of a nasal aspirator to remove mucus and aid breathing may be of some value during this period.

Colic

Many babies suffer from "colic" or fussiness of an undetermined origin. Most infants seem to have a "fussy period" every day, and there is no evidence that the breast-fed baby is any more frequently or severely affected. The mother should be assured that this is natural and does not reflect hunger or dissatisfaction with feedings.

Relactation

Many cases have documented relactation in women who have adopted a baby years after their own last pregnancy, even when they never lactated before (p. 142). Considerable perseverance and a strong desire to breast-feed are required, but success is not so uncommon as to preclude an attempt if the woman sincerely wants to try. Sucking is the chief stimulus for prolactin secretion, and adequate stimulation will generally produce milk flow. A device whereby the infant receives formula from a tube placed alongside the nipple has been developed* and seems to encourage the infant's sucking on the nipple so that sufficient milk flow can be established.

COMMON REASONS FOR FAILURE OF LACTATION

Probably the chief reason for failure of breast-feeding is poor maternal attitude toward lactation in the first place. The mother who does not sincerely want to breast-feed her infant but agrees to do so to placate her family, friends, or nurse will

---

*Lact-Aid Nursing Supplementer, manufactured by J. J. Avery, Inc., P.O. Box 6459, Denver, Colo. 80206.

have a difficult time. As Newton and Newton[20] pointed out, fear, worry, distraction, anger, and other such emotions have a potent effect on the let-down reflex. When this reflex functions poorly, the infant receives only a portion of the milk supply; the bulk of the milk stored in the alveoli is not released. The infant cries from hunger and eventually fails to gain weight. This provides negative feedback to the mother, and a vicious circle begins.

Failure to establish adequate milk supply by frequent feeding on demand is a great deterrent to successful lactation. The ways that inappropriate hospital routine can contribute to this problem have been discussed. Other problems can stem from the use of supplements too soon and too frequently and early introductions of solids.

Another common reason for failure of lactation is lack of information and lack of support for the mother. Many women do not have the support of friends or relatives who have successfully breast-fed infants. These women are often poorly informed about the physiology of lactation and about the virtually foolproof method of meeting the infant's nutritional needs. New breast-feeding mothers may have fears of the milk supply being too low in quality or quantity to support the infant's growth requirements. They may become discouraged when the infant does not feed well because he has been sedated during labor and birth. Or they may be discouraged by nipple discomfort or engorgement, common complaints during the first few days of breast-feeding. Often a new mother feels mildly depressed around the fourth or fifth day post partum, and any new problems with the beginning of lactation will be magnified out of proportion at this time. This is particularly true if the mother does not see these occurrences as normal. If the parents have had adequate prenatal instruction and good instruction during the hospital stay, the chances of weathering these storms are greatly increased. If the breast-feeding mother has the support of her husband and of understanding professionals, she will feel she has a place to turn for help and advice when things go badly. These same important supporters in her environment can provide kind words to bolster her confidence when things are going fine, and under such circumstances problems that cannot be avoided will be more easily overcome.

REFERENCES

1. American Hospital Association: Personal communication.
2. Applebaum, R. M.: The modern management of successful breastfeeding, Child Family, vol. 9, no. 2, 1970.
3. Archavsky, I. A.: Immediate breastfeeding of newborn infant in the prophylaxis of the so-called physiological loss of weight. (Text in Russian.) Vopr. Pediatri. **20:**45, 1953; abst. in Courrier **3:** 170.
4. Berg, A.: The nutrition factor, Washington, D.C., 1973, Brookings Institution.
5. Ewy, D., and Ewy, R.: Preparation for breastfeeding, New York, 1975, Dolphin Books, Doubleday & Co., Inc.
6. Graber, T.: Muscles, malformation and malocclusion, Am. J. Orthod. **49:**429, 1963.
7. Greiner, T.: The promotion of bottle feedings by multinational corporations: how advertising and the health professions have contributed, Cornell Int. Nutr. Monogr. Series No. 2, 1975.
8. Gryborski, J.: Gastrointestinal milk allergy in infants, Pediatrics **40:**354, 1967.
9. Haire, D.: Instructions for nursing your baby, New York, 1969, International Childbirth Education Association.
10. Haire, D., and Haire, J.: The nurse's contribution to successful breastfeeding. In Haire, D., and Haire, J.: Implementing family-centered maternity care with a central nursery, Hillside, N.J., 1974, International Childbirth Education Association.
11. Haire, D., and Haire, J.: The medical value of breastfeeding. In Haire, D., and Haire, J.: Implementing family-centered maternity care with a central nursery, Hillside, N.J., 1974, International Childbirth Education Association.
12. Harfunche, J. K.: The importance of breast feeding. Monograph issued in conjunction with the J. Trop. Pediatr. vol. 16, no. 3, 1970.
13. Iffrig, M.: Early breastfeeding with alternate massage, Int. J. Stud. **4:**193, 1967.
14. Jelliffe, D. B., and Jelliffe, E. F. P.: Approaches to village level infant feeding, Environmental Child Health, June, 1971.
15. Kenny, J., Boesman, M., and Michaels, R.: Bac-

terial and viral coproantibodies in breastfed infants, Pediatrics **39:**202, 1967.

16. Kimball, E. R.: Personal communication.
16a. Mother's milk: pure enough for baby? Medical World News, p. 34, Oct. 18, 1976.
17. MacKeith, R., and Wood, C.: Infant feeding and feeding difficulties, ed. 4, London, 1971, J. & A. Churchill, Ltd.
18. Meyer, H.: Infant foods and feeding practice, Springfield, Ill., 1960, Charles C Thomas, Publisher.
18a. La Leche League News, vol. 18, Nov.-Dec., 1976.
19. Newton, N.: Breastfeeding, Psychol. Today June, 1968.
20. Newton, M., and Newton, N.: The normal course and management of lactation, Child Family, vol. 9, no. 1, 1970.
21. Olmstead, R., and Jackson, E.: Self-demand feeding in the first week of life, Pediatrics **6:**396, 1950.
22. Robinson, M.: Infant morbidity and mortality: a study of 3266 infants, Lancet **260:**788, 1951.
23. Svirsky-Gross, S.: Pathogenic strains of coli (0,111) among prematures and the use of human milk in controlling the outbreak of diarrhea, Ann. Pediatr. **190:**109, 1958.

SUGGESTED READINGS

Eiger, M. S., and Olds, S. W.: The complete book of breastfeeding, New York, 1972, The Workman Publishing Co., Inc.

Ewy, D., and Ewy, R.: Preparation for breastfeeding, New York, 1975, Dolphin Books, Doubleday & Co., Inc.

Haire, D., and Haire, J.: I. The nurse's contribution to successful breastfeeding. II. The medical value of breastfeeding (Chapter V on Implementing Family Centered Maternity Care with a Central Nursery), The International Childbirth Education Association (available from Publication Distribution Center, P.O. Box 9316, Midtown Plaza, Rochester, N.Y. 14604).

Pryor, K.: Nursing your baby, New York, 1973, Harper & Row, Publishers.

9
Nutrition and family planning

Bonnie S. Worthington and Roscius N. Doan

One of the major concerns of mature women in all societies is the regulation of family size through planned contraception. Many approaches to family planning can be identified around the world, and observed practices relate largely to cultural patterns and also reflect, to some extent, socioeconomic status and availability of "modern devices." In general terms, approaches to birth control differ markedly between industrialized developed countries on the one hand and malnourished developing nations on the other. In the former circumstance, limitation in family size is widely accepted, but in the latter, where infant mortality is high and where family "manpower" determines productivity and income, birth control seems ludicrous as a means of improving happiness and survival. In discussing the topic of nutrition and family planning therefore, effort will be made to focus briefly on each of these situations with the intent that an appreciation might be developed for nutritional concerns as they relate to the process of fertility regulation.

BIRTH CONTROL AND NUTRITION: GENERAL CONSIDERATIONS

Birth control achieves its greatest impact on nutrition by preventing pregnancies among women at high risk for obstetrical complications and poor pregnancy outcome. Such a high-risk group includes teenage women,[64] women of high parity and late maternal age,[30] and chronically malnourished women of any age.[29] Birth control allows parents to space pregnancies at greater intervals. Longer intervals improve the prospects for a favorable pregnancy outcome and allow the mother to make a fuller physical and nutritional recovery between childbirths.

In many parts of the world uncontrolled fertility and malnutrition coexist.[21] These phenomena are highly interactive. High fertility means more babies to feed and more malnutrition if the availability of adequate food does not keep pace. Chronically malnourished mothers living under marginal economic conditions have a high rate of fetal loss. Yet this ill-nourished group has a high net rate of reproduction.[60] Birth control can partially alleviate this vicious circle by reducing the nutritional stress of high fertility on the malnourished mother and her family. Under such circumstances birth control may especially enhance the nutritional status of the youngest child as yet unweaned. By delaying the arrival of a new baby who would preempt the breast milk supply, the mother protects her youngest from inferior substitute feeding and the risks of gastrointestinal infections.[4,35]

Birth control and nutrition impinge on the most fundamental of human social behaviors, sexual activity and eating. Limiting one's fertility and choosing well what one eats are highly personal events. They require accurate knowledge and a sustained commitment to act on that knowledge. Birth control and good nutrition are total participatory activities for which the individual takes full personal responsibility.

Appropriate education and access to birth control methods and a good diet are essential but not sufficient without the motivation to act. Couples typically do not accept family planning when infant mortality is high and they see fewer of their children surviving. Moreover, as long as parents perceive a large family size as advantageous, they are not inclined to practice birth control. Large populations in many parts of the world find themselves in such a marginal economic position that even the argument of fertility control to avoid having more mouths to feed has little meaning. Their life experiences tell them that producing fewer babies does not necessarily mitigate their hunger. In this cli-

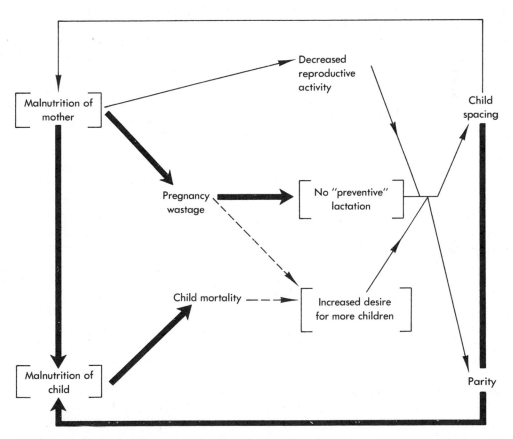

Fig. 9-1. Nutrition-fertility relationships. Width of line indicates relative impact; dotted lines indicate uncertain interaction; items enclosed in boxes indicate points appropriate for intervention. (Modified from Subcommittee on Nutrition and Fertility, Food and Nutrition Board, National Research Council, National Academy of Sciences: Nutrition and fertility interrelationships: implications for policy and action, Washington, D.C., 1975, Government Printing Office.)

mate of hunger and concern about child mortality, protection of the pregnancy-free period is highly unlikely, and focus of the family is typically placed on maintenance of the surviving infant at substantial risk for illness or death. The relationships outlined in Fig. 9-1 provide an appreciation for the complexity of the issues here described. Nutrition and fertility are closely related, and this relationship needs constant attention in all efforts to solve problems in either arena.

If programs are established to provide appropriate education and socioeconomic improvements to needy families, parents might recognize that smaller family size enhances the family's opportunities. If attitudes like this are developed, birth control may assume a level of significant acceptance. Improved maternal and child nutrition itself can encourage this acceptance by reducing infant and child mortality. If survival of offspring is noted to improve, family planning will ultimately become more desirable. Thus it can be said that better nutrition favors the adoption of fertility control.

EFFECTS OF FERTILITY ON NUTRITION

Fertility influences the nutritional status of the mother and her unborn child in a variety of ways, depending on the frequency, timing, and circumstances of childbearing.[60] Establishing the relationship between pregnancy outcome and maternal nutriture is highly problematical for the human population because both are conditioned by a number of variables.[30] Hence, poverty commonly dictates food supply and the accessibility of medical care. The level of education and cultural identity may influence the direction of prenatal care and illness management. Previous experience with child rearing and earlier pregnancies may shape maternal behavior during the current pregnancy.[26] Some, none, or all of these factors may be important influences on maternal nu-

triture and pregnancy outcome for a given mother.

Pregnancy in adolescence

The pregnant teenager is confronted with a number of special risks and stresses that may influence the outcome of the pregnancy and the well-being of the mother (Chapter 6). The nutritional stresses for the pregnant teenager are superimposed on the nutritional needs associated with significant growth and maturation.[7,17] Although childbirth among women in their late teens has constantly become less hazardous in "modern settings," a greater risk of difficulty persists among those under 20 years of age in developing countries. The specific reasons for the observed differences are not completely understood, but better obstetrical care and improved socioeconomic conditions likely account for much of the disparity. In an investigation in Hawaii a number of years ago, first births among mothers 15 to 19 years of age were recorded and followed for the degree of pregnancy wastage.[60] A comparison was made between married and unmarried mothers, with the finding of a threefold differential in pregnancy wastage after the first trimester and a sevenfold differential in their quality of antepartum care. It was clear from these observations that the circumstance of "illegitimacy" carried with it distinct barriers to acquisition of satisfactory health care support at that time. Unfortunately, this circumstance still exists in many communities around the world, with the end result that both young women and their offspring are automatically subject to malnutrition, suboptimal development, and chronic poor health.

This adverse situation is especially prominent in less developed countries of the world because early marriage and immediate pregnancy routinely occur. Often the family of the young couple counts the months that elapse between consummated alliance and pregnancy, which ultimately proves the bride's worth. It is even the case in some countries that pregnancy is a prerequisite to marriage, as is frequently observed for legitimization in modern societies. In any case, because of the obvious tendency toward early conception in many parts of the world, serious attention must be given to optimizing the nutritional status of adolescent girls. Ideally, trends toward delay in the first pregnancy can be promoted so that the quality of health of both mother and infant will not be compromised by poor nutritional support.

Pregnancy in late maternal age

Pregnancy in the immediate premenopausal years is correlated consistently with obstetrical complications and unfavorable outcomes.[30] The older woman may also be the woman of highest parity; women of high parity are susceptible to anemia and low weight to height ratio.[60] High parity is associated with greater fetal wastage.[30] Thus the late pregnancy may represent a risk for unfavorable outcome on two counts.

Close birth spacing

Pregnancy stimulates an adjustment of the mother, fetus, and placenta to a new physiological state. After birth the process reverses and a readjustment takes place. It is undesirable for another pregnancy to occur before the readjustment is complete.[60]

A reduced interval between pregnancies is one of several factors related to prematurity and low birth weight. In one study 18% of newborns born within twelve months of the previous child were of low birth weight.[7] In cases where the child spacing was increased up to twenty-three months, 10.3% of the newborns were of low birth weight. However, when the interval between births was twenty-three months or more, only 7.8% of the newborns were of low birth weight.

The interval during pregnancy and between successive conceptions has been usefully divided into three parts in a recent publication of the National Academy of Sciences entitled *Nutrition and Fertility Interrelationships: Implications for Policy and Action.*[60] The first stage of the process is pregnancy. After the birth of the infant, the mother enters an anovulatory period during which she is amenorrheic. With the postpartum physiological readjustment, ovulation is reestablished and the mother is again at risk for pregnancy. Table 9-1 illustrates factors that shorten each of the components of the interconceptional interval and interventions that may lengthen the interval. Factors that foreshorten the pregnancy are those which jeopardize a favorable reproductive outcome. Measures that enhance a favorable outcome tend to restore the gestational length. The anovulatory period will be shortened if the pregnancy was shortened by a fetal death or a premature birth. Death of a young breast-fed infant or the absence of curtailment of breast-feeding eliminates the anovulatory effect of prolactin and other anterior pituitary hormones released by the stimulus of the baby's sucking.[33] In many traditional cultures abstinence from sexual intercourse was practiced during lactation. As this practice of sexual abstinence has eroded, other effective birth control methods may not be substituted. The result may be an early conception. The encouragement of breast-feeding together with effective use of alternative birth control methods and better medical care may maximize the duration of the anovulatory period. Effective birth control techniques can prolong the pregnancy-free interval after ovulation resumes, according to the desires of the parents.

In places where high fertility prevails and modern birth control techniques are unavailable, the usual interval of child spacing is between two and one-half and three years.[60] This interval includes the extension of amenorrhea achieved by lactation and the traditional sexual abstinence practiced in many parts of the world during that period. When artificial feeding replaces breast-feeding and lactation, sexual

Table 9-1. Three major components of the interval between conceptions*

		Factors that shorten the interval	Interventions that lengthen the inverval
Pregnancy	Conception	Interruption of pregnancy or prematurity	Adequate nutrition enhances favorable outcome Improved socioeconomic status Better medical care
Anovulatory period and amenorrhea	Delivery	Fetal death or death of infant Absence or curtailment of breast-feeding	Breast-feeding may delay return of ovulation Birth control can replace failure to practice traditional postpartum (lactation) abstinence Nutrition education in breast-feeding Better medical care
At risk for pregnancy	Return of ovulation	Failure of modern birth control Failure of postpartum abstinence Infant death may motivate conception	Birth control Better medical care
	Conception		

*Modified from Subcommittee on Nutrition and Fertility, Food and Nutrition Board, National Research Council, National Academy of Sciences: Nutrition and fertility interrelationships: implications for policy and action, Washington, D.C., 1975, Government Printing Office.

taboos may also be removed and the interval of child spacing is shortened by at least six months. The pregnancy-free interval is also drastically shortened after a fetal or neonatal death. Although a well-nourished, healthy woman in an affluent society may not be threatened by a shortened interconceptional period, a chronically malnourished woman in marginal socioeconomic circumstances may find her health seriously compromised by a shortened interval.

BIRTH CONTROL AND BREAST-FEEDING

Traditionally, it has been believed that unsupplemented breast-feeding provides a contraceptive–child spacing effect in the early weeks after childbirth. Recent studies indicate that this phenomenon is real and is related to the anovulatory effect of prolactin and other hormones which are secreted by the anterior pituitary in response to the baby's sucking.[33] The existence of this biological mechanism indeed seems sensible and, in fact, resembles the spacing of offspring that is seen in other mammals as a consequence of the defined "mating seasons."

The onset of ovulation and menstruation in the lactating mother is delayed for at least ten weeks, provided breast-feeding is complete, successful, and unrestricted.[18,34] This pattern is the routine mode of breast-feeding for most mother-infant pairs in a supportive environment; babies begin sucking after birth and continue thereafter at short intervals. The contraceptive effect of lactation is greatly reduced if breast-feeding is *partial* and *supplemented* early with other feeds of cow's milk formula or semisolids; provision of these foods leads to reduced need for breast milk by the infant, which thereby reduces sucking stimulus and prolactin secretion in the mother.[43,55]

Evidence regarding the suppression of ovulation and extension of postpartum amenorrhea resulting from lactation is available from body temperature studies, endometrial biopsies, and field observations in various developing countries. In the Philippines, a study of the Catholic population in representative areas demonstrated achievement of a twenty-four to thirty-five month birth spacing interval by 51% of mothers who breast-fed their infants for seven to twelve months. Only 30% of mothers whose infants were artificially fed achieved spacing of a twenty-four month period.[20] In Rwanda, Central Africa, prolonged lactation reportedly produced amenorrhea in 50% of women for over twelve months and was also responsible for an overall delay in pregnancy of fifteen months. Since sexual intercourse in this community was culturally permitted from eight days after birth, the contraceptive effect of lactation is indeed impressive.[8]

Looking at populations of the world as a whole, lactation contraception has been estimated to provide a greater rate of protection from pregnancy than reportedly has been achieved by many "technical devices." The numerical extent of this protective effect has been computed in areas of high fertility and unrestricted, prolonged lactation. It has been estimated that lactation is responsible for a reduction of as much as 20% of expected births.[31] If these estimates are correct, the decline in breast-feeding in urban areas in developing countries clearly has an anticontraceptive effect. In these regions statistical data reveal an augmentation in birth rate accompanied by an ever-increasing problem of food shortage.

EFFECT OF SPECIFIC BIRTH CONTROL METHODS ON MATERNAL NUTRITIONAL STATUS
Oral contraceptives

One of the most common forms of birth control in use today is the oral contraceptive (O.C.). Recent estimates suggest that over 18 million women around the world are utilizing "the pill" and find it to be a desirable method of contraception because of its ease and proved effectiveness. The oral agents that typically are employed consist of a synthetic estrogen (ethinyl estradiol or mestranol) and one of several synthetic progestogens taken either in combination or in sequence (Table 9-2). Combinations of estrogens and progesterones were first marketed in 1957 for correction of menstrual disorders, and by 1960 the drugs were approved as oral contraceptive agents.[28]

Oral contraceptive preparations available in the United States are primarily of two types (Fig. 9-2): the combination type, which contains both estrogenic and progestional substances in all tablets, and the sequential type, which contains estrogenic substances in tablets taken during the first portion of the menstrual cycle and estrogen plus progestational compounds in tablets taken during the latter part of the cycle. Some brands also provide an iron supplement in tablet form for the five to seven days at the end of the cycle. Research data and clinical reports suggest that the combination type of contraceptive pills are much more effective in the prevention of contraception but are, at the same time, substantially more likely to cause side effects, metabolic disorders, and serious complications. The trend over the past decade in Great Britain and the United States has been toward reduction in dosage of both estrogenic and progestational substances, and with this trend has come a reduced incidence of recognized side reactions and metabolic alterations.

The mechanism of action of oral contraceptives was originally assumed to be

Table 9-2. Relative estrogenic activity of the combined oral contraceptive agents*

Drug	Estrogen (mg/tab)				Progestogen (mg/tab)		
	Mes-tranol	Ethinyl estradiol	Nor-gestrel	Ethnodiol diacetate	Noreth-indrone acetate	Noreth-indrone	Norethy-nodrel
Strongly estrogenic							
Enovid 5	0.075						5.0
Enovid E	0.1						2.5
Moderately estrogenic							
Norinyl 1 + 50—Ortho-Novum 1/50	0.05					1.0	
Norinyl 1 +80—Ortho-Novum 1/80	0.08					1.0	
Norinyl 2—Ortho-Novum 2	0.1					2.0	
Ovulen	0.1					1.0	
Minimally estrogenic							
Brevicon—Modicon†		0.035					
Demulen		0.05		1.0			
Loestrin—Zorane†		0.02		1.0			
Lo/Ovral†		0.03	0.3				
Norlestrin 2.5 mg		0.05			2.5		
Ortho-Novum 2	0.1					2.0	
Ortho-Novum 10	0.06					10.0	
Ovral		0.05	0.5				

*From Rauh, J. L., Burket, R. L., and Brookman, R. R.: Contraception for the teenager, Med. Clin. North Am. **59:**1407, 1975.
†The frequency of breakthrough bleeding and "patient failure," pregnancy, from missed days contraindicate their use in adolescents.

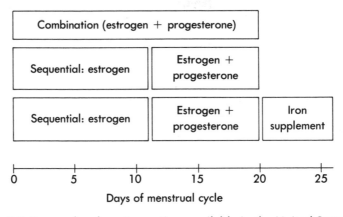

Fig. 9-2. Types of oral contraceptives available in the United States.

simple suppression of ovulation. Indeed, the original combination type of preparation, norethynodrel (Enovid), contained relatively high doses of both estrins and progestins and *did* suppress ovulation most of the time. Careful evaluation has shown, however, that preparations containing smaller doses, especially those of sequential type, frequently do not suppress ovulation, but they are still effective in preventing conception. The proposed mechanism of action is that the hormones promote changes in the chemical and physical characteristics of the cervical mucus and endometrium which render the uterine environment less favorable for implantation of the ovum.[54]

Since widespread use of oral contraceptives has developed, observed side effects and metabolic complications resulting from prolonged usage have received increasing attention by both basic science and clinical researchers. The complications reported as a result of taking "the pill" can be divided roughly into those which are merely annoying and those which are serious or potentially fatal. Many of the reported problems are also seen in women during the time of pregnancy. Minor complications of pill usage include nausea, vomiting, emotional changes, facial pigmentation, slight loss of hair, and headaches. With regard to the latter, there is some evidence to suggest that women who have suffered from migraine or similar vascular headaches may be unable to use this form of contraceptive.[25]

Of considerable interest is the observation that oral contraceptives were in use for nearly eight years before medical science presented conclusive evidence that serious and even fatal complications could result. Major complications are of four types: hypertension and its sequelae,[33] thromboembolic phenomena with and without premature myocardial infarction,[41,47,58,65] hepatic hemorrhage and tumors,[42,46] and metabolic disorders, in particular diabetes mellitus.[3,24] The problem of hypertension secondary to oral contraceptive use generally occurs in women who have a familial trait or actually have had hypertension prior to using the pill. The same can be said for diabetes. Deaths resulting from pulmonary embolism, coronary occlusion, and stroke, however, have been reported with an unusually high frequency in young women who have used oral contraceptives for at least six

months. Repeated observations have now shown clearly that women on the pill develop increased coagulability of the blood accompanied by an increase in concentration of certain lipid fractions.[2,51]

The high interest in metabolic dyscrasias associated with oral contraceptive use has been accompanied by concern about effects of the pill on nutritional status. Early observations of women using the pill revealed its stimulation of moderate weight gain (3 to 6 pounds), fluid retention, minor impairment of carbohydrate metabolism, and slight to moderate increase in nitrogen balance.[9,33] Recent attention, however, has focused primarily on vitamin and mineral status, and some research in this area has been completed during the past five years. Evaluation of circulating levels of specific vitamins and minerals in oral contraceptive users has revealed increased serum concentration of vitamin A,[63] copper,[14] iron,[13] and tryptophan intermediates[12] and decreased concentrations of folate,[45,48,56,57,59] vitamin B_{12},[6,10,19,61] riboflavin,[53] vitamin C,[11,50] zinc,[27,40,49] and certain amino acids.[33] Additional observations of urinary excretion patterns have revealed increased urinary xanthurenic acid excretion after an oral test dose of tryptophan; such a finding implies an increased need for vitamin B_6 in individuals taking synthetic estrogens.[12,16,19,36,52]

By far the most attention to vitamin status in women using oral contraceptives has been given to the issue of tryptophan metabolism and vitamin B_6 requirements. Luhby and co-workers,[38] in a 1971 study of oral contraceptive users, reported increased urinary excretion of xanthurenic acid after a test dose of tryptophan. This observation is believed to indicate vitamin B_6 deficiency, since a deficit of this vitamin metabolically prevents normal conversion of 3-hydroxykynurenine to N-methylnicotinamide so that accumulation of xanthurenic acid and other preliminary breakdown products of tryptophan takes place (Fig. 9-3). Since the initial reports of abnormal

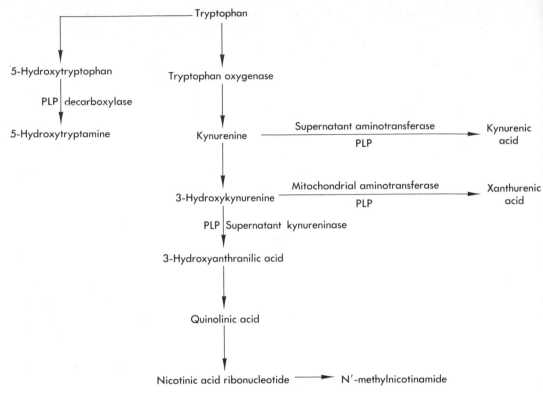

Fig. 9-3. Major pathways of tryptophan metabolism. *PLP* indicates the known pyridoxal phosphate-dependent enzyme reactions.

tryptophan metabolism in oral contraceptive users, Lumeng and associates[39] have substantiated these early findings and, on the basis of their extensive studies, proposed that tryptophan metabolism is abnormal in approximately 80% of oral contraceptive users.

Research data seem to suggest that oral contraceptives increase the metabolism of tryptophan down the nicotinic acid–ribonucleotide pathway because of the induction of the rate limiting enzyme hepatic tryptophan oxygenase by the estrogen.[1] This apparently leads to an increased urinary excretion of intermediate tryptophan metabolites and to a secondary vitamin B_6 deficiency. Pyridoxal phosphate, the coenzyme form of vitamin B_6 constituting a substantial portion of B_6-containing compounds present in the blood of humans, is required as a cofactor for several enzymatic reactions in this pathway (Fig. 9-3). Thus it seems justifiable to suggest that oral contraceptives increase the requirements for pyridoxal phosphate.

The issue is muddied, however, by the later observation of Leklem and co-workers[36,37] that other measures of vitamin B_6 metabolism, like urinary 4-pyridoxic acid, plasma pyridoxal phosphate, and erythrocyte alanine aminotransferase, seem to be maintained at normal levels in oral contraceptive users ingesting the Recommended Dietary Allowance (RDA) of vitamin B_6. These researchers proposed that since altered tryptophan metabolism persisted in oral contraceptive users even when other indices of vitamin B_6 status were normal, oral contraceptives must specifically affect tryptophan metabolism by some means other than through a vitamin B_6 deficiency.

Of considerable interest is a recent report

by Adams and colleagues[1] that oral contraceptive–induced depression in women can be alleviated by vitamin B_6 therapy in those depressed women with biochemical evidence of an absolute deficiency of vitamin B_6. In this study 22 depressed women using oral contraceptives were found whose symptoms were judged to be due to the effects of the pill. Eleven of the women demonstrated clear-cut biochemical evidence of vitamin B_6 deficiency, as judged by lower urinary excretion of 4-pyridoxic acid (a major excretory product of vitamin B_6), increased urinary 3-hydroxykynurenine/3-hydroxyanthranilic acid (HK/HA) ratios, and decreased activity of pyridoxal phosphate–dependent erythrocyte aspartate and alanine aminotransferase enzymes. In a double-blind crossover trial, these deficient women responded favorably to the administration of pyridoxine hydrochloride; the remaining eleven women without absolute vitamin B_6 deficit demonstrated no such clinical response to the pyridoxine supplement, and placebo administration was without effect.

Possible explanations for oral contraceptive–induced depression have been proposed by Adams and colleagues[1] and involve disturbance in brain-amine metabolism. Defective synthesis of brain 5-hydroxytryptamine (5-HT) is implicated, and low levels of 5-HT metabolite have been found in the cerebrospinal fluid of depressed patients. Additionally, there is evidence of low 5-HT and 5-hydroxyindolacetic acid (5-HIAA) in the hindbrains of depressive suicide victims. Finally, the administration of the 5-HT precursor L-tryptophan may be effective in the treatment of depression.[1]

There are three ways in which the changes in tryptophan metabolism may lead to reduced formation of 5-HT in the brain and therefore to depression. First, increased metabolism of tryptophan along the nicotinic acid–ribonucleotide pathway may result in an inadequate supply of precursor for 5-HT synthesis. Second, there is experimental evidence that the metabolites of tryptophan, kynurenine and 3-hydroxykynurenine, inhibit the transport of tryptophan across the blood-brain barrier. This mechanism could apply to women using oral contraceptives because of increased formation of these metabolites. Third, increased requirements of vitamin B_6 in women using oral contraceptives because of increased pyridoxal phosphate–dependent enzyme activity may result in inadequate amounts of this coenzyme for normal 5-hydroxytryptophan decarboxylase activity in the brain. Although decarboxylation is not the rate limiting step in 5 HT synthesis in rats, there is some evidence that it may be in humans.[1,36,37]

Early suggestions that vitamin B_6 administration might relieve depression due to oral contraceptives were made by Winston in 1969.[22] Baumblatt and Winston subsequently reported that the administration of pyridoxine to 58 women using oral contraceptives relieved premenstrual depression in 18 women and caused some improvement in 26 others. In these studies, however, no double-blind, placebo-controlled trials of pyridoxine therapy were instituted, and the original vitamin B_6 status of the women was unknown.

It is proposed therefore that the administration of vitamin B_6 can correct two of the possible mechanisms whereby abnormal tryptophan metabolism develops in response to oral contraceptive use. Vitamin B_6 might thus prevent the accumulation of tryptophan metabolites that inhibit tryptophan transport into the brain, and it could also restore normal activity to 5-hydroxytryptophan decarboxylase. The preliminary findings of Adams and associates[1] support the effectiveness of vitamin B_6 therapy in improving clinical symptomatology in some women with oral contraceptive–induced depression. Overall, then, it must be accepted that prolonged use of oral contraceptive agents interferes with normal tryptophan metabolism and thus alters metabolic requirements for vitamin B_6.

Whether or not routine low-level pyridoxine supplementation should be recommended for women using the pill is still a question that cannot be answered. As a result of the work of Adams and associates,[1] however, it seems reasonable to explore the value of supplementation in women with significant tendencies toward pessimism, dissatisfaction, crying, and tension related very clearly to oral contraceptive use.

Another vitamin of relevance in this discussion is folic acid, since the use of oral contraceptive agents reportedly promotes a reduction in blood concentration of this vitamin.[45,48,56,57,59] Originally, this finding was disturbing, since the developing fetus is known to require folic acid during early stages of cell division; thus if a woman became pregnant soon after discontinuing the pill, the fetus might thereby be exposed to a folic acid–deficient environment. Initially, the observed reduction in circulating folic acid level was believed to be due to a reduced ability to absorb the vitamin. In one study a physiological dose of polyglutamic folic acid was given by mouth to

two groups of women.[59] Serum folic acid (folate) rose significantly less in the women who were taking the contraceptive pill than in those who were not. When "free folate" was given orally, no significant difference in the rise in scrum folate was noted between the two groups. The effect on polyglutamate folate absorption was ascribed to an inhibition of the intestinal "deconjugase" enzyme system by the pill (Fig. 9-4). Of interest, however, is a subsequent study of the same problem in which estradiol, progesterone, and estrone were not found to inhibit the activity of folate "deconjugase."[57]

If oral contraceptives *do* interfere with folate metabolism and do not impair deconjugation and absorption of folic acid folate, it is possible that they increase the rate of clearance of folate from plasma to tissues as occurs during pregnancy. A recent study by Shojania and colleagues[56] supports this concept, since increased plasma clearance and urinary excretion of folate were observed in contraceptive users when compared with control subjects. It has

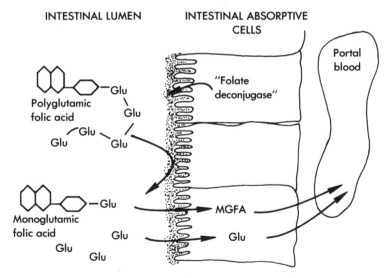

Fig. 9-4. Diagrammatic representation of polyglutamic folic acid digestion and absorption in the upper small intestine. Food folate in the form of polyglutamic folic acid is deconjugated by folate deconjugase, which is located in the brush border of the absorptive cells. Monoglutamic folic acid and glutamic acid can be absorbed into the absorptive cells and subsequently transported into the portal blood.

also been suggested that oral contraceptives act by acceleration of folate metabolism through induction of hepatic enzymes; some evidence for this mechanism has been provided by Stephens and associates.[57]

Of interest, however, is a recent study involving 526 women attending a family planning clinic in Louisiana.[48] In this population no correlation between serum folate level and length of time using contraceptives could be demonstrated; no evidence could be found of macrocytosis or hypersegmentation of polymorphonuclear leukocytes, and no case of macrocytic anemia was identified. It is obvious therefore that the effects of the pill on folate metabolism are still unclear; whether or not folic acid supplementation should accompany oral contraceptive usage is still open to much debate.

Vitamin B_{12} status in oral contraceptive users has received limited attention overall, but Bianchine and colleagues[6] reported that serum vitamin B_{12} binding capacity was significantly increased in women using oral contraceptives. Wertalik[61] found a significantly lower serum vitamin B_{12} level in women taking oral contraceptives, and 15% of these women were clearly deficient. Decreased vitamin B_{12} absorption was not observed, and folate therapy did not increase vitamin B_{12} levels to suggest an existent folic acid deficiency. No anemia or evidence of tissue depletion of vitamin B_{12} was detected, and thus it has been proposed that enhanced tissue avidity for vitamin B_{12} is most likely the cause of its reduced serum concentration. Whether or not this circumstance is detrimental to the health of the oral contraceptive user is currently under investigation.

Riboflavin status of oral contraceptive users may also be compromised by the use of this "drug." Erythrocyte glutathione reductase (EGR) activity has been used as a measure of riboflavin availability, since flavin adenine dinucleotide (FAD) is needed as a coenzyme by EGR. In a study

by Sanpitak and Chayutimonkul,[53] mean EGR activity was significantly lower in the oral contraceptive group when compared with the control group. Efforts to stimulate EGR activity by provision of FAD revealed a stimulation response of the oral contraceptive users which was twice as great as that of the control group. These results suggest that the original difference in EGR activity between the two groups was due to lower saturation of EGR with FAD in the women using oral contraceptives. It has also been proposed that oral contraceptives may interfere with the absorption of riboflavin, its metabolic conversion to FAD, or the binding of FAD to the enzyme. Evidence supportive of any of these hypotheses is currently lacking.

Ascorbic acid status of oral contraceptive users was studied by Briggs and Briggs[11] in the early 1970s. Evaluation of four groups of women revealed that ascorbic acid levels in both leukocytes and platelets were lower in women using the pill than in untreated control subjects, pregnant women, or women receiving an injectable contraceptive (Depo-Provera) every three months. In addition, animal experiments clearly indicate that estrogens increase the rate of ascorbic acid destruction and additionally reduce tissue levels of this vitamin. It has also been proposed that oral contraceptives may increase the breakdown of ascorbic acid, perhaps by their stimulant action on liver release of ceruloplasmin, a copper-containing protein with ascorbate oxidase activity. It is *possible* therefore that some women ingesting the pill may exist in a hypovitaminotic C condition and may benefit from a dietary supplement.

Serum vitamin A levels in women fluctuate in a cyclic pattern during the menstrual cycle, suggesting an interplay between the hormones secreted during the cycle and serum vitamin A levels. Estrogen administration induces a large increase in plasma vitamin A–binding globulin, which leads to an increase in plasma vitamin A (retinol).[63] This discovery of increased serum vitamin A levels in oral contraceptive users led to fears that a pregnancy following the arrest of contraception might be associated with malformation in the fetus, since vitamin A is known to be teratogenic in large doses.[5] Attention to this possibility by Wild and colleagues,[62] however, revealed no significant difference in vitamin A levels in the first trimester of pregnancy between women who had never taken oral contraceptives and women who discontinued them shortly before conceiving. Those women who conceived within twenty weeks of discontinuing oral contraceptives had no increase in the incidence of abortion or abnormalities in their babies. The significance of the observed effect of oral contraceptives on serum vitamin A level is unknown, but available data strongly suggest that the phenomenon is not detrimental to the health of the woman or to future offspring.

As far as trace minerals are concerned, few thorough investigations in this area have yet been completed. Serum iron levels and iron-binding capacity are both increased by oral contraceptives,[13] and diminution of menstrual blood loss frequently accompanies cyclic hormonal therapy; these observations suggest that iron needs may be slightly reduced in oral contraceptive users. Reduction of circulating zinc levels has been observed in women taking the pill, and the potential effect of this alteration on the health of women and the development of future babies is the subject of considerable speculation and research at the present time.[40,49] Estrogen is associated with a significant elevation of serum copper and ceruloplasmin[14] without changes in urinary copper excretion; this observation, like those related to iron, is suggestive of a reduced requirement for copper while a woman is using the pill.

A final issue of concern dealing with prolonged use of oral contraceptives relates to the possible problems associated with their use by women who are malnourished. Normal use of the daily hormone-containing oral contraceptive tablet as a means of preventing conception is recommended with the assumption that liver "detoxification capabilities" are working well and that all other aspects of physiological and metabolic behavior are normal. Since fatty infiltration of the liver and/or liver dysfunction have frequently been reported in recognized cases of "malnutrition," one must question the potential safety of introducing into such a patient hormones that are known themselves to promote changes in liver lipid concentration in animals placed on a high sucrose diet.[32] Additionally, it has been shown that both protein-calorie malnutrition and estrogen-progesterone administration tend to modify cortisol metabolism so that a significant rise in circulating corticosteroid level is apparent. The general catabolic effects of corticosteroids are well recognized, and the potential adverse consequences for malnourished oral contraceptive users are largely unknown. Overall, it is clear in surveying the literature that little information or data are available concerning the wisdom of oral contraceptive use by women in suboptimal nutritional status. Attention to this question is certainly warranted if widespread use of oral contraceptive agents is to be recommended for women from disadvantaged, as well as prosperous, situations.

It is obvious from the information available on oral contraceptives and nutritional status that a number of observations have been made and reported in this area, but little clear understanding of the meaning of the observations has yet been developed. According to the Food and Nutrition Board of the National Academy of Sciences,[23] the most pressing need at the present time is for additional research directed at more precise delineation of the metabolic effects of oral contraceptives and correlation of these parameters with clinical sequelae. By and large, such research should be prospective in nature and take into account variations in nutritional status related to general health and socioeconomic, cultural and geographical factors. Well-designed research should involve assessment of the different dosages and components of oral contraceptive agents, and studies with relatively long-term longitudinal focus should be included. In all cases appropriate control observations should be recorded, and subjective effects of oral contraceptive usage should be evaluated using controlled double-blind experiments for best results.

Other contraceptive methods

Effects of other contraceptive "agents" on nutritional status have received relatively little attention by the scientific community. The intrauterine device (IUD) has become popular in some parts of the world, but its mechanism of contraceptive action is unclear other than that it appears to involve, in part, the potent antifertility properties of metallic copper in the uterine environment. Of interest are recent studies from several laboratories that revealed significant variations in the concentrations of copper, zinc, and other trace elements in the endometrium during the menstrual cycle. Repetitive biopsies indicated that late secretory endometrium contained relatively high concentrations of copper and zinc, whereas lower concentrations were found during the prolifcrative phase. These same changes were reflected in analyses of cervical mucus. After the insertion of a copper-containing IUD, sequential biopsies indicated an increased concentration of copper in both the proliferative and secretory endometrium. After about one year with the IUD in place, only the secretory endometrium had a significant increase in copper content. When the device was removed after one year, the endometrial copper levels rapidly returned to normal.

The copper content of the cervical mucus is clearly increased by the presence of the copper device. This increase is eight to ten times the normal amount during the proliferative phase and twice the normal amount during the secretory phase. Uterine fluid copper is increased during both phases of the cycle for as long as the copper device is within the uterine cavity. Copper levels in the myometrium may be slightly elevated in the areas adjacent to the copper, but no change in circulating copper concentration has been observed. Thus it would appear that whereas the IUD promotes distinct changes in the "nutritional environment" in the uterus, the influence on overall nutritional status of the user is minimal, with the exception of its well-known production of increased blood (and iron) loss during menstruation. Those women exhibiting substantial blood loss each month (more than 50 ml) should be advised to supplement their diet with absorbable iron salts (i.e., ferrous sulfate, ferrous gluconate).

Patient counseling

Because of the recognized effects that oral contraceptives and IUDs have on nutritional status, dietary counseling should be a routine part of the management of women on either "device." Since oral contraceptives tend to reduce the body's ability to use certain nutrients, it is imperative that an adequate diet be consumed. Following is a list of sources of selected nutrients:

Folic acid (folacin)
  Dark green leafy vegetables
  Lettuce
  Lima beans
  Cauliflower
  Liver
  Meats
  Eggs
  Nuts
Vitamin B_6 (pyridoxine)
  Liver
  Meats
  Cabbage
  Banana
  Eggs
  Corn
  Whole wheat
  Fish
  Rolled oats

Ascorbic acid (vitamin C)
  Oranges
  Tomatoes
  Grapefruit
  Raw cabbage
  Green pepper
  Dark green leafy vegetables
  Selected fortified products (read labels)
Riboflavin (vitamin B_2)
  Milk
  Cheese
  Eggs
  Meats
  Bread
  Dark green leafy vegetables
  Lettuce
  Green peas
Iron
  Meats
  Egg yolk
  Whole wheat (or fortified products)
  Seafood
  Green leafy vegetables
  Nuts
  Legumes

If the diet is inadequate and the oral contraceptive reduces absorption and increases the need for certain nutrients, a "double inadequacy" situation then develops. Since the interconceptual period is a crucial time for recouping one's nutrition stores and stamina for support of a future fetus, it is extremely important to prevent the double inadequacy from occurring in women who have just given birth. The most helpful recommendation for the woman with an IUD is to provide for iron needs in relation to menstrual blood losses. Improvement in iron intake through dietary modification can be suggested as sufficient in itself to meet iron needs, but supplementation with iron salts may be appropriate for those women with excessive menstrual bleeding.

CONCLUSION

It seems clear from the discussions presented in this chapter that nutrition, fertility and family planning are issues with considerable interrelationship in developed as well as developing societies. Future planning with regard to nutrition policy and programs must focus on the specific needs and problems in given communities. The decline in the trend toward breast-feeding should be aggressively countered whenever possible. Integrated programs involving birth control services and nutritional maintenance should be developed with special attention to the protection of adolescent, pregnant, and lactating women, as well as the young children they care for. The potential consequences of long-term use of oral contraceptives should be further evaluated in human populations, and an effort should be made to judge their suitability for malnourished women in breast-feeding and nonbreast-feeding situations. Interrelationships among nutritional status, fertility rates, socioeconomic levels, and population growth should be thoroughly evaluated by interdisciplinary teams on an ongoing basis. Intervention programs with educational components should be systematically established with periodic evaluation to determine if they are improving the health and happiness of the families they serve while reducing the trend in uncontrolled population expansion.

REFERENCES

1. Adams, P. W., Rose, D. P., Folkard, J., Wynn, V., Seed, M., and Strong, R.: Effect of pyridoxine hydrochloride (vitamin B_6) upon depression associated with oral contraception, Lancet **1:**897, 1973.
2. Aftergood, L., Alexander, A. R., and Alfin-Slater, R. B.: Effect of oral contraceptives on plasma lipoproteins, cholesterol and α-tocopherol levels in young women, Nutr. Rep. Int. **11:**295, 1975.
3. Beck, P.: Contraceptive steroids: modifications of carbohydrate and lipid metabolism, Metabolism **22:**841, 1973.
4. Berg, A.: The nutrition factor, Washington, D.C., 1973, Brookings Institution.
5. Bernhardt, I. B., and Dorsey, D. J.: Hypervitaminosis A and congenital renal anomalies in a human infant, Obstet. Gynecol. **43:**750, 1974.
6. Bianchine, J. R., Bonnlander, B., Macaraeg, P. V., Jr., et al.: Serum vitamin B_{12} binding capacity and oral contraceptive hormones, J. Clin. Endocrinol. **29:**1425, 1969.

7. Bishop, E. H.: Prevention of premature labor. In Proceedings of the National Conference for the Prevention of Mental Retardation Through Improved Maternal Care, Washington, D.C., U.S. Children's Bureau, 1968, Government Printing Office.

8. Bonté, M., and Van Balne, H. J.: Prolonged lactation and family spacing in Rwanda, J. Biosoc. Sci. **1:**97, 1969.

9. Briggs, M., and Briggs, M.: Contraceptives and serum proteins, Br. Med. J. **3:**521, 1970.

10. Briggs, M., and Briggs, M.: Endocrine effects on serum vitamin B_{12}, Lancet **2:**1037, 1972.

11. Briggs, M., and Briggs, M.: Vitamin C requirements and oral contraceptives, Nature **238:**277, 1972.

12. Brown, R. R., Rose, D. P., Leklum, J. E., Linkswiler, H., and Anaud, R.: Urinary 4-pyridoxic acid, plasma pyridoxal phosphate and erythrocyte aminotransferase levels in oral contraceptive users receiving controlled intakes of vitamin B_6, Am. J. Clin. Nutr. **28:**10, 1975.

13. Burton, J. L.: Effect of oral contraceptives on hemoglobin, packed cell volume, serum iron and total iron-binding capacity in healthy women, Lancet **1:**978, 1967.

14. Carruthers, M. E., Hobbs, C. B., and Warren, R. L.: Raised serum copper and ceruloplasmin levels in subjects taking oral contraceptives, J. Clin. Pathol. **19:**498, 1966.

15. Chopra, J. G.: Effect of steroid contraceptives on lactation, Am. J. Clin. Nutr. **25:**1202, 1972.

16. Cleary, R. E., Lumeng, L., and Li, T. L.: Maternal and fetal plasma levels of pyridoxal phosphate at term: adequacy of vitamin B_6 supplementation during pregnancy, Am. J. Obstet. Gynecol. **121:**25, 1975.

17. Committee on Maternal Nutrition, Food and Nutrition Board, National Research Council, National Academy of Sciences: Maternal nutrition and the course of pregnancy, Washington, D.C., 1970, Government Printing Office.

18. Cronin, T. J.: Influence of lactation upon ovulation, Lancet **2:**422, 1968.

19. Davis, R. E., and Smith, B. K.: Pyridoxal, vitamin B_{12} and folate metabolism in women taking oral contraceptive agents, South Afr. Med. J. **48:**1937, 1974.

20. Del Mundo, F., and Adiao, A.: Lactation and child spacing as observed among 2,102 rural Filipino mothers, J. Pediatr. **19:**128, 1969.

21. Echols, J. R.: Population vs. environment: a crisis of too many people, Am. Sci. **64:**165, 1976.

22. Ferreira, A. J.: Prenatal environment, Springfield, Ill., 1969, Charles C Thomas, Publisher.

23. Food and Nutrition Board, National Academy of Sciences: Oral contraceptives and nutrition, Washington, D.C., 1975, Government Printing Office.

24. Gershberg, H., Javier, H., and Hulse, M.: Glucose tolerance in women receiving an ovulatory suppressant, Diabetes **13:**378, 1964.

25. Goldzieher, J. W.: Oral contraceptives: a review of certain metabolic effects and an examination of the question of safety, Fed. Proc. **29:**1220, 1970.

26. Gordon, J. E.: Nutritional individuality, Am. J. Dis. Child. **129:**422, 1975.

27. Halstead, J. A., and Smith, J. C.: Plasma zinc in health and disease, Lancet **1:**322, 1970.

28. Hodges, R. E.: Nutrition and "the pill," J. Am. Diet. Assoc. **59:**212, 1971.

29. Hunscher, H. A., and Tompkins, W. T.: The influence of maternal nutrition on the immediate and long-term outcome of pregnancy, Clin. Obstet. Gynecol. **13:**130, 1970.

30. Illsley, L., and Kincaid, J. C.: Social correlations of perinatal mortality. In Butler, N. R., and Bonham, D. G., editors: Perinatal mortality: the first report of the 1958 British Perinatal Mortality Survey, Edinburgh and London, 1963, E. & S. Livingstone, Ltd.

31. Jain, A. K., Hsu, T. C., Freedman, R., and Chang M. C.: Demographic aspects of lactation and postpartum amenorrhea, Demography **7:**255, 1970.

32. Jeffreys, D. B., and White, I. R.: Influence of a combined oral contraceptive on rats fed low protein/high carbohydrate diets, Nutr. Metab. **16:**155, 1974.

33. Jelliffe, D. B., and Jelliffe, E. F. P.: Lactation, conception and the nutrition of the nursing mother and child, J. Pediatr. **81:**829, 1972.

34. Jelliffe, D. B., and Jelliffe, E. F. P.: Human milk, nutrition and the world resource crisis, Science **188:**557, 1975.

35. Latham, M. C.: Nutrition and infection in national development, Science **188:**561, 1975.

36. Leklem, J. E., Brown, R. R., Rose, D. P., Linkswiler, H., and Arend, R. A.: Metabolism of tryptophan and niacin in oral contraceptive users receiving controlled intakes of vitamin B_6, Am. J. Clin. Nutr. **28:**146, 1975.

37. Leklem, J. E., Brown, R. R., Rose, D. P., and Linkswiler, H. M.: Vitamin B_6 requirements of women using oral contraceptives, Am. J. Clin. Nutr. **28:**535, 1975.

38. Luhby, A. L., Brin, M., Gordon, M., Davis, P., Murphy, M., and Spiegel, H.: Vitamin B_6 metabolism in users of oral contraceptive agents: abnormal urinary xanthurenic acid excretion and its correction by pyridoxine, Am. J. Clin. Nutr. **24:**684, 1971.

39. Lumeng, L., Cleary, R. E., and Li, T.: Effect of oral contraceptives on the plasma concentration of pyridoxal phosphate, Am. J. Clin. Nutr. **27:**326, 1974.

40. Margen, S., and King, J. C.: Effect of oral contra-

ceptive agents on the metabolism of some trace minerals, Am. J. Clin. Nutr. **28:**392, 1975.

41. Masi, A. T., and Dugdale, M.: Cerebrovascular diseases associated with the use of oral contraceptives, Ann. Intern. Med. **72:**111, 1970.

42. Mays, E. T., Christopherson, W. M., Mahr, M. M., and Williams, H. C.: Hepatic changes in young women ingesting contraceptive steroids: hepatic hemorrhage and primary hepatic tumors. J.A.M.A. **235:**730, 1976.

43. McKeown, T., and Gibson, J. R.: A note on menstruation and conception during lactation, J. Obstet. Gynecol. **61:**824, 1954.

44. McLaren, D. S.: A study of factors underlying the special incidence of keratomalacia in Oriya children, J. Trop. Pediatr. **2:**135, 1956.

45. Meguid, M. M., and Loebl, W. Y.: Megaloblastic anemia associated with the oral contraceptive pill, Postgrad. Med. J. **50:**470, 1974.

46. Metreau, J. M., Dhumeaux, D., and Berthelot, P.: Oral contraceptives and the liver, Digestion **7:** 318, 1972.

47. Oliver, M. F.: Oral contraceptives and myocardial infarction, Br. Med. J. **2:**210, 1970.

48. Paine, C. J., Grafton, W. D., Dickson, V. L., and Eichner, E. R.: Oral contraceptives, serum folate and hematologic status, J.A.M.A. **231:**731, 1975.

49. Prasad, A. S., Oberleas, D., Lei, K. Y., Moghissi, K. S., Stryker, J. C.: Effect of oral contraceptive agents on nutrients. I. Minerals, Am. J. Clin. Nutr. **28:**377, 1975.

50. Rivers, J. M., and Devine, M. M.: Plasma ascorbic acid concentrations and oral contraceptives, Am. J. Clin. Nutr. **25:**684, 1972.

51. Rossner, S., Larsson-Cohn, U., Carlson, L. S., and Boberg, J.: Effects of an oral contraceptive agent on plasma lipids, plasma lipoproteins, the intravenous fat tolerance and post-heparin lipoprotein lipase activity, Acta Med. Scand. **190:**301, 1971.

52. Salkeld, R. M., Knorr, K., and Korner, W. F.: The effect of oral contraceptives on vitamin B_6 status, Clin. Chim. Acta **201:**195, 1973.

53. Sanpitak, N., and Chayutimonkul, L.: Oral contraceptives and riboflavin nutrition, Lancet **1:**836, 1974.

54. Saunders, F. J.: Endocrine aspects and mechanisms of action of oral contraceptives, Fed. Proc. **29:**1211, 1970.

55. Sharman, A.: Ovulation after pregnancy, Fertil. Steril. **2:**371, 1951.

56. Shojania, A. M., Hornady, G. J., and Scaletta, D.: The effect of oral contraceptives on folate metabolism. III. Plasma clearance and urinary folate excretion, Am. J. Obstet. Gynecol. **111:**782, 1971.

57. Stephens, M. E. M., Craft, I., Peters, T. J., and Hoffbrand, A. V.: Oral contraceptives and folate metabolism, Clin. Sci. **42:**405, 1972.

58. Stolley, P. D., Tonascia, J. A., Tockman, M. S., Sartwell, P. E., Rutledge, A. H., and Jacobs, M. P.: Thrombosis with low-estrogen oral contraceptives, Am. J. Epidemiol. **102:**197, 1975.

59. Streiff, R. R.: Folate deficiency and oral contraceptives, J.A.M.A. **214:**40, 1970.

60. Subcommittee on Nutrition and Fertility, Food and Nutrition Board, National Research Council, National Academy of Sciences: Nutrition and fertility interrelationships: implications for policy and action, Washington, D.C., 1975, Government Printing Office.

61. Wertalik, L. F.: Decreased serum B_{12} levels with oral contraceptive use, J.A.M.A. **221:**1371, 1972.

62. Wild, J., Schorah, C. J., and Smithells, R. W.: Vitamin A, pregnancy, and oral contraceptives, Br. J. Med. **1:**57, 1974.

63. Yeung, D. L.: Effects of oral contraceptives on vitamin A metabolism in the human and the rat, Am. J. Clin. Nutr. **27:**125, 1974.

64. Zackler, J., Andelman, S. L., and Bauer, F.: The young adolescent as an obstetric risk, Am. J. Obstet. Gynecol. **103:**305, 1969.

65. Zilkha, K. J.: Cerebrovascular accidents in women taking oral contraceptives, Am. Heart J. **70:** 280, 1965.

10

Nutritional environment in which reproduction takes place

Jane M. Rees and Bonnie S. Worthington

OPPORTUNITIES FOR NUTRITION COUNSELING

Nutritional counseling to promote successful reproduction appropriately should begin long before childbearing is undertaken.[2,11,12] It logically must be directed at persons in all stages of the life cycle, not just expectant young parents whose motivation to change may temporarily be great. Traditional nutritional counseling as it is routinely provided in the prenatal period occasionally serves to promote minor changes in dietary patterns and may correct certain acute nutritional deficiencies the woman manifests. Promotion of *significant* changes in eating patterns, however, is difficult at best and rarely is done effectively without substantial motivation on the part of the individual involved. Therefore dependence on prenatal nutrition counseling *alone* to "prepare" the woman adequately for successful reproduction is a naive approach to the objective at hand. Only with continuous appropriate nutritional support through childhood and adolescence can the mature woman enter pregnancy in optimum nutritional condition to provide for the development of a healthy infant without undue stress to herself.

Dietary habits of any pregnant woman are influenced by many aspects of her life. The building of dietary patterns during early life can appropriately be described as pyramidal in nature (Fig. 10-1). The lower part of the pyramid represents those factors such as culture and individual family patterns which provide the basis in any family setting for the establishment of food preferences and eating habits of the children. Onto these basic food habits is added the multitude of individual feeding experiences in which every child participates. Finally, the apex of the triangle represents the special food-related experiences a person engages in at the time of pregnancy. The chosen diet of the pregnant woman therefore is a synthesis of many influences that have demonstrated significant impact on her feeding pattern since infancy. For this reason it is clear that health professionals who expect to change dietary patterns of the pregnant woman must direct energy toward the more basic parameters which influence food habit formation in early life.

Priority for attention should therefore be

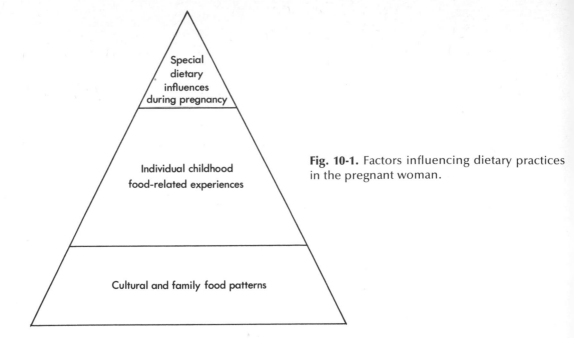

Fig. 10-1. Factors influencing dietary practices in the pregnant woman.

given to the development of high quality nutrition education materials for children as well as adults. Increased emphasis should also be placed on the improvement of programs and materials for all professionals in the health sciences.[8] Acquisition of required nourishment is a survival skill that today demands education to accomplish successfully. For this reason the provision of appropriate nutrition education justifiably deserves a position of priority in the United States educational system; formal as well as informal mechanisms of information transmission need to be stimulated if future generations in this society are to develop normally and survive in good health.

POPULATIONS TO REACH

The improvement of maternal health and fetal well-being may be partially achieved by dietary counseling and nutrition education to special subgroups with unique food habits or economic disadvantages.[19] The identifiable persons with a special need for nutrition education fall into groups of the type listed in Table 1-3. Significant risk fac-

tors in reproduction include poverty, lack of education, very young or old age (<17 or >35 years), first pregnancy or high parity, prior obstetrical complications or fetal wastage, and lack of supportive spouse or family. It should be recognized that both males and females are candidates for educational efforts; both have significant influence on dietary habits of young women. Consequently, it is essential to plan programs with this aim in mind and to address both sexes when any topic related to health, nutrition, and reproduction is covered. Excluding the male in such educational activities is ignoring his influence on the behaviors of females as well as his role in the process of reproduction. Strangely enough, the simple logic and obvious need of "preparing" the male for a normal and happy experience with "pregnancy" has largely been ignored in health and nutrition education programs for adolescents.

To emphasize further the need for nutrition education of boys and men in the United States, it is pertinent to point out the significant role that is assumed by the father in a typical family. The father, by way of his activities in the home, has a great influence on what, when, and how the children (and the mother) will eat.[14] Most fathers contribute significantly to decisions related to how much money will be spent on food, where the money will be spent, what it will be spent for, and how much food will be purchased and consumed outside the home. Recent trends have clearly shown that men are assuming greater responsibility for planning, shopping, and preparing meals. Many of these skills are currently being developed in adolescence, with carry-over and continued exposure in the period of single adulthood, and later in the life-style of the typical young family.

The sharing of influence on dietary habits alone is sufficient reason to include an appeal to men in nutritional counseling and educational campaigns. Although men may not always accompany their wives on clinic visits during pregnancy, a consideration of their food patterns and related behaviors is imperative for a concerned clinician who intends to be effective in recommendations for individual women. Similarly, it goes without saying that educational materials and techniques which are used should be directed to both men and women if improvement of the nutritive climate is deemed appropriate for all people of reproductive age.

SUBJECT MATTER
General considerations

The provision of realistic dietary guidance necessitates a thorough consideration of the woman's economic resources, ethnic or social associations, life-style, and age. During the prenatal period a wealth of nutritional advice and specific guidelines can be provided to expectant families as part of overall prenatal care. Additionally, however, the principles of normal nutrition as they relate to reproduction should be presented as part of the total health education process, and pertinent topics should be thoroughly discussed in logical sequence through the school years. New emphasis ought to be placed on specific issues that have been largely ignored in the past. The advantages of breast-feeding, for example, should be clearly presented to the population as a whole, ideally before and/or during adolescence, when attitudes begin to solidify.[22] Since breast-feeding is relatively unpopular in United States culture at the present time,[17] a vigorous effort at reeducation is necessary to establish this process as a viable alternative for the young family today. In all efforts aimed at health education of today's children, it should be kept in mind that attitudes toward infant feeding techniques and child care practices are molded long before conception ever occurs. If one waits until the time of pregnancy to educate young people about issues related to reproduction and child rearing, it may be too late to have a major impact on behavior and attitudes at that time.

Another issue that has received minimal attention in the past is the need for women to replenish their nutritional state after childbirth. The usual postpartum guidance in most clinic settings is directed toward infant feeding and infant care without regard for the needs of the mother unless she breast-feeds. In all cases attention should be given to the nutritional status of the mother after childbirth, and emphasis should be placed on the inclusion of nourishing food in her diet and the management of weight adjustment by reasonable diet planning. If this type of sensible dietary program is instituted, the new mother can more rapidly gain strength for the demands of parenting and/or employment and additionally will be better prepared to support future pregnancies should these occur.

Weight management

An aspect of total preconceptual and interconceptual care that influences the success of pregnancy is the successful management of body weight. Obesity is a problem in pregnancy in several respects.

First, there is a greater physiological stress placed on the obese woman during pregnancy that predisposes her to a high risk of pregnancy complications.[33] Second, the poor eating habits that caused the obesity problem before pregnancy may continue through the prenatal period with possible adverse effects on the development of the fetus.[2]

Since it is inappropriate to attempt weight reduction during pregnancy,[24] the problem of overweight or obesity requires attention on a long-term basis. Effective weight management should begin in childhood and be emphasized repeatedly throughout the life cycle. Reasonable programs concerned with the total physical and emotional well-being of the individual are required if weight management is to be successful. These programs ideally should be interdisciplinary, where professionals of the psychosocial sciences work with physicians and nutritionists to formulate sensible recommendations for the treatment of individual obese persons.

Because the condition of obesity is recognized as extremely complex, it is obvious that representatives from one discipline alone cannot deal with the problem.[4] Physicians and nutritionists are needed to screen the patients to separate those who would be most likely to lose weight from those who are likely to remain obese. The course of further management then should be based on the results of initial assessments. Subsequent plans should involve a carefully taken history of dietary parameters, growth, physical activity, and behavioral patterns. The physician may also evaluate endocrine status to ascertain the normality of hormonal patterns and to assess overall physical health.

The psychological and social aspects of the obese patient's situation are best assessed by psychologists and social workers who attend especially to feelings of self-worth, body image, and family and social interactions. After the assessment by individuals in these disciplines, trained specialists should involve themselves in the counseling of patients when issues in this category need attention. Appropriate therapists may come from the ranks of social workers, psychologists, or nurses with specialized training; experts in behavior modification programs may also make important contributions. Changes in food habits will occasionally proceed after adequate attention has been given to the psychosocial aspects of the problem. The nutritionist should help the client find an appropriate caloric level over the course of therapy and aid in planning suitable menus that will include foods that provide for nutritional needs. Ultimately, the client should assume full responsibility for diet management on a long-term basis. The objective in terms of nutrition should always be to improve the dietary intake regardless of the probability of weight loss. The overall goal of the team endeavor should be to attend to all aspects of the nutritional, physical, and emotional patterns of the client's life. Ultimately, the healthful patterns of living developed by the overweight woman as a result of appropriate management will be highly beneficial to her at a later date in preparation for successful reproduction.

In the absence of organized interdisciplinary programs for weight management, the health professional can be very helpful in guiding clients away from the potential harm of short-term measures, where the emphasis is on quick weight loss without consideration for maintenance of adequate nutritional status. Emphasis should be placed on gradual loss of body weight with maintenance of weight loss once the goal has been achieved. Attempts should be made whenever possible to refer patients to available programs and professionals who provide in their routine services a sound approach to weight management that considers the unique problems of individual patients in the planning for effective therapy.

TECHNIQUES
General considerations

A wide variety of techniques can be employed in the effort to improve nutritional status of the population and ultimately its readiness for the reproductive experience. Moralistic descriptions of "good" and "bad" food habits appropriately should be replaced by communication centering on the relationship of food intake to health and optimum body functions. No single mode of presentation is adequate for all audiences encountered, and consequently, pertinent information must be organized in an understandable form for persons of several intellectual levels.[53]

To communicate effectively with an audience, it is essential to maximize interaction with the participants by the use of appropriate techniques developed by professionals in the fields of psychology, social work, and anthropology. Nutritionists can profit from the creation of active working relationships with these practitioners for the purpose of keeping abreast of developments in teaching and communication methodology. Dietitians or nutritionists, as well as other involved professionals, need to be familiar with advanced techniques in interviewing.[10] The therapeutic process revolves around establishing a dialogue with the patient or client so that a meaningful exchange of nutrition information can take place. A couple, for example, who is coping with an unexpected pregnancy, financial problems, and a recent move to a strange city may accept nutritional guidance only if it is done in the spirit of exchange, where the opportunity is provided for thinking through solutions to a variety of problems. This approach to nutrition counseling necessitates the establishment of a conversational exchange of information so that recommendations for modifications can be done in line with the recognized ability of the client to receive and utilize new ideas. The success of the interchange between patient and professional depends largely on the communication skills of the interviewer and his or her ability to facilitate effective discussion. In direct opposition to this method is the rigid approach in which the professional has a fixed agenda and presents information in formal fashion without regard for the client's input or ability to assimilate information that is provided.

Behavioral scientists can assist in improving the abilities of nutritionists to facilitate changes in the behavior of clients. Persons often express the desire to alter their habits but are unable to do so without aid. The obese adolescent, near the age of reproduction, who knows her eating habits are unhealthful but is powerless to resist the high calorie foods in her social milieu, is a striking example of a situation where nutritionists require the use of special techniques developed by other professionals to assist in modifying human behavior.

Motivating entire populations of people to change established eating habits in relation to a changing food supply is a difficult task requiring the expertise, and often the historical perspective, of anthropologists. Increased consultation with representatives of this profession may help in the future to design reasonable methods of coping with the challenge. The Expanded Nutrition Program of the U.S. Department of Agriculture makes use of a special training technique involving the preparation of qualified lay persons to act as conveyors of updated information to members of their own communities.[49] Since the origin of this system in 1968, many trained homemakers have taught other homemakers to improve their skills in providing for the nutritional needs of their families. This technique of nutrition education takes advantage of the superior communication that is established between persons of the same culture and socioeconomic groupings. There is a special need for such peer consultation techniques where significant differences in native language or basic cultural values exist.[40]

Mass media

Nutrition educators should recognize the potential of utilizing mass media in a comprehensive manner to reach millions of persons in all stages of the reproductive cycle.[3] The effect could be positive in many circumstances as opposed to the present situation where media use to promote nutrition issues has been co-opted by commercial interests. The latter is especially true in the case of television.[48] The influence of television is heavily weighted in favor of foods with low nutrient content in relation to calorie level. These "foods," which provide only empty calories, are the ones most frequently advocated in daily advertising.[26] These same types of food seem to receive considerable emphasis in programming for cooking schools and other similar activities; high calorie foods outnumber significantly all other food items selected for such occasions, and clarification of nutritional information (including calorie value) is rarely included. Such a "food experience" alone creates for the participant a feeling of familiarity with "empty foods," promotes positive feelings about them, and supports, as a result, their continued use.[29]

For a variety of reasons it is appropriate to claim that television advertising is a distinct detriment to promoting healthful food habits in both children and adults. Not only are nonnutritious foods heavily emphasized, but an effort is made to promote the notion that today's life-style provides limited time for food preparation and thus the frequent use of "time-saving" prepared products is essential. This practice of dependence on convenience foods may tend to eliminate more nutritious foods from the diet. Recent data on consumption trends in the United States *do* tend to reveal a decrease in the purchase of foods such as fresh vegetables and fruits and whole grain cereals, which require greater preparation time than packaged products.[13] Although families may, in fact, have limited time for meal preparation when schedules are busy, many people are influenced to believe that they have less time than they actually do by repeated television messages supporting this idea.

Manoff[26,27] describes strategies by which nutritionists can magnify their influence using television and comprehensive "advertising" campaigns. Initially the plan would utilize that time allotted by stations for public service announcements. A campaign could be based on an issue related to maternal nutrition, such as need for iron-rich foods in the diet, and could be planned specifically for the population where the messages would be aired. Time would be arranged for the selected broadcasts through the station managers who are required under the terms of their licenses to accept a certain number of public service announcements. An effective educational campaign of this sort requires a great deal of careful planning and, as Manoff[27] points out, a commitment to competence in fields beyond those in which nutritionists normally have expertise. Nevertheless, television is an effective medium and should not be overlooked as a potential source of worthwhile nutrition information for all age groups.

Telecourses are a well-established type of programming on both public and commercial television at the present time. A visual presentation of this type is an effective means of reaching a relatively motivated section of the population. A videotaped course on nutritional considerations in human reproduction could be developed and distributed widely with the intention of reaching a sizable audience and increasing appreciation for the role of nutrition in supporting a healthy pregnancy.

A variety of well-planned television programs have clearly demonstrated that children as well as adults can be effectively educated when the format selected is appealing and clever. "Sesame Street" provides basic educational material to young children and does so with such skill that learning is fun for the viewers. "All About

You" and "Feeling Good"[25] have focused on themes related to health and body function. "Mulligan Stew,"[21] produced by the U.S. Department of Agriculture, has been aired on television to promote healthful eating habits in children. It is evident therefore that prototypes have appeared with some success, and these should stimulate the modern educator to consider the potential of various television projects to present important nutritional messages which support improvement in health.

Health workers can and should be effective advocates for change in the commercial media where saturation techniques are most frequently used by promoters of unhealthful food habits.[23] Health professionals must first perceive the sizable influence of mass media on living patterns. They must then recognize the legitimate need for attention to this problem and allocate professional time to its solution. The strong influence of the media in comparison with the weakness of professionals who may contact a limited number of persons a year is convincing proof to any professional that the system must be changed. Groups of professionals with similar goals can frequently work together for common results. Affiliation with an organization like Action for Children's Television* may maximize the level of accomplishment of the individuals by focusing group attention on specific issues of concern and planning a systematic means of dealing with them.

Radio campaigns are less expensive than those designed for the television medium. Radio messages have the additional advantage of reaching large numbers of people and should not be overlooked as potentially powerful tools of nutrition education. Often short messages related to nutrition and health can be worked into the time allotted for public service announcements. "Talk shows" and "magazine-of-the-air" formats allow for greater depth in discussion of complex and controversial subjects. It is clear in observing recent trends that health educators in developing countries make significantly more use of radio presentations than similar educators in the United States.[40]

Audiovisual materials

Presentations consisting of a series of slides or a filmstrip with audio accompaniment have great potential adaptability for nutrition education. An example of an organized slide presentation is "Inside My Mom"[39] featuring the cartoon character illustrated in Fig. 10-2. In this presentation a light approach to the subject of fetal dependence on maternal nutrition provides an effective stimulant for discussing with an adolescent audience. Compared with

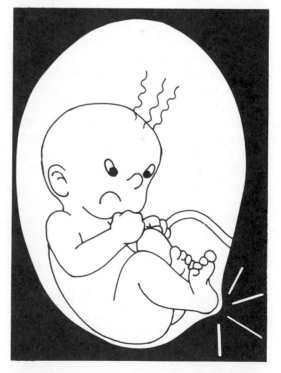

Fig. 10-2. "At coffee break she only had some pop. I was so mad I gave her a great big kick." An example of a light approach to the subject of fetal dependence on maternal nutrition from "Inside My Mom."

---

*Action for Children's Television, a nationwide organization advocating reform in television for children, 46 Austin St., Newtonville, Mass. 02160.

the motion picture format, this method is much less expensive, entailing in the simplest form, still photographs and a script that is read by the presenter as the photographs change. A more sophisticated form of slide presentation is the programmed slide or filmstrip show with equipment that changes the photographs automatically in coordination with the recorded audio portion. Flexibility can be achieved with the slide format by revising the slides and the script as appropriate to the changing situation. For example, in accordance with the idea that education should be language specific, "Inside My Mom" has been set in the Chicano culture of the western United States. In this presentation, called "Dentro de Mi Mamá",[38] not only language but also story, food, and characters were modified to create a presentation relevant to this population.

To create a slide presentation of this type, one needs to develop a plan carefully, since even the simplest forms require a relatively large expenditure of funds. Explicit objectives based on the intended use of the final product will provide an overall guide to organization. Analysis of the age and character of the audience is an important preliminary step in that these data largely determine the manner in which the material will be presented. For greatest success, project consultants should be acquired who are familiar with, or members of, the target audience. With defined objectives and audience analysis as background, the story idea and specific plans can be formulated. A combination of photographs and graphics can be used to achieve the end result. The ratio of each will depend on the desired effect and on the availability of funds for the project.

If a complex presentation is necessary or if distribution is proposed to be extensive, it is advisable to consult professional media personnel. Such a production will necessitate the preparation of projected budgets, production schedules, actors, sets, field testing, legal coverage, and instructional materials. Each of these issues requires, in most cases, substantial preliminary organization; the experience and production knowledge of skilled media personnel can dramatically affect the progress in final slide show synthesis and its effectiveness in achieving its intended function.

A fresh approach can often be achieved in a slide show with themes that are simple but effectively presented. This format is well suited to the needs of the individual nutritionist or nurse who can analyze the audience and organize the material into a presentation that appeals specifically to the defined group. The images a professional can employ to enhance the effectiveness of a message are virtually unlimited when photographs and drawings are used. Under all circumstances where minimal media assistance is available, slide show preparation should be seriously considered as a useful mechanism of greatly improving the quality of communication in the area of nutrition.

Movies, of course, are highly effective in assisting in a variety of educational efforts. As the capabilities of nutritionists improve and their familiarity with audiovisual production becomes more widespread, the expenditure of time and funds in this medium may be justified. Several projects using this method have recently been completed, and preliminary evaluations of their effectiveness suggest that they have been well received.[35,45]

Whatever the scope of the defined project might be, careful evaluation of the final product is essential; this exercise serves to judge if the specific objectives and needs of the audience have been met; it also provides feedback to the producers, who stand to improve with criticism. Communication by way of audiovisual material is a complex art, and only in the testing phase can one understand the process in its entirety. Since additional expenditure of energy and funds is involved for product evaluation, this step is often overlooked by educators, with the result that there is little understanding of the relative effectiveness of the completed materials which have received so much time and effort in preparation.[6]

Nutrition education aids that have been developed in the past have often followed the familiar pattern in which an overabundance of material is presented rather than a specific theme with a clearly defined single purpose. Often, related principles are added to the extent that the impact of the basic thrust is diluted for the audience. With greater numbers of audiovisual aids now becoming available, a growing sophistication in preparation will allow for development within the field of nutrition of a variety of presentations suitable for different types of audiences with diverse needs. The existent body of nutritional knowledge is much too complex to present adequately the "whole story" in one package.

It is now apparent that people in the United States and other developed countries are accustomed to sophisticated audiovisual communication and, in fact, expect it in any high-quality educational production. Nutrition education must therefore include its share of such productions if attention to this field is to be stimulated and maintained. The Society of Nutrition Education has recently compiled an invaluable listing (with discussion) or relevant teaching aids that are available from various sources in the United States and Canada.[43,44]

Printed materials

Printed materials are the most commonly used educational aid available at the present time. Use of this medium generally takes the form of short printed pamphlets or mimeographed sheets. In actuality, however, a tremendous range of different formats exists. Popular magazines provide one possible forum for health education, including nutrition. Indeed, relevant topics like nutrition, reproduction, and infant feeding are frequently considered in articles and advertising in a variety of magazines, but seldom are trained health professionals involved in their preparation. The overall effect is sometimes detrimental when erroneous or poorly justified recommendations are made. Opportunities to reach millions of readers are lost by the neglect of this source of communication with the public. For this reason it seems justifiable, in fact necessary, that trained health educators focus more attention on this important mechanism of educating both children and adults. An article, for example, about the dangers of weight loss during pregnancy could be extremely interesting and effective if written in popular style. Such an article could be developed specifically to appeal to readers of particular magazines, thus reaching groups at high risk for complications in pregnancy.

Magazine or comic book materials have proved to be a rewarding approach to the presentation of pertinent topics to children. A magazine like "Ranger Rick"[31] demonstrates that biological subjects can be made very interesting to children of specific ages. It would be advantageous to treat nutrition in the same manner, searching out an existent method for publication or pursuing funds for a new system or vehicle of distribution. The comic book format has been explored by the creators of "Butter and Boop"[9] and "Mulligan Stew."[21] Nutritionists and other interested professionals could develop many more of these materials with likely success in widespread distribution. Effectiveness in presentation would no doubt increase to the point where principles of nutrition could compete with other interests in the popular culture of today's children.

Nutritionists are infrequently involved in the preparation of books that are interesting and understandable to lay persons. The majority of popular books that have been written on nutrition topics have been presented by authors who are seeking to exploit the market by providing spectacular ideas about dietary preventions or cures. Frequently, these special diets or ideas have not been subjected to the traditional

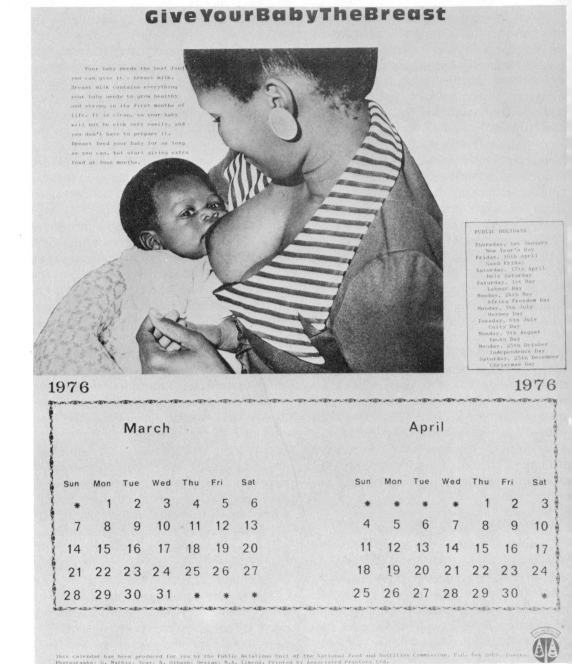

Fig. 10-3. Example of graphics used as an effective promotion of a nutritional message. A calendar produced by the Zambian National Food and Nutrition Commission, Lusaka, Zambia.

scientific process of evaluation, and often their bases are at variance with the widely accepted body of scientific information. Authoritative books written by knowledgeable nutritionists in interesting styles about a variety of topics are desperately needed.

Newspapers publish an abundance of material about food but very little about nutrition. The few articles that are written often represent dubious interpretations of poorly trained "science editors."[3] A welcome exception is the column written by Jean Mayer,[28] which deals with contemporary nutrition issues and questions from the public in a practical and authoritative way. There is a need for additional columns or presentations of this type in local newspapers. A well-informed public might encourage such a service, and assertive professionals should take advantage of opportunities to contribute nutrition information to this popular form of communication.

Photographs and graphics can be utilized in various settings to promote nutrition-related ideas to the general public. At present, budgets of most nutrition education programs do not allot sufficient funds for such projects. The lack of attention to graphics in many circumstances is short-sighted, since this form of communication is frequently employed in preventive campaigns, which save the public's money in the long run if they decrease the need for costly crisis-oriented treatment. An example of such a project appears in Fig. 10-3, where a calendar becomes a vehicle for nutritional messages.

In general, professionals have disdained the use of mass media, spending the major portion of their time communicating with each other or with individual clients.[3] The result of this behavior is a loss of influence over health matters in the lives of most people, with great influence left in the hands of those who tend to exploit rather than aid the population.

APPLICATION

Opportunities for nutritional counseling and education present themselves through-out the life cycle. The idea of nutrition education is an exciting prospect at the present time because of increasing desires on the parts of many people to know about this aspect of their lives. Table 10-1 provides a summary of the kind of situations in which such programs can be included, expanded, and/or improved if they now exist; many of the techniques that were described previously can be utilized to make the applications that are proposed.

Schools

In *day care centers* and in *preschools*, food experiences built around nutritious foods influence the food habits of very young children.[7,16,20,37] Learning about the taste, feel, color, and texture of a certain vegetable with an enthusiastic teacher and with peers can encourage interest in nutrition and enjoyment in eating. Positive experiences such as these can be much more effective in their educational merit than the parents' constant admonishment about "what not to eat." Under appropriate classroom circumstances, children become more involved in the learning experience and, as a result, are much more familiar with foods; projects that frequently prove worth while include growing fruits and vegetables, washing and peeling these same items, watching cooking demonstrations, participating in preparation thereafter, and finally tasting the finished product and serving it to friends.

Snack time in any school setting is a good opportunity to influence food habits to a significant degree. Enjoyment of a refreshing fruit after active play sessions can have a positive influence on the development of healthful habits. Sweets used in these same experiences become "treats," with the obvious result that food is taken out of context and not associated with maintaining health.

The use of food as a reinforcement is a technique that should be avoided if at all possible, since it distorts the meaning of food to a child.[34] When food is used as a reward over a period of time, a person can

Table 10-1. Situations in which nutrition education can be brought to persons at all stages in the life cycle leading to reproduction

Schools	
Day care and preschool	Meaningful, nutritious food experiences included
	Nonnourishing food excluded; food reinforcement excluded
Public schools, K through 12	Appropriate school lunches with accompanying education provided
	Nutrition education specifically planned to all intellectual levels and integrated into various classes provided
University, community college, and vocational schools	Nutritional counseling and educational campaigns made available through campus health services
	Basic nutrition courses made available without prerequisite
	Appropriate nutrition information included in curricula of training for vocations that will influence food habits of others
Professional training and advanced education in medicine, nursing, occupational therapy, dentistry, dental hygiene, etc.	Thorough education in the principles of nutrition provided; interdisciplinary experience in utilizing the capabilities of nutritionists provided
	Training in counseling patients and disseminating information provided
Clinical settings	
Pediatrician, adolescent specialist, nutritionist, nurse, and other clinicians	Professional knowledge and skill to disseminate nutrition education mandated
	Prevention rather than acute care emphasized
	Nutritional aspects of health care emphasized with time given to answer questions of parents and/or children
	Relationship of nutritional health to successful future life including reproduction emphasized
Health-related agencies	
Public (federal, state, local) and private (commercial, voluntary) organizations combating disease and disability	Nutrition education and consulting services provided
	Emphasis on nutrition in programs dealing with family planning and reproduction provided
	Nutritionists in sufficient numbers to act as impetus for expanded programs provided

develop a dependency on food for a sense of pleasure or security. Excessive and unbalanced dietary intakes may result as a child matures. Any number of less harmful material rewards such as books, art materials, and special privileges can be utilized. In behavior modification programs for severe situations where only primary reinforcement will be effective, food rewards should always be paired with a secondary reinforcer and faded out as quickly as possible when the secondary reinforcer is established.

In the public schools, kindergarten through Grade 12, further impact on eating patterns can be achieved by appropriate school lunches accompanied by an educational component. Such programs have been organized, instituted, and described in nutrition education literature.[53] The best efforts required cooperation and energy on the part of school lunch personnel, administrators, teachers, and often parents and students. Effective programs contribute significantly to the establishment of good health and sensible eating habits, which should help in the maintenance of health in the future.

Key components of successful school lunch programs seem to be the creation of an interesting atmosphere, the offering of several choices of food to students, the provision of information to students about the nutritional values enabling them to make wise choices, the coordinating of experiences at school lunch programs with classroom and home experiences, and the overall establishment of a pleasant and interesting learning experience.

Another means of improving dietary patterns of children is to encourage parents, teachers, and other school personnel to guard against the widespread availability of non-nutritive, high calorie foods in the school setting. Such foods may be sold as part of fund-raising schemes to the extent that various organizations are dependent on them. A bit of imagination should generate ideas as to nutritious foods or other useful items or services that could be substituted. The resulting change of influence on dietary habits of young people would be most beneficial to the general state of health. It is worth the effort of health workers to act as advocates for optimum nutrition, whether they be school employees, parents, or simply members of the community. Efforts can frequently be spearheaded by nutrition education specialists at the state level.[36]

Nutrition education can be specifically planned for various cognitive levels and integrated into the general academic curriculum.[46] A beginning science lesson for the primary grades, for example, could be built around cells and how they are nourished. An experiment for high school students could focus on more complex situations such as variation of animal nutrient intake with the observation of detrimental effects on growth, development, reproduction, and

other anatomical and physiological characteristics of representative "parents" and their "offspring."

In *university settings* the typical health service for students is an appropriate opportunity to reach young women and men close to the age of reproduction. Personnel in these clinics need the specific communication skills that foster a relationship of trust in which information provided by the "counselor" can be meaningful in the life of a busy, often newly independent individual. Nordquest and Medved[32] have described an interesting program in which nutritional counseling was provided in connection with a birth control clinic for college women. Problem issues were identified in a pretest with discussion on a one-to-one basis revolving around those identified topics of concern. The authors suggest that this type of situation would be an appropriate setting to test and utilize various educational techniques, including those for group instruction.

In many respects persons in *community colleges* and *vocational schools* may be more accepting of guidance than traditional university students; this may be related largely to the motivation provided by a limitation of funds, time, and facilities for preparation of meals. The need for nutrition information may be especially great in the inner city schools, where students are frequently "nontraditional" in terms of age, life-style, and degree of responsibility for themselves and others.[42]

Public polls have strongly suggested that courses which teach the basic principles of nutrition with much emphasis on practical application need to be made available without prerequisites for persons from a variety of backgrounds. Such forms of education are essential for the development of a well-informed lay public that can face the proliferation or propaganda and myth and can decipher truth from fallacy. Many popular issues based on nutrition fact or nonsense are debated on the front pages of newspapers and on television interview shows with claimed "experts"; unfortunately, the average person feels inadequate in his ability to evaluate the merit of statements that are made and to decide whether or not proposed "nutritional remedies" are justly supported by scientific data or even common sense.

Whether it be in a university, college, or vocational school setting, persons preparing for careers in which work and attitudes will directly influence the eating habits of others should be educated in the basic principles of nutrition. Blank and Wilder[5] describe a situation where food service personnel were involved in a training experience that allowed them to learn nutrition concepts in a real life setting. During this experience participants were taught how to deal effectively with parents and children in a day care center. They were required, along with regular course work, to be involved in planning and execution of the food service and nutrition education program for children, parents, and staff of the center. The students' skills in assuming responsibility were thought to be significantly enhanced by their participation in this type of program, to the extent that on completion of the course they acted as community advocates for strong nutrition programs in day care settings and demonstrated increased effectiveness in their individual situations of employment. A similar experience would be useful in training food service workers, licensed practical nurses, health education teachers, teachers of special classes (such as those for pregnant adolescents), and persons in similar positions who are responsible for menu planning or food purchasing for institutions or business establishments.

For persons receiving *advanced education in professions,* such as dentistry, medicine, nursing, occupational therapy, and dental hygiene, study of the principles of nutrition and application to their particular field is of prime importance if the public is going to have access to holistic care.[1,51,52] Nutrition is a basic aspect of the environ-ment, and health workers must be cognizant of its relationship to their area of expertise and additionally must be able to teach their clients how to apply basic principles of nutrition in the maintenance of physical well-being.

As well as studying nutrition in a didactic format, health professionals should be provided with opportunities to work with capable nutritionists for the purpose of comprehending their functions more fully.[36] Such experiences would improve the skills and confidence of health care workers to assess problem situations and make more appropriate referrals. Professionals who will ultimately be responsible for planning health care programs and facilities require experience with effective nutritionists to become sufficiently committed to the provision of adequate funding and resources for such services in their institutions.

Finally, professionals must be trained in the art of sharing knowledge with the public; they also must be stimulated to do so. Partly because of a rising cry by consumerist groups, educators of health professionals are beginning to give greater attention to the idea that their trainees learn to educate, not simply treat.[30] When professionals learn to communicate to lay persons the important aspects of health maintenance, nutrition should be a major thrust in the messages they impart. This educational approach seems an ideal means of administration of health care, that is, strong emphasis on prevention of difficulties before they occur so that aggressive management is unnecessary.

Clinical settings

In this era when professionals are being urged to practice preventive rather than curative medicine,[15,30,40,47,50] a great deal of nutrition information can be communicated to the public by health professionals who see patients in a clinical setting for family care. Relating nutritional health to successful future life, including reproduction, is a contribution health professionals can make toward improved reproductive status. Each clinician's effectiveness could be magnified in a situation where various professionals are sufficiently atuned to providing nutrition information that they support each other in the messages they deliver.[30]

In this family care setting, time should be allocated to present the nutrition aspects of health and to answer questions of parents and/or children. Professionals in these settings should keep abreast of the best available research regarding nutritional issues. There is evidence that health workers at present rely heavily on information provided through consultative services, seminars, and printed promotional materials prepared by food-oriented companies.[22] Such information resources should be replaced, or at least accompanied, by materials that provide sound ideas about practical applications of scientifically accepted theories. New systems of communication may be necessary to make desirable information readily available.

Health-related agencies: general

Specific responsibility for maternal and child nutrition falls in the purview of those agencies directly serving the public. Comprehensive medical care plans organized around the philosophy of providing total care for the individual offer an optimum setting for nutritional education. In these situations nutrition education would appropriately function as one focus in the effort to prevent illness, its complications, and the need for costly hospital care. Nutritionists should provide not only impetus for nutrition education but also ongoing consultation throughout the system with special attention to the area of reproduction.

Insurance companies, such as Blue Cross, have a vested interest in supplying consumers with information to help them maintain their health.[30] Nutrition is among topics addressed by educational materials distributed by these companies. Newspaper, radio, and television campaigns on behalf of improving nutritional status would also be effective, and use of funds allotted for communication and education might legitimately be considered for this purpose.

Labor unions and businesses are beginning to sense the importance of health education for their members and employees.[30] Distribution of written materials and organizations of events such as seminars, lectures, and films would provide personnel with another opportunity to improve their understanding of important alternatives in life-style that might assist them in their efforts to maintain health.[30]

Privately financed voluntary organizations, such as the International Childbirth Education Association* and La Leche League† have continuous contact with persons involved in reproduction. These groups have substantial influence over nutritional patterns of their trainees. Disseminating the most up-to-date information on nutrition is well within the scope of the organizational objectives; significant community benefit can be realized from the nutrition education activities of these voluntary organizations concerned with family health.

State agencies

A special importance must be placed on the provision of nutrition services within public health agencies. State governments have a responsibility to establish communication among their population, their health professionals, and their governing agencies with the goal of providing a health care system that includes health education. It has been postulated that an individual state can accomplish this task more effectively for the typical living patterns of its citizens than can the recognized bodies of the fed-

---

*International Childbirth Education Association, Inc., an organization devoted to educating persons about childbearing, P.O. Box 20852, Milwaukee, Wis. 53220.
†La Leche League International, Inc., an organization devoted to educating persons about breast-feeding, 9616 Minneapolis Ave., Franklin Park, Ill. 60131.

eral government.[15] A network for the delivery of health care in many cases can be designed to utilize existing facilities so that monetary expenditures for new buildings and other facilities may be unnecessary. Various health resources could be tied together to deliver improved health care to a greater number of the population. At the present time many needy individuals are virtually unserved.

Nutritional services are an integral part of such a health care system. Advisory groups can act in a liaison role between legislative bodies and health agencies to examine decisions that will have an impact on the nutritional environment of the state; additionally, such groups can make recommendations regarding the direction that health education should assume. Nutritionists should be delegated at the state level to plan programs and provide consultation to the networks of nutritionists throughout the state in individual county and city health departments. These local level nutritionists should have the responsibility for surveillance, consultative, and educational functions as well as delivery of health care to the population. Further development of state systems to provide sensible health care would improve the nutritional status of the population and ultimately their preparation for successful reproduction.

Federal agencies

In a discussion of how health education, including nutrition services, can be realistically integrated into the system of health care, the federal government generally is accepted as providing at least an advisory contribution. In 1971 government leaders proposed that a national center for health education be established to act as a center of communication for all agencies, public and private, involved in educational activities.[50] As an initial step, the Bureau of Health Education was established by the U.S. Department of Health, Education, and Welfare in an attempt to coordinate the various education components within that agency. One of its initial projects was to survey health education divisions of public and private agencies nationwide.[30] Hopefully, the activities of this agency will be further developed so that ultimately the chosen mechanism of health care delivery will be clearly organized and understood by all, and the involvement of nutrition services in the total package will be recognized as highly significant.

Other existent federal agencies have seen the need for educational programs that are instigated at the national level.[41] The Food and Drug Administration (FDA) has initiated nutritional labeling as part of a policy that regulatory bodies should take an energetic hand in the education of the public. The U.S. Department of Agriculture (USDA) has developed a network of personnel and a wide range of materials that provide nutritional information to the public. The Expanded Nutrition Program is part of this agency's efforts to meet educational needs in the area of nutrition.

A federally sponsored, USDA–managed food supplementation program for Women, Infants and Children (WIC) has been designed to upgrade the nutritional status of high-risk individuals in the population during pregnancy, lactation, and infancy. Although the level of funding for nutritional education in the WIC program is limited, the philosophy behind it is sound.[18] Through this program a nationwide network of health workers has been established which can contact needy persons and provide nutrition guidance and food so that support of optimal nutritional environment during early development can be accomplished. A basic level of nutritional training is provided to the staff involved with WIC so that many project workers have now become valuable consultants to the clients who appear in the clinical setting for progress assessment and food vouchers. With the focus on teaching people to care for themselves, nutrition educators will have the opportunity to utilize vital new techniques to meet the challenge of facilitating an improvement of nutritional status of the reproductive population in the United States. Throughout the system, although messages regarding nutrition may be delivered by any number of professional disciplines, the ultimate source of nutrition information is highly trained nutritionists. Only persons educated in this specialized field are able to aid other professionals and lay persons to sort through the maze of products and evaluate conflicting theories. Nutritionists may also generate the basic research that attempts to answer an ever-increasing list of questions regarding the influence of nutrition on the quality of life.

CONCLUSION

The preparation of today's youth for successful reproductive experience of necessity requires attention to this goal from early childhood. Health education, including a strong nutrition component, should be presented in well-organized, stimulating formats to children at all levels of educational activity. Health education efforts within the schools should be accompanied by the continual support of community organizations, clinics, mass media, and family environment. A wide variety of educational tools and techniques should be employed with the intent of arousing and maintaining sincere interest in health status from early childhood through maturity. If a health-oriented climate of this type can be created in the majority of communities in the world today, it is highly likely that unnecessary maternal and infant mortality can be greatly reduced and that overall complications of reproduction can be minimized.

REFERENCES

1. American Dietetic Association: Position paper on nutrition education, J. Am. Diet. Assoc. **62**:429, 1973.
2. Aubry, R. H., Roberts, A., and Cuenca, V. G.: The assessment of maternal nutrition. In Barnes, L. A., and Pitkin, R. M., editors: Clinics in perinatology, symposium on nutrition, Philadelphia, 1975, W. B. Saunders Co.
3. Barnum, H. J.: Mass media and health communications, J. Med. Educ. **50**:24, 1975.
4. Bjorntorp, P.: Renaissance of a new frontier in obesity research, Acta Med. Scand. **196**:145, 1974.
5. Blank, H., and Wilder, S. M.: Training dietetic technicians in preschool child nutrition, J. Nutr. Educ. **6**:15, 1974.
6. Braza, J., and Kreuter, M. W.: A comparison of experiential and traditional learning models in studying health problems of the poor, J. Sch. Health **45**:353, 1975.
7. Cohl, V.: Science experiments you can eat, Philadelphia, 1973, J. B. Lippincott Co.
8. Committee on Maternal Nutrition, Food and Nutrition Board, National Research Council, National Academy of Sciences: Maternal nutrition and the course of pregnancy, Washington, D.C., 1970, Government Printing Office.
9. Cooperative Extension Service: Food facts and fun, Rutgers, New Brunswick, 1973.
10. De Schweinitz, E., and De Schweinitz, K.: Interviewing in the social services, National Council of Social Service No. 636, London, 1962.
11. Dwyer, J. T., Jacobson, H. N., and Mayer, J.: Nutrition-related problems in pregnancy, Postgrad. Med. **48**:285, 1970.
12. Dwyer, J. T., Jacobson, H. N., Hutchins, B. K., and Mayer, J.: Management of weight in pregnancy, Postgrad. Med. **48**:208, 1970.
13. Economic Research Service, United States Department of Agriculture: National food situation, Washington, D.C., 1976, Government Printing Office.
14. Eppright, E. S., Fox, H. M., Fryer, B. A., Lamkin, G. H., Vivian, V. M., and Fuller, E. S.: Nutrition of infants and preschool children in the north central region of the United States of America. XIV. Eating behavior, World Rev. Nutr. Diet. **14**:322, 1972.
15. Evans, D. J.: The role of the state governments in educating the public about health, J. Med. Educ. **50**:130, 1975.
16. Ferrerra, N.: The mother-child cookbook, Menlo Park, Calif., Pacific Coast Pubs.
17. Fomon, S.: Infant nutrition, ed. 2, Philadelphia, W. B. Saunders Co.
18. Food and Nutrition Service, United States Department of Agriculture: WIC program regulations: Title 7 Agriculture, Washington, D.C., 1976, Government Printing Office.
19. Galli, N.: The influence of cultural heritage on the health status of Puerto Ricans, J. Sch. Health **45**:10, 1975.
20. Goodwin, M. T., and Poll, G.: Creative food experiences for children, Washington, D.C., 1974, Center for Science in the Public Interest.

21. Great Plains National ITV Library: Mulligan stew, Lincoln, Nebr. 1972.

22. Greiner, R.: The promotion of bottle feeding by multinational corporations: how advertising and the health professions have contributed, Cornell International Nutrition Monograph Series No. 2, Ithaca, N.Y., 1975.

23. Gussow, J.: Counternutritional messages of TV ads aimed at children, J. Nutr. Educ. **4:**48, 1972.

24. Jacobson, H. N.: Nutrition and pregnancy. In Wallace, H. M., Gold, E. G., and Lis, E. F., editors: Maternal and child health practices, Springfield, Ill., 1973, Charles C Thomas, Publisher.

25. Kobin, W. H.: Encouraging better health through television, J. Med. Educ. **50:**143, 1975.

26. Manoff, R. K.: Potential uses of mass media in nutrition programs, J. Nutr. Educ. **5:**125, 1973.

27. Manoff, R. K.: Toward a new "American mentality," J. Nutr. Educ. **7:**139, 1975.

28. Mayer, J.: Food for thought, New York News, Inc., current.

29. McArthur, L. Z., and Resko, B. G.: The portrayal of man and woman in American television commercials, J. Soc. Psychol. **97:**209, 1975.

30. McNerney, W. J.: The missing link in health services, J. Med. Educ. **50:**11, 1975.

31. The National Wildlife Federation: Ranger Rick's Nature Magazine, Washington, D.C., current.

32. Nordquest, M., and Medved, E.: A nutrition counselling session for college women on the pill, J. Nutr. Educ. **7:**29, 1975.

33. Oakes, G. K., and Chez, R. A.: Nutrition during pregnancy, Contemp. Obstet. Gynecol. **4:**147, 1974.

34. O'Neil, S.: Behavior management of feeding. In Pipes, P. L.: Nutrition in infancy and childhood, St. Louis, 1977, The C. V. Mosby Co.

35. Oxford Films: The real talking, singing, action movie about nutrition, Los Angeles, Calif., 1972.

36. Peck, E. B.: Nutrition education specialists: time for action, J. Nutr. Educ. **8:**11, 1976.

37. Project Headstart, Rainbow Series: 3F, Nutrition Education for Young Children; 3B, Nutrition Instructors Guide for Training Leaders; 3C, Leader's Guide for a Nutrition and Food Course, Office of Child Development, Washington, D.C., 1969, United States Department of Health, Education and Welfare.

38. Rees, J., and Doan, R.: Dentro de Mi Mamá: presentation audio-visual con manual de ensenaza, Puget Sound Chapter, Seattle, 1975, National Foundation, March of Dimes.

39. Rees, J.: Inside my mom: audio-visual with teaching manual, White Plains, 1975, National Foundation, March of Dimes.

40. Sanford, T.: The role of formal education, J. Med. Educ. **50:**3, 1975.

41. Schmidt, A. M.: The role of regulation in educating the public about health, J. Med. Educ. **50:**124, 1975.

42. Seattle Central Community College: Non-traditional student seminar, Seattle, 1975.

43. Society for Nutrition Education: Audio-visuals for nutrition education. Nutrition Education Resources Series, No. 9, Berkeley, Calif., 1975.

44. Society for Nutrition Education: Pregnancy and nutrition, Nutrition Education Resource Series, No. 2, Berkeley, Calif., 1975.

45. Society for Nutrition Education: Great expectations, Berkeley, Calif., 1975.

46. Society for Nutrition Education: Nutrition education, K-12 teacher references: concepts, theories, and guides, Berkeley, Calif., 1976.

47. Tosteson, D. C.: The right to know: public education for health, J. Med. Educ. **50:**117, 1975.

48. United States' Senate, Hearings of Select Committee on Nutrition and Human Needs: TV advertising of food to children, 93rd Cong., Washington, D.C., March 6, 1973, Government Printing Office.

49. Wang, V. L., and Ephross, P. H.: ENEP evaluated, J. Nutr. Educ. **2:**148, 1971.

50. Weinberger, C. W.: The role of the federal government in educating the public about health, J. Med. Educ. **50:**138, 1975.

51. Wen, C., Weerasinghe, H., and Dwyer, J.: Nutrition education in U.S. medical schools, J. Am. Diet. Assoc. **63:**408, 1973.

52. White House Conference on Food, Nutrition and Health: final report, Washington, D.C., 1970, Government Printing Office.

53. Wilson, C. S., and Knox, S.: Methods and kinds of nutrition education (1961-1972): a selected annotated bibliography, J. Nutr. Educ. **5:**75, 1973.

Index